Updates in Surgery

Ugo Boggi
Editor

Minimally Invasive Surgery of the Pancreas

In collaboration with
Fabio Vistoli, Vittorio G. Perrone,
and Carlo Lombardo

Forewords by
Marco Montorsi
John L. Cameron

Springer

Editor
Ugo Boggi
Department of Translational Research and of New Surgical and Medical Technologies
University of Pisa
Division of General and Transplant Surgery
Azienda Ospedaliero-Universitaria Pisana
Pisa, Italy

The publication and the distribution of this volume have been supported by the Italian Society of Surgery

ISSN 2280-9848 ISSN 2281-0854 (electronic)
Updates in Surgery
ISBN 978-88-470-3957-5 ISBN 978-88-470-3958-2 (eBook)

DOI 10.1007/978-88-470-3958-2

Library of Congress Control Number: 2017947913

Figures 8.1–8.3, 9.1 (bottom), 9.2, 10.1–10.3, 18.1, 18.2, 19.1, 19.2, 21.1, 21.2, 22.1–22.4, 25.1, 25.4, 26.1–26.10, 27.1–27.4, 28.1–28.6, 29.1–29.4 by Cristina Cati, Sonia Giubertoni, Luca Guerriero (Biographia studio grafico, Turin, Italy)

Cover design: eStudio Calamar S.L.
External publishing product development: Scienzaperta, Novate Milanese (Milan), Italy
Typesetting: Graphostudio, Milan, Italy

This Springer imprint is published by Springer Nature
The registered company is Springer-Verlag Italia S.r.l.
The registered company address is Via Decembrio 28, I-20137 Milan

To the loving memory of my wonderful father
To my mother, who raised three boys
To my wife, who shared with me the heavy weight of "a surgeon's life"
To my daughters, who make every day a brighter day

Foreword

It's with great pleasure that I have accepted to introduce this important and exhaustive monograph by Ugo Boggi and coworkers dealing with a hot and current topic as the minimally invasive approach to pancreatic surgery is.

After the first anesthesia performed in 1846 by Bigelow and the spread of antiseptic procedures due to the work of Joseph Lister in the second half of the 19th century, surgeons were finally able to extend their "invasivity" and perform new and more complex types of resections, further pushing the limit of surgical trauma.

After having managed the most difficult and unthinkable procedures with a traditional laparotomic approach, surgeons faced a new revolution with the beginning of the laparoscopic era. In the early 1990s, after the increasing adoption of laparoscopic surgery, a minimally invasive approach to pancreatic diseases began to be performed and progressively utilized. In 1994, Cuschieri reported the first laparoscopic distal resection and, in the same year, Gagner and Pomp reported the first laparoscopic pancreatoduodenectomy.

Pancreatic surgery has greatly improved in recent years leading to reduced operative mortality, at least in high-volume centers, and more effective treatment of postoperative morbidity and complications, unfortunately still common, with a consequent reduction in reoperation rate.

Despite this, a report from Italian national database demonstrated that pancreatic surgery still remains a demanding field for surgeons, with many unsolved problems. In this scenario, the role of the laparoscopic approach, above all in major resective pancreatic surgery, is still debated. New fire was added to the already hot discussion with the introduction of the da Vinci robotic system, which gave some Italian authors the opportunity to become real innovators, reaching remarkable results and significant experiences.

Ugo Boggi has to be commended for having put together a great number of distinguished authors from all over the world to discuss the most controversial topics in this field.

In an era of "enhanced postoperative recovery" this monograph can help us refine our insight into this intriguing topic, thanks to the great efforts, meticulous research and extensive experience of some of the leading international groups.

Milan, September 2017

Marco Montorsi
President, Italian Society of Surgery

Foreword

The first successful local resection of a periampullary tumor was performed by Halsted in 1898. A German surgeon from Berlin, Kausch, performed the first regional resection of a periampullary cancer and reported it in 1912. Whipple in 1935 popularized the operation. However, for the next 50 years the operation was performed only infrequently because of a hospital mortality rate in the range of 25%. In the middle 1980's, several high-volume centers developed, that reported mortality rates for pancreatoduodenectomy of less than 5%. Now the operation is performed with substantial frequency throughout the world. The first laparoscopic pancreatoduodenectomy was performed by Gagner in 1994. Little more was accomplished with minimally invasive surgery for pancreatic diseases, however, until the last decade.

During the last decade, there has been surprisingly rapid growth in many institutions throughout the world. The current status of minimally invasive surgery on the pancreas is very nicely documented in this current text that is edited by Professor Ugo Boggi from the University of Pisa. The text is comprised of international contributors, but the majority are Italians, many of whom have made important contributions to this field. All topics from evolving technologies, to training in simulation laboratories, to documenting a variety of important outcome measures in pancreatic surgery are discussed. A variety of minimally invasive procedures are described varying from thoracoscopic splanchnicectomy for severe pancreatic pain, biliary bypass, gastric bypass, to percutaneous necrosectomy and sinus tract endoscopy for infected pancreatic necrosis. The main procedures for pancreatic neoplasms, pancreatoduodenectomy, the variety of distal pancreatectomies, and central pancreatectomy performed minimally invasively are also discussed in detail. Many of the chapters have outstanding illustrations that complement the written text very nicely. Not only laparoscopic, but also robotic minimally invasive procedures are covered.

In our institution, we do approximately 500 pancreatectomies per year, including pancreatoduodenectomy (350) and distal pancreatectomies (150). Fifteen percent are done minimally invasively. Both laparoscopic and robotic techniques are utilized. For the young surgeon in training, and just starting his or her career, who is interested in pancreatic surgery, it is essential that they learn minimally invasive techniques. Even though today the vast majority are done open, ten years from now the majority will be done with minimally invasive techniques.

This book is an ideal text for surgeons of all stages to be brought up to date on the various techniques for all pancreatic procedures using minimally invasive techniques. It will be the reference text for many years to come. It is to be recommended for all individuals who are interested in pancreatic diseases.

Baltimore, September 2017

John L. Cameron, MD
Alfred Blalock Distinguished Professor of Surgery
Johns Hopkins University, School of Medicine

Preface

This book comes five years after the text edited by Fulvio Calise and Luciano Casciola on minimally invasive surgery of the liver and published in the same editorial series promoted by the Italian Society of Surgery. Like its predecessor, this monograph is meant to provide an overview of current knowledge and future developments of minimally invasive techniques for pancreatic surgery, a surgical branch considered until recently the realm of open surgery.

The challenges posed by minimally invasive pancreatic surgery (MIPS), however, are unique. Indeed, in most abdominal procedures including liver resections, implementation of minimally invasive surgery was confronted by the safety of open operations, but could also rely on the lessons learned from open procedures, for which standardized techniques had been developed. MIPS, instead, is confronted by the unique challenge of improving the outcome of still imperfect open procedures, with little agreement, and low level of evidence, on which techniques should be preferred. Additionally, MIPS requires extensive and meticulous dissection in the deep and narrow retroperitoneal space with its large and fragile vasculature, and it may require complex digestive reconstructions, making the inherent technical limitations of laparoscopy even more evident. The aggressive biologic behavior of most pancreatic tumors also poses concerns about the oncologic adequacy of MIPS.

The Italian contribution to the development of pancreatic surgery has deep historical roots in the contributions of Giuseppe Ruggi (1889: pancreatic tumor enucleation), Domenico Biondi (1894: duodenum-sparing partial head resection), and Alessandro Codivilla (1898: pancreatoduodenectomy), and was recently revived by Pier Cristoforo Giulianotti (2003: robotic pancreatoduodenectomy) and Ugo Boggi (2010: robotic pancreas transplantation). The current generation of Italian pancreatic surgeons has a high international reputation thanks to the demonstrated ability to couple excellent levels of clinical practice with a somewhat "new" scientific mentality that has produced hundreds of scientific papers published in high-impact journals and has brought some of us to play major roles in international hepato-pancreato-biliary societies.

The high reputation of Italian pancreatic surgery is also witnessed by the list of international authors who have contributed to this text. All of them are acknowledged authorities in the field in which they have written.

The book provides an overview of MIPS starting with a summary of the recent State of the Art Conference held on April 20th, 2016 in São Paulo (Brazil) and going all the way through every aspect of MIPS, including robotic pancreas transplantation, an operation that until recently would probably have been considered impossible. Indeed, there is probably no pancreatic operation that cannot be duplicated using minimally invasive techniques, and there is now little doubt that MIPS has a role in the treatment of pancreatic diseases. What remains to be clarified are the indications to MIPS in terms of which pancreatic diseases could be treated and which patients should be selected. Indications are also expected to vary with the type of pancreatic resection, being probably more restrictive for pancreatoduodenectomy and more permissive for distal pancreatectomy. Training and credentialing are other challenges that pancreatic surgeons will face in the near future. This renewed effort towards education, although demanding, will result in an additional improvement in the competency and proficiency of the future generations of pancreatic surgeons. Indeed, if pancreatic surgery in general accepts no compromise on education, MIPS requires even higher educational levels. Pancreatic surgery, perhaps more than any other surgical branch, requires knowledge, dedication and specific practical training. The real hazard of MIPS is that non-dedicated surgeons could embrace it too enthusiastically, potentially ending up with poor, or sometimes even embarrassing, outcomes that could compromise the still fragile reputation of MIPS and slow down its final development and wider use.

Finally, I wish to thank the Italian Society of Surgery for the honor of editing this book and sincerely hope our readers will be inspired from reading this monograph.

Pisa, September 2017 Ugo Boggi

Contents

All web addresses have been checked and were correct at time of printing.

Contributors

Francesca Aleotti Pancreas Translational and Clinical Research Center, Università Vita e Salute, San Raffaele Scientific Institute, Milan, Italy

Sergio Alfieri Chirurgia Digestiva, Fondazione Policlinico Universitario Agostino Gemelli, Università Cattolica del Sacro Cuore, Rome, Italy

Gabriella Amorese Division of Anesthesia and Intensive Care, Azienda Ospedaliero-Universitaria Pisana, Pisa, Italy

Enrico Andolfi Department of Surgery, Division of General Surgery, Hospital of Arezzo, Arezzo, Italy

Valentina Andreasi Pancreas Translational and Clinical Research Center, Università Vita e Salute, San Raffaele Scientific Institute, Milan, Italy

Stefano Andrianello General and Pancreatic Surgery, The Pancreas Institute, University of Verona Hospital Trust, Verona, Italy

Pierluigi Angelini Department of General Surgery, Center of Laparoscopic and Robotic Surgery, V. Monaldi Hospital, AORN dei Colli, Naples, Italy

Mario Annecchiarico Division of Oncological and Robotic General Surgery, Careggi University Hospital, Florence, Italy

Riccardo Ariotti Pancreas Translational and Clinical Research Center, Università Vita e Salute, San Raffaele Scientific Institute, Milan, Italy

Fabio Bagante Department of Surgery, Unit of Hepato-Pancreato-Biliary Surgery, University of Verona, School of Medicine, Verona, Italy

Gianpaolo Balzano Pancreas Translational and Clinical Research Center, Università Vita e Salute, San Raffaele Scientific Institute, Milan, Italy

Courtney E. Barrows Pancreas and Liver Institute, Beth Israel Deaconess Medical Center, Harvard Medical School, Boston, Massachusetts, USA

Claudio Bassi General and Pancreatic Surgery, The Pancreas Institute, University of Verona Hospital Trust, Verona, Italy

Dirk Bausch Klinik für Chirurgie, Universitätsklinikum Schleswig-Hosltein, Campus Lübeck, Lübeck, Germany

Andrea Belli Division of Surgical Oncology, Department of Abdominal Oncology, Istituto Nazionale Tumori - IRCCS Fondazione G. Pascale, Naples, Italy

Giulio Belli Gastrointestinal General and Hepato-Pancreato-Biliary Surgery, S.M. Loreto Nuovo Hospital, Naples, Italy

Stefano Berti Department of Surgery, S. Andrea Hospital, POLL-ASL5, La Spezia, Italy

Marc G. Besselink Department of Surgery, Academic Medical Center, Amsterdam, The Netherlands

Ugo Boggi Division of General and Transplant Surgery, University of Pisa, Pisa, Italy

Giovanni Butturini HPB Surgery, Casa di Cura Pederzoli, Peschiera del Garda, Verona, Italy

Fulvio Calise Centre of Hepatobiliarypancreatic Surgery, Pineta Grande Hospital, Castelvolturno, Caserta, Italy

Carla Cappelli Diagnostic and Interventional Radiology, Department of Translational Research and New Technologies in Medicine and Surgery, University of Pisa, Pisa, Italy

Damiano Caputo Department of Surgery, Campus Biomedico, University of Rome, Rome, Italy

Davide Caramella Diagnostic and Interventional Radiology, Department of Translational Research and New Technologies in Medicine and Surgery, University of Pisa, Pisa, Italy

Riccardo Casadei Department of Medical and Surgical Sciences (DIMEC), University of Bologna, S.Orsola-Malpighi Hospital, Bologna, Italy

Luca Casetti General and Pancreatic Surgery, The Pancreas Institute, University of Verona Hospital Trust, Verona, Italy

Emma Cavazzi Department of Surgery, Fondazione IRCCS Policlinico San Matteo, Pavia, Italy

Graziano Ceccarelli Department of Surgery, Division of General Surgery, Hospital of Arezzo, Arezzo, Italy

Rosa Cervelli Diagnostic and Interventional Radiology, Department of Translational Research and New Technologies in Medicine and Surgery, University of Pisa, Pisa, Italy

Kevin C. Conlon Professorial Surgical Unit, Surgery Deparment, Tallaght Hospital Trinity College Dublin, Dublin, Ireland

Alessandro Coppola Hepato-Biliary Surgery Unit, Fondazione Policlinico Universitario Agostino Gemelli, Università Cattolica del Sacro Cuore, Rome, Italy

Roberto Coppola Department of Surgery, Campus Biomedico, University of Rome, Rome, Italy

Andrea Coratti Division of Oncological and Robotic General Surgery, Careggi University Hospital, Florence, Italy

Francesco Corcione Department of General Surgery, Center of Laparoscopic and Robotic Surgery, V. Monaldi Hospital, AORN dei Colli, Naples, Italy

Diego Cuccurullo Department of General Surgery, Center of Laparoscopic and Robotic Surgery, V. Monaldi Hospital, AORN dei Colli, Naples, Italy

Isacco Damoli Department of Surgery, Pancreas Institute, Verona University Hospital, Verona, Italy

Thijs de Rooij Department of Surgery, Academic Medical Center, Amsterdam, The Netherlands

Alessandro Esposito General and Pancreatic Surgery, The Pancreas Institute, University of Verona Hospital Trust, Verona, Italy

Massimo Falconi Pancreas Translational and Clinical Research Center, Università Vita e Salute, San Raffaele Scientific Institute, Milan, Italy

Laureano Fernández-Cruz Department of HPB Surgery and Transplantation, ICMDiM, Hospital Clínic de Barcelona, Barcelona, Spain

Antonello Forgione Department of General Surgical Oncology and Minimally Invasive Surgery, Ospedale Niguarda Ca' Granda, Milan, Italy

Elisa Francone Department of Surgery, S. Andrea Hospital, POLL-ASL5, La Spezia, Italy

Isabella Frigerio HPB Surgery, Casa di Cura Pederzoli, Peschiera del Garda, Verona, Italy

Andrea Gennai Department of Surgery, S. Andrea Hospital, POLL-ASL5, La Spezia, Italy

Alessandro Giardino HPB Surgery, Casa di Cura Pederzoli, Peschiera del Garda, Verona, Italy

Antonio Giuliani Department of Transplantation, Unit of Hepatobiliary Surgery and Liver Transplant Center, A. Cardarelli Hospital, Naples, Italy

Felice Giuliante Hepato-Biliary Surgery Unit, Fondazione Policlinico Universitario Agostino Gemelli, Università Cattolica del Sacro Cuore, Rome, Italy

Alfredo Guglielmi Department of Surgery, Unit of Hepato-Pancreato-Biliary Surgery, University of Verona, School of Medicine, Verona, Italy

Ahmad Hamad Department of Surgical Oncology, University of Pittsburgh Medical Center, Pittsburgh, Pennsylvania, USA

Calogero Iacono Department of Surgery, Unit of Hepato-Pancreato-Biliary Surgery, University of Verona, School of Medicine, Verona, Italy

Tobias Keck Klinik für Chirurgie, Universitätsklinikum Schleswig-Hosltein, Campus Lübeck, Lübeck, Germany

Sjors Klompmaker Department of Surgery, Academic Medical Center, Amsterdam, The Netherlands

David A. Kooby Emory University School of Medicine, Emory Saint Joseph's Hospital, Atlanta, Georgia, USA

Luca Landoni General and Pancreatic Surgery, The Pancreas Institute, University of Verona Hospital Trust, Verona, Italy

Carlo Lombardo Division of General and Transplant Surgery, University of Pisa, Pisa, Italy

Paola Maffi Department of Transplantational Medicine, IRCCS San Raffaele Scientific Institute, Milan, Italy

Robert Memba Professorial Surgical Unit, Surgery Deparment, Tallaght Hospital Trinity College Dublin, Dublin, Ireland

Roberta Menghi Chirurgia Digestiva, Fondazione Policlinico Universitario Agostino Gemelli, Rome, Italy

Francesco Minni Department of Medical and Surgical Sciences (DIMEC), University of Bologna, S.Orsola-Malpighi Hospital, Bologna, Italy

Andrea Moglia EndoCAS - Center for Computer Assisted Surgery, University of Pisa, Pisa, Italy

A. James Moser Pancreas and Liver Institute, Beth Israel Deaconess Medical Center, Harvard Medical School, Boston, Massachusetts, USA

Francesca Muffatti Pancreas Translational and Clinical Research Center, Università Vita e Salute, San Raffaele Scientific Institute, Milan, Italy

Rita Nano Diabetes Research Institute, IRCCS San Raffaele Scientific Institute, Milan, Italy

Niccolò Napoli Division of General and Transplant Surgery, University of Pisa, Pisa, Italy

Donal B. O'Connor Professorial Surgical Unit, Surgery Deparment, Tallaght Hospital Trinity College Dublin, Dublin, Ireland

Ana Sofia Ore Pancreas and Liver Institute, Beth Israel Deaconess Medical Center, Harvard Medical School, Boston, Massachusetts, USA

Carlo Alberto Pacilio Department of Medical and Surgical Sciences (DIMEC), University of Bologna, S.Orsola-Malpighi Hospital, Bologna, Italy

Stefano Partelli Pancreas Translational and Clinical Research Center, Università Vita e Salute, San Raffaele Scientific Institute, Milan, Italy

Andrea Peri Department of Surgery, Fondazione IRCCS Policlinico San Matteo, Pavia, Italy

Vittorio G. Perrone Division of General and Transplant Surgery, University of Pisa, Pisa, Italy

Lorenzo Piemonti Diabetes Research Institute, IRCCS San Raffaele Scientific Institute, Milan, Italy

Andrea Pietrabissa Department of Surgery, Fondazione IRCCS Policlinico San Matteo, Pavia, Italy

Luigi Pugliese Department of Surgery, Fondazione IRCCS Policlinico San Matteo, Pavia, Italy

Marco Ramera Department of Surgery, Pancreas Institute, Verona University Hospital, Verona, Italy

Claudio Ricci Department of Medical and Surgical Sciences (DIMEC), University of Bologna, S.Orsola-Malpighi Hospital, Bologna, Italy

Aldo Rocca Department of Surgery, Division of General Surgery, Hospital of Arezzo, Arezzo, Italy

Andrea Ruzzenente Department of Surgery, Unit of Hepato-Pancreato-Biliary Surgery, University of Verona, School of Medicine, Verona, Italy

Roberto Salvia General and Pancreatic Surgery, The Pancreas Institute, University of Verona Hospital Trust, Verona, Italy

Santiago Sánchez Cabús Department of HPB Surgery and Transplantation, ICMDiM, Hospital Clínic de Barcelona, Barcelona, Spain

Monica Solis Velasco Pancreas and Liver Institute, Beth Israel Deaconess Medical Center, Harvard Medical School, Boston, Massachusetts, USA

Greg Strowig Fujifilm Medical Systems USA, TeraMedica Division, Milwaukee, Wisconsin, USA

Giovanni Taffurelli Department of Medical and Surgical Sciences (DIMEC), University of Bologna, S.Orsola-Malpighi Hospital, Bologna, Italy

Antonio Pio Tortorelli Chirurgia Digestiva, Fondazione Policlinico Universitario Agostino Gemelli, Rome, Italy

Fara Uccelli Pancreatic Surgery Unit, Humanitas University, Humanitas Research Hospital, Rozzano, Milan, Italy

Jony van Hilst Department of Surgery, Academic Medical Center, Amsterdam, The Netherlands

Fabio Vistoli Division of General and Transplant Surgery, University of Pisa, Pisa, Italy

Charles M. Vollmer University of Pennsylvania, Perelman School of Medicine, Philadelphia, Pennsylvania, USA

Herbert J. Zeh III Department of Surgical Oncology, University of Pittsburgh Medical Center, Pittsburgh, Pennsylvania, USA

Alessandro Zerbi Pancreatic Surgery Unit, Humanitas University, Humanitas Research Hospital, Rozzano, Milan, Italy

Amer H. Zureikat Department of Surgical Oncology, University of Pittsburgh Medical Center, Pittsburgh, Pennsylvania, USA

Acknowledgements

The volume editor and the publisher gratefully acknowledge the educational contribution offered by:

– Associazione Per Donare la Vita Onlus (http://www.perdonarelavitaonlus.it/)
– Invernizzi S.p.A. Forniture Ospedaliere
– Karl Storz
– ab medica S.p.A.

1 State of the Art on Minimally Invasive Pancreatic Resection: IHPBA 2016 Conference

David A. Kooby and Charles M. Vollmer

1.1 Introduction

After a slow start, minimally invasive pancreatic resection (MIPR) is now performed frequently around the world. The first description of laparoscopic pancreatoduodenectomy (PD) was in 1994 [1] and distal pancreatectomy in 1996 [2], yet explosive growth of these procedures followed more than a decade later. Obstacles to wide application of MIPR include: the organs' retroperitoneal location, technical complexity due to the intimate relationship of the pancreas with the major mesenteric vasculature, concerns regarding oncologic efficacy of such approaches, and challenges in training for these relatively low-volume, moderate- to high-risk operations. Improvements in training and technology (such as surgical robotics), correlate with a surge MIPRs, yet some aspects of this field remain controversial among the pancreatic surgical community. It was time to examine the status and progress in MIPR, and the potential directions for future research and development of this field.

In March 2014, President Palepu Jagannath, MD, FRCS from Mumbai, India, the International Hepato-Pancreato-Biliary Association (IHPBA) conducted a strategic planning meeting at their World Congress held in Seoul, Korea. The Association held a conference that stressed the educational goal for its membership. The IHPBA Research Committee was asked to develop and stage an educational "Consensus Conference" at the World Congress in 2016. MIPR was chosen as the topic due to its topical appeal and developing controversies. This chapter describes the origins, preparation, execution and deliverables from this landmark event, held in São Paulo, Brazil on April 20th, 2016.

D.A. Kooby (✉)
Emory University School of Medicine
Atlanta, Georgia, USA
e-mail: dkooby@emory.edu

U. Boggi (Ed), *Minimally Invasive Surgery of the Pancreas*,
Updates in Surgery
DOI: 10.1007/978-88-470-3958-2_1,

1.2 Conference Development

An organizing committee was developed eighteen months prior to the planned 10th World Congress of the IHPBA to be held in April 2016. Two co-Chairmen were appointed: David Kooby, MD, FACS, of Emory University (Atlanta, USA) was chosen to represent the IHPBA Research Committee, and Charles Vollmer, MD, FACS, from the University of Pennsylvania (Philadelphia, USA) represented the interests of the Scientific Program Committee. Attention was first given to selection of an international steering group of acclaimed pancreatic surgeons, which balanced the various regions of the world (Americas, Europe/Africa, and Asian/Pacific). Consideration was given to assuring that the group was composed of both open- and minimally invasive surgery (MIS)-based pancreatic specialists. Members were chosen for their expertise in certain topics (i.e., research design, outcomes assessment, health care economics, educational innovation), or prior experience in directing similar conferences.

The 16-member steering committee consisted of: Co-Chair: David A. Kooby - Emory University, USA; Co-Chair: Charles M. Vollmer - University of Pennsylvania, USA; Horacio J. Asbun - Mayo Clinic Florida, USA; Jeffrey Barkun - McGill University, Canada; Marc GH Besselink - Academic Medical Center, University of Amsterdam, the Netherlands; Ugo Boggi - University of Pisa, Italy; Kevin CP Conlon - The University of Dublin, Trinity College, Ireland; Ho-Seong Han - Seoul National University Bundang Hospital, South Korea; Paul D. Hansen - Portland Providence Cancer Center, USA; Michael Kendrick - The Mayo Clinic, Rochester, USA; Andre L. Montagnini - Universidade de Sao Paulo, Brazil; C Palanivelu - GEM Hospital & Research Center Coimbatore, India; Bård I. Røsok - Oslo University Hospital, Norway; Shailesh V. Shrikhande - Tata Memorial Centre, India; Go Wakabayashi - Ageo Central General Hospital, Japan; and Herbert Zeh - University of Pittsburgh, USA.

The working group met by video-conference monthly for a year to develop the conference format and content, and continued to convene for eight months thereafter for manuscript development. Logistical support was provided by the society's management group – ACS Global.

Each of the regional (Americas, Europe/Africa/Middle East, and Asia/Pacific) societies under the umbrella of the IHPBA (AHPBA, E-AHPBA, and A-PHPBA), provided endorsement, as did The Pancreas Club and patient advocacy groups The National Pancreas Foundation (USA) and The Pancreatic Cancer Action Network (PanCAN, USA). Funding was generously provided by the IHPBA and the AHPBA (the regional co-host for the World Congress). Association with the IHPBA World Congress simplified logistics and costs for conducting this international conference. April 20th, 2016, the day preceding the Congress, was selected. External commercial support was forbidden to minimize bias to any conclusions drawn.

1.3 Conference Design and Content

The initial intent was to create a consensus conference in MIPR. The steering committee considered this plan and following deliberation, concluded that there was not enough high-level data to support a true consensus model. A "State-of-the Art" format was adopted and focused on incorporation of surgical innovation relating to MIPR. The committee decided to avoid technique-heavy presentations and concentrated on the following issues: 1) defining key metrics in pancreatic resection; 2) clarifying terminology in MIPR; 3) comparing outcomes for open and minimally invasive distal pancreatectomy (MIDP), 2) comparing outcomes for open and minimally invasive pancreatoduodenectomy(MIPD); 3) examining cost/value/quality of life issues in MIPR, 4) exploring concepts in training/education/credentialing; and 5) proposing strategies for research development in MIPR.

As a parallel effort to gain more insight on current trends, the steering committee conceived and initiated an international survey on MIPR themes. This was developed under the leadership of Marc Besselink, MD and his pancreatic outcomes research group from Amsterdam, the Netherlands. Once constructed and vetted through several iterations by the steering committee, the survey was globally distributed to the memberships of the IHPBA, AHPBA, E-AHPBA, A-PHPBA and Pancreas Club six-months prior to the meeting. Results obtained served as a foundation for development of the meeting's themes.

Two prominent laypersons (Julie Fleshman, JD, MBA, CEO of the Pancreatic Cancer Action Network and Jane Holt, co-founder of the National Pancreas Foundation) were invited to provide their unique perspectives –regarding patient-advocacy concerns. Faculty were invited to give focused presentations, and panels were developed to solicit opinions from experienced pancreatic surgeons.

Four panel discussions focused on 1) MIDP, 2) MIPD, 3) training/education, and 4) future research, were led by members of the organizing committee. Panelists were a mix of surgeons in academic practices around the world; some who prefer open pancreatectomy and others who prefer MIPR. Audience response technology allowed for audience participation. This meeting was intended to spark future international MIPR endeavors. The day was video recorded, and the videos can be watched on myHPB.org.

1.3.1 Systematic Data Review

An essential element of the meeting was scrutiny of existing MIPR evidence published up to 45 days prior to the meeting. Drs. Jony van Hilst, MD and Thijs de Rooij, MD, from Academic Medical Center, Amsterdam, Netherlands, conducted systematic reviews of perioperative and oncologic outcomes comparing open versus MIPR approaches for both distal and proximal pancreatic resections. A review of published economic outcomes for MIPR was conducted. Their search and inclusion strategies are described in the corresponding manuscripts [3–5].

1.3.2 Overview of the Day

On April 20th, 2016, over 400 surgeons, from 52 countries, attended the day-long event held in the WTC Theater of the Sheraton Hotel in downtown São Paulo, Brazil.

1.3.2.1 Opening Session

The meeting began with introductions from the program co-Chairs, informing attendees of the genesis of the conference (Vollmer) and of the day's structure and content (Kooby). Professor Jagannath emphasized the importance of the topic to the HPB community and indicated the IHPBA's essential commitment to advancing progress in the field.

Conference content commenced with a special talk by Claudio Bassi, MD from Verona, Italy, who identified the key outcome metrics in pancreatic resection most important to surgeons and patients [6]. These included: center-specific criteria, such as a need for 24-hour availability of interventional radiology care; procedure-specific criteria, such as pancreatic remnant texture and duct size; and outcome-specific criteria, such as risk-adjusted mortality and use of enhanced recovery protocols (Table 1.1). This presentation helped "frame" ensuing presentations and panel discussions.

Andre Montagnini from São Paulo, Brazil presented a framework clarifying terminology for MIPR. Existing literature is replete with vague terms such as "hybrid" and "laparoscopic-assisted", making it difficult to compare results of one study to another. Some groups define "laparoscopic pancreatoduodenectomy" as a laparoscopic resection with an open reconstruction through a small laparotomy incision. The potential risks and benefits of this approach may differ from performance of the procedure laparoscopically from start to end, and yet these studies may be included in the same meta-analyses.

Using Delphi methodology, the steering committee voted on a strategy for common parlance in MIPR surgery [7]. The anticipation is that this will allow for more precise definitions to be used in future research studies and publications on MIPR. A summary of this framework is provided in Table 1.2.

The opening session concluded with a presentation by Marc Besselink from Amsterdam, the Netherlands, who provided results of the first international survey on MIPR, which included responses of 435 surgeons from 50 countries (Fig. 1.1) [8]. This 60-question survey explored experience with and attitude towards MIPR with respect to specific procedures [pancreatoduodenectomy (PD) and distal pancreatectomy (DP)] and concepts such as training, education, cost,

Table 1.1 Main indicators of quality in pancreatic surgery

Center-specific	Interventional radiology no-stop service on site
	Endoscopy no-stop service on site
	Intensive care unit on site
	Dedicated pathology
	Multidisciplinary meeting
	Nuclear medicine
	Dedicated medical and radiation oncology
	Dedicated endocrinology
	Acute and chronic pain services
	Duration of waiting list
Procedure-specific	EBL assessment
	Pancreatic stump texture assessment
	MPD size assessment
	Case load
Outcome-specific	Risk-adjusted mortality
	Pancreatic surgery-specific definitions
	ERAS protocols application
	Use of blood transfusions
	PMI assessment
	Health-care related costs reduction

EBL, estimated blood loss; *MPD*, main pancreatic duct; *ERAS*, enhanced recovery after surgery; *PMI*, postoperative morbidity index.

Table 1.2 Strategy for labeling the minimally invasive pancreatic resection (MIPR) approach

Method	Approaches	Type of resection
Open **Minimally invasive** – Laparoscopic – Hand-assisted – Single-port laparoscopic – Robot-assisted	**Single approach** (approach + resection) **Combined approaches** – ***Intended*** 1st approach + to + 2nd approach + resection *or* 1st approach + resection + to/with + 2nd approach + resection or reconstruction – ***Conversion*** 1st approach + converted to + 2nd approach + resection	– Pancreatoduodenectomy – Left/distal pancreatectomy – Central pancreatectomy – Uncinate process resection – Enucleation – Total pancreatectomy (Other organ resection/ Vascular resection + reconstruction)

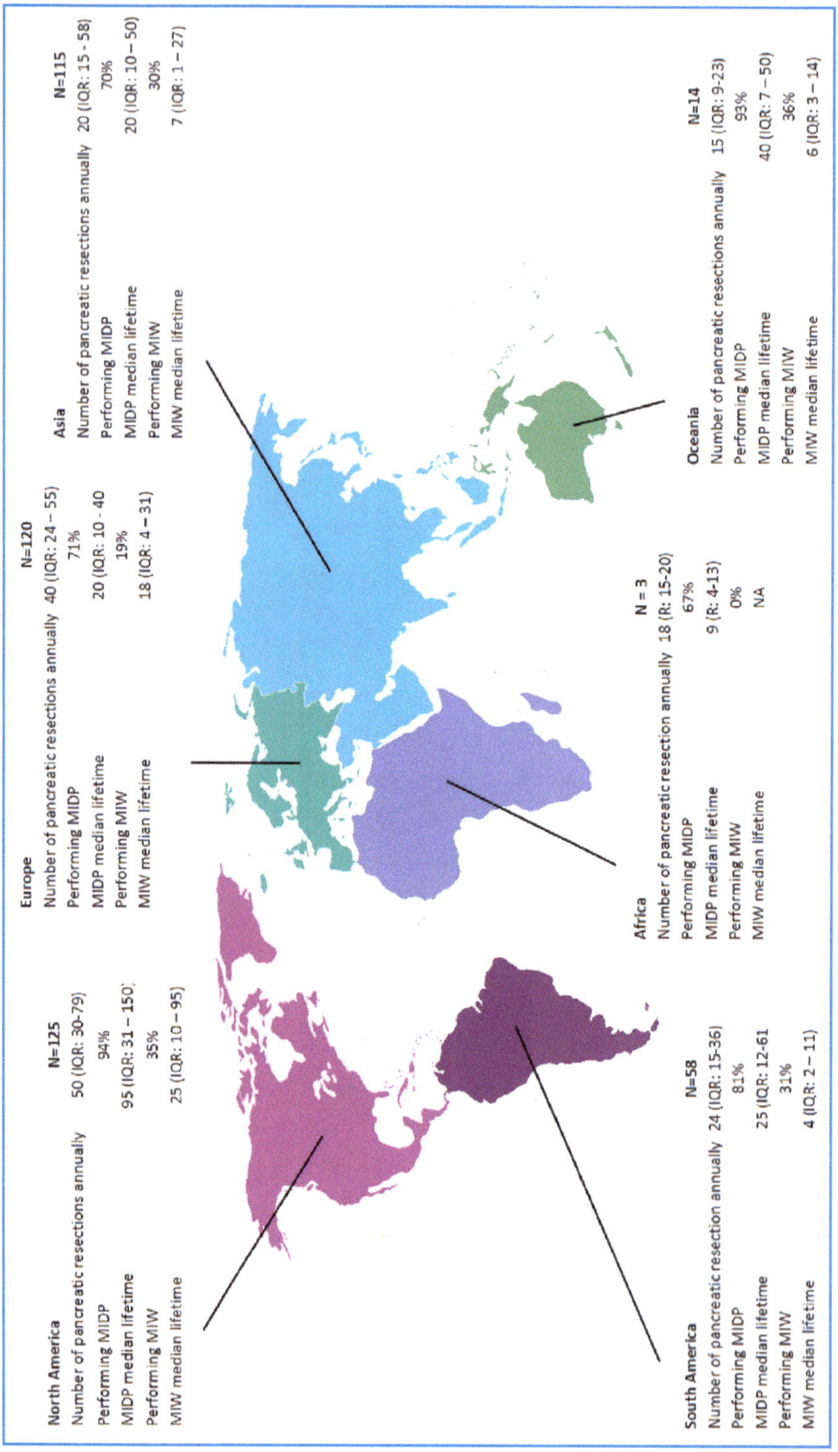

Fig. 1.1 Location of responses to the first worldwide survey on minimally invasive pancreatic resection (reproduced with permission from [8])

value, and future research planning. These results provided an early snapshot of existing impressions on the current state of MIPR.

Some of the key findings included: 345 surgeons (79%) reported performing MIDP, while only 124 (29%) reported performing MIPD, despite PD being a more commonly performed operation than DP. Lack of specific training in MIDP and MIPD was cited as the most common reason for not performing a minimally invasive approach. Fifty-eight responders felt MIDP was beneficial, while 42% felt that MIPD was potentially beneficial. The survey also explores what the benefits are perceived to be and what hurdles exist to adopting MIPR. Please refer to the published survey for further details.

1.3.2.2 Minimally Invasive Distal Pancreatectomy (MIDP)

The next module, chaired by Bård Røsok, MD from Oslo, Norway, focused on MIDP [5]. Compared with minimally invasive pancreatoduodenectomy, MIDP is more widely accessible to a greater number of surgeons and patients, given the inherently less complex nature of this operation, which typically does not require reconstruction. There are more existing data regarding MIDP compared with open distal pancreatectomy than are available for pancreatoduodenectomy, but the data quality is still low. Objective outcomes presentations, reflecting results from the pre-conference systematic reviews, were given by Markus Diener from Heidelberg, Germany (perioperative results) and Dave Kooby from the Atlanta, USA (oncologic efficacy). This was followed by an opinion talk by Peter Allen from New York's Memorial Sloan Kettering Cancer Center regarding optimal patient selection for MIDP.

Understanding the quality limitations, summary perioperative findings included: as compared with open distal pancreatectomy, MIDP is associated with similar operative times (235 vs. 221 minutes), but lower blood loss (263 vs. 552 cc), lower morbidity (12 vs. 17%), and shorter hospital stays (8 vs. 12 days). As for cancer outcomes, there were no substantial differences between margin status, lymph node harvest or overall survival for either cohort.

Shailesh Shrikhande from Mumbai, India led a spirited panel discussion which probed controversies and selection criteria for MIDP. This panel included recognized experts in both open pancreatic resection and MIPR techniques: Peter Allen, MD (New York, USA); Patrick Pessaux, MD (Paris, France); Nicholas O'Rourke, MD (Adelaide, Australia); Ho-Seong Han, MD (Seoul, Korea); Masafumi Nakamura, MD (Japan); and Nipun Merchant, MD (Miami, USA).

While superiority of MIDP over open DP is not proven, equipoise for further comparison exists. As surgeons continue to negotiate the learning curve and technology gets more refined, laparoscopic DP will be more widely applied in the future.

1.3.2.3 Minimally Invasive Pancreatoduodenectomy (MIPD)

Ugo Boggi from Pisa, Italy, led a similar outcomes assessment module on the more controversial topic of pancreatoduodenectomy [3]. Matthew Walsh from the Cleveland Clinic provided an overview of the generally low-level evidence for MIPD as compared to open PD. This was followed by a similar overview of oncologic outcomes provided by Michael Kendrick from the Mayo Clinic. Observational reports show longer operative times with lower blood loss for MIPD over open PD. Effects on hospital length of stay are inconsistent.

Four brief presentations focused on benefits and disadvantages of various approaches to pancreatoduodenectomy. Herbert Zeh from Pittsburgh, USA, discussed how robotic pancreatectomy represents a new paradigm of "computerized surgery". Steven Hughes of Gainesville, USA, discussed his trials and tribulations overcoming the learning curve for laparoscopic PD. This was followed by a nice discussion of the merits of using a "hybrid" approach, presented by Yoshiharu Nakamura from Tokyo, Japan. Finally, Charles Vollmer from Philadelphia, USA, explained how open PD remains the standard to which MIPR techniques must still be compared.

1.3.2.4 Cost, Value, and Quality of Life Considerations

The third major theme probed during the conference was the importance of cost and value when assessing emerging technologies like MIPR [4]. Kevin Conlon from Dublin, Ireland, led this session and suggested that major concerns linger about the expense of MIPR, particularly in a more cost-conscious health-care sector. Comparative studies which have thus-far assessed cost outcomes between MIPR and open approaches were reviewed by Mo Abu-Hilal from Southampton, United Kingdom. Next, Tsafrir Vanounou, from Montreal, Canada, informed us of the inadequacies of current economic analyses and proposed other models to pursue when comparing various surgical approaches. He stressed the importance of "value", rather than generic cost assessments of the various surgical approaches. The perspective of the health-care leadership was probed by Mark Talamonti (Chicago, USA) who shared his unique perspective as a department chairman. He outlined what it takes to properly implement a "program" in MIPR surgery, such as assessing the institutional need, resources, and market. The next step is to prepare your team and select ideal patients (educated, lean patients, with tumors away from major vasculature), followed by team debrief and process improvement. Finally, outcomes should be assessed and charted over time to assess for continued support of the program, much like any significant business plan. This was followed by a thought-provoking presentation by Vic Velanovich (Tampa, USA) who provided insight on how patient quality-of-life assessment needs to be developed as we continue to assess the potential value of MIPR. He challenged the audience to consider what degree of improvement MIPR needs to show over traditional open outcomes to become a new standard of care. A sobering talk was provided by Julie Fleshman, JD, MBA (Los Angeles, USA), the Executive Director of the patient advocacy group PanCAN. She shared with us her understandings of how patients are sizing up MIPR as an option for their care. She reported that cancer patients are less concerned with technique and are more concerned with survival from pancreatic cancer. The take-away message was to perform safe surgery and focus energy on early detection and therapy of cancer. This was not an indictment of the MIPR meeting, but a reminder that cancer patients may be subject to different motivations from non-cancer patients.

1.3.2.5 Combined Panel Discussion – MIPD and Cost/Value Issues

A 90-minute panel discussion on MIPD and cost/value was then led by Horacio Asbun, from the Mayo Clinic-Jacksonville, USA [3]. Six invited experts in both MIPR and open pancreatic resection participated, including: Herb Zeh, MD (Pittsburgh, USA); Michael Farnell, MD (Rochester, USA); C. Palanivelu, MD (Coimbatore, India); Thilo Hackert, MD (Heidelberg, Germany); Richard Schulick, MD (Aurora, USA); Mark Callery, MD (Boston, USA); and John Martinie, MD (Charlotte, USA). Questions addressed included, among others: 1) is MIPD here to stay, 2) how important is it to have a substantial experience with open PD before embarking on MIPD, 3) how do I get started with MIPD, 4) when and how should I convert to an open approach. This session can be reviewed in the cited manuscript and watched on myHPB.org.

1.3.2.6 Training and Credentialing in MIPR

A topic identified by the organizing committee to be of utmost importance is how experience in MIPR is being taught, acquired, and certified [9]. Herbert Zeh (Pittsburgh, USA) and Paul Hansen (Portland, USA) developed and led a robust section on training, education and credentialing, which Dr. Hansen initiated by sharing current statistics on exposure of HPB trainees to MIPR during fellowship training in the United States. He indicated that current exposure to MIDP is reasonable (although varied by approach with only a few centers using a robotic approach; while MIPD is not being taught at most centers (Fig. 1.2).

This was followed by a progressive approach on "organized dissemination" of MIPR training where Marc Besselink shared a novel training paradigm developed in the Netherlands, where 17 hospitals participated in LAELAPS (Longitudinal Assessment and Realization of Minimally Invasive Pancreatic Surgery) training program [10], and then worked together to begin coordinated clinical trials. Melissa Hogg from the United States followed with insights about how robotic training might be best accomplished through a novel 5-step learning approach. This approach originated at the University of Pittsburgh and includes: 1) a simulation curriculum, 2) a biotissue curriculum, 3) a video curriculum, 4) an operative curriculum, and 5) a skills maintenance and ongoing assessment component (Fig. 1.3)

Oliver Varban, MD, a bariatric surgeon from Ann Arbor, USA, discussed the role of operative video-assessment as a tool for performance improvement. This was followed by a review by Henry Pitt (Philadelphia, USA) from the American College of Surgeons National Surgical Quality Improvement Program (ACS-NSQIP), who illustrated the potential for HPB-NSQIP to contribute to quality assessment in MIPR surgery. Finally, James Moser from Harvard University (Boston, USA) discussed the contentious subject of credentialing for MIPR, and stressed the need for new approaches to credentialing.

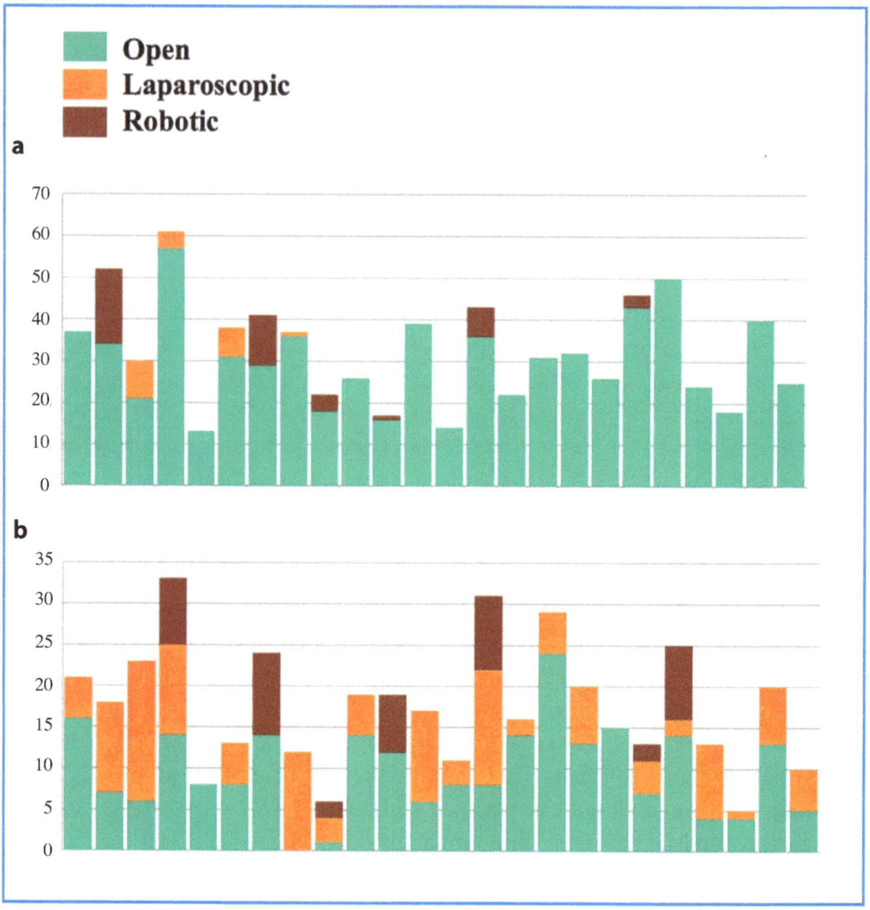

Fig. 1.2 Minimally invasive pancreatic resection (MIPR) experience of HPB trainees in North America (2014-2015). **a** Number of pancreatoduodenectomies performed by at each HPB training center in one academic year, with respect to approach. **b** Number of distal pancreatectomies performed by at each HPB training center in one academic year, with respect to approach (reproduced with permission from [9])

Dr. Hansen then led a lively panel discussion on these topics that completed the section on education and training. Panelists included the following recognized HPB surgical-educators: Pierre Clavien, MD (Geneva, Switzerland); Rohan Jeyarajah, MD (Dallas, USA); Abe Fingerhut, MD (Austria); Herb Zeh, MD (Pittsburgh, USA); James Moser, MD (Boston, USA); and Henry Pitt, MD (Philadelphia, USA).

1.3.2.7 Research Considerations for MIPR

Rounding out the day was a section on future research considerations in MIPR. Jeff Barkun, MD, moderated a collection of talks and a panel discussion on how

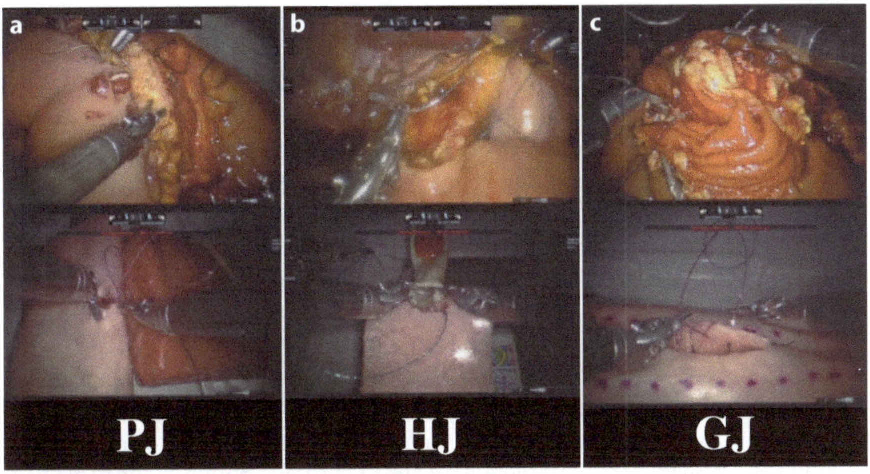

Fig. 1.3 Side-by-side images comparing biotissue and operative components of robotic pancreatoduodenectomy from the University of Pittsburgh 5-step training curriculum in MIPR. These panels demonstrate use of biotissue models (lower half of each panel) to mimic the steps of completing the three anastomotic connections: **a** pancreatojejunostomy (*PJ*), **b** hepaticojejunostomy (*HJ*), and **c** gastrojejunostomy (*GJ*) (reproduced with permission from [9])

to optimally conduct future research endeavors on MIPR [11]. The strengths and weaknesses of randomized control trials (RCTs) and registries to study MIPR were examined during this module. The session began with Bill Fisher, MD from Houston, USA, contemplating whether conducting highest-level evidence RCTs comparing efficacy of MIPR to open resection is feasible. Steven Strasberg, MD, discussed how properly conducted observational studies can still provide value in lieu of RCTs, which may be impractical. An alternative approach would be through registry development. Giana Davidson, an accomplished healthcare outcomes researcher from Seattle, USA, provided a nice overview of the power and pitfalls of surgical registries. This talk was augmented by the insights of Jane Holt, the Executive Director and founder of the National Pancreas Foundation, a patient advocacy group based in Boston, USA. She illustrated the function and substance of a powerful patient-driven registry her organization has conceived, developed, and launched. It was recognized that there is great potential for surgical outcomes to be merged with their data.

The session was concluded with a panel discussion on the feasibility of creating an international registry for MIPR. Dr. Barkun led a discussion between panelists Go Wakabayashi, MD (Saitama, Japan), Henry Pitt, MD (Philadelphia, USA), and Jane Holt (Boston, USA). The main point expressed in this session was that attendees were interested in participating in an international effort to define the role and value of MIPR for our patients and our healthcare systems.

1.3.3 Key points

Comprehensive content from each element of the meeting follows in separate manuscripts in this volume, but major points of emphasis are summarized here:

1. Current terminology describing pancreatic resection is confusing and imprecise. A new framework for thinking about this is proposed by the MIPR steering group.
2. Assessment of, and improvement in, MIPR surgery should be predicated focusing on certain outcomes, beyond the traditional metrics of mortality and major morbidity.
3. An international survey of pancreatic surgeons indicates that MIDP is an accessible procedure that appears to provide similar value to open distal pancreatectomy, but that MIPD is yet unproven for the general population
4. Outcomes data comparing open to minimally invasive distal pancreatectomy are fairly robust at this point and have thus far shown both perioperative and oncologic equivalence.
5. On the other hand, the data regarding proximal MIPR is less developed and too preliminary to endorse its relevance.
6. Cost assessment of this new technology is in its infancy and probably relies on ineffective analyses. Properly designed quality-of-life investigations are desperately needed.
7. How best to learn (and teach) MIPR is not well understood, but there are several promising educational approaches in development.
8. Randomized controlled trials will potentially provide the best evidence for or against MIPR. Despite their strengths, RCTs have limitations which may be further address through development and implementation of prospective national and international data registries.

1.4 Conclusions

This formative event allowed some of the brightest minds in pancreatic surgery to gather and consider the impact of MIPR on the field of pancreatic surgery. The accumulated MIPR experience was critically assessed, and current perceptions by surgeons were obtained. Potential benefits of MIPR were considered through the prism of cost and value assessments. New training paradigms were explored, and enthusiasm for collective, high-impact research efforts was generated. The conference was specifically conducted in a bias-free manner with international contributions by surgeons who perform both open and MIS pancreatectomy. The output of this event, including its numerous descriptive publications, should serve as a platform for better understanding the role of MIPR, as well as improving its future development.

References

1. Gagner M, Pomp A (1994) Laparoscopic pylorus-preserving pancreatoduodenectomy. Surg Endosc 8(5):408–410
2. Gagner M, Pomp A, Herrera MF (1996) Early experience with laparoscopic resections of islet cell tumors. Surgery 120(6):1051–1054
3. Kendrick ML, van Hilst J, Boggi U et al (2017) Minimally invasive pancreatoduodenectomy. HPB (Oxford) 19(3):215–224
4. Conlon KC, de Rooij T, van Hilst J et al (2017) Minimally invasive pancreatic resections: cost and value perspectives. HPB (Oxford) 19(3):225–233
5. Røsok BI, de Rooij T, van Hilst J et al (2017) Minimally invasive distal pancreatectomy. HPB (Oxford) 19(3):205–214
6. Bassi C, Andrianello S (2017) Identifying key outcome metrics in pancreatic surgery, and how to optimally achieve them. HPB (Oxford) 19(3):178–181
7. Montagnini AL, Røsok BI, Asbun HJ et al (2017) Standardizing terminology for minimally invasive pancreatic resection. HPB (Oxford) 19(3):182–189
8. van Hilst J, de Rooij T, Abu Hilal M et al (2017) Worldwide survey on opinions and use of minimally invasive pancreatic resection. HPB (Oxford) 19(3):190–204
9. Hogg ME, Besselink MG, Clavien PA et al (2017) Training in minimally invasive pancreatic resections: a paradigm shift away from "See one, Do one, Teach one". HPB (Oxford) 19(3):234–245
10. de Rooij T, van Hilst J, Boerma D et al (2016) Impact of a nationwide training program in minimally invasive distal pancreatectomy (LAELAPS). Ann Surg 264(5):754–762
11. Barkun J, Fisher W, Davidson G et al (2017) Research considerations in the evaluation of minimally invasive pancreatic resection (MIPR). HPB (Oxford) 19(3):246–253

2 Evolving Technologies in the Operating Room for Minimally Invasive Pancreatic Surgery

Graziano Ceccarelli, Antonello Forgione, Enrico Andolfi, Aldo Rocca, Antonio Giuliani, and Fulvio Calise

2.1 Improvements in Minimally Invasive Vision

Since the beginning of the laparoscopic era, the surgeon has had to work in a three-dimensional (3D) space through a two-dimensional (2D) projection on a monitor, with a difficulty in depth perception. Moreover, the first optic (camera and monitor) devices on the market were actually analogic, with a low definition (4:3 aspect ratio, 640 by 480 horizontal and vertical lines) and poor lighting performance. The move towards digital technology, with the adoption of CCD (charged couplet device) microsensors and LED (light emitting diode) light sources and monitors, started a real revolution in vision quality. Endoscopes, first equipped with a single CCD mounted on the camera head, are now supplied with three tip-mounted CCDs. Newer, powerful LED light sources and full-HD monitors provide clear and well-defined images with a 16:9 aspect ratio, 1280 by 720 horizontal and vertical lines.

Wider monitors provide a peripheral vision that allows for safer access to the peritoneal cavity. A newer image sensor technology, the complementary metal-oxide semiconductor (CMOS), has widely replaced CCD in the commercial camera market and will probably do the same in future surgical endoscopy, promising further improvements in image quality. The most recent monitor technology, the so-called 4K standard, is recently available in the medical devices market. It improves horizontal resolution to approximately 4,000 pixels and vertical resolution to approximately 2,000 pixels with nearly a four-fold improvement of the actual best definition (Fig. 2.1a).

G. Ceccarelli (✉)
General Surgery Unit, San Donato Hospital
Arezzo, Italy
e-mail: g.cecca2003@libero.it

U. Boggi (Ed), *Minimally Invasive Surgery of the Pancreas*,
Updates in Surgery
DOI: 10.1007/978-88-470-3958-2_2,

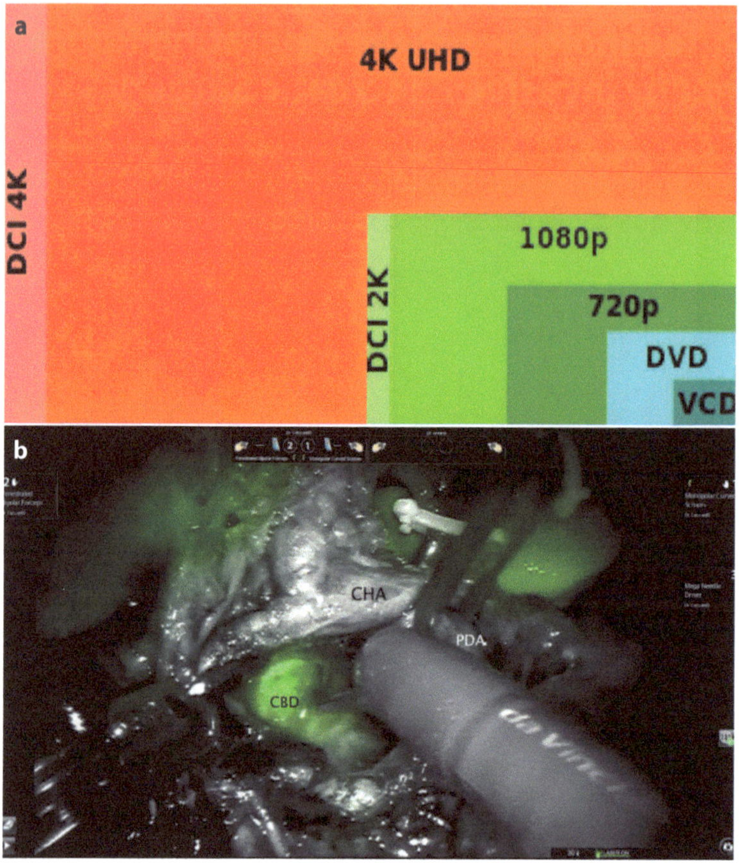

Fig. 2.1 **a** Comparison of common broadcast resolutions. **b** Indocyanine green fluorescence (IGF) at hepatobiliary liver pedicle

Better image quality undoubtedly improves depth perception, but the recent introduction of HD-3D vision in laparoscopy has probably filled the gap. Initially limited by the associated discomforts (commonly headache, dizziness and strain) due to single-lens technology, the diffusion of 3D systems has been accelerated by the introduction of modern lightweight passive, polarized dual-lens glasses to perceive images in 3D. This technology allows a real "surgical immersion", very similar to the one already offered by robotic surgery, providing enhanced space perception.

A systematic review by Sorensen et al. analyzing 31 randomized clinical trials (RCT) shows how in the majority of cases HD-3D vision reduces the operative time and number of mistakes during the operation [1]. Moreover, Spille et al. demonstrate how HD-3D vision versus HD-2D may improve the surgical skill of 277 either residents or specialized surgeons. Results consisted of a better handling, better view sensation and faster approach to technical findings in both groups [2]. Velayutham et al. in a retrospective study found only a reduction of surgical time using 3D technology versus 2D in hepatobiliary surgery [3].

In summary, RCTs and case series report that HD-3D vision improves surgical performance, shortens operative time and the learning curve and minimizes technical errors. The lower costs of HD-3D versus the higher costs of robotic platforms will probably favor the spread of the former.

2.2 The Role of Indocyanine Green Fluorescence Imaging

Another fairly new innovation in vision technology is notably the so-called near-infrared (NIR) indocyanine green (ICG) fluorescence imaging. ICG is a sterile water-soluble dye that, once injected, binds to plasma proteins and is rapidly extracted and excreted by the liver. It becomes fluorescent once exited by a laser beam or NIR and can be detected using specifically designated scopes and camera. It affords a "virtual" real-time angiography as soon as injected, and later, about 45 minutes after the injection, a "virtual" cholangiography (Fig. 2.1b). The applications of this technology are multiple and probably still not completely exploited. It could help to understand the vascular and biliary anatomy in complex cases [4] and evaluate organ perfusion/ischemia in digestive surgery. Furthermore, extravascular injection allows for a lymphoscintigraphy that opens new frontiers in sentinel node surgery and fluorescence-guided lymphadenectomy.

In minimally invasive pancreatic surgery there is still a long way to go to assess the reliability and efficacy of ICG. A first report by Subar et al. assessed the utility of ICG in evaluating the viability of the margin of the remnant pancreas in a Whipple's procedure. The ICG is visualized in the viable areas but not in the ischemic areas that can therefore be resected before anastomosis [4]. In another paper, ICG was tested to assess, after resection of bile duct, viability of margins or bile leakage after anastomosis [5].

2.3 The New da Vinci Xi Surgical System

Still today the vast majority of pancreatic surgery is performed in an open fashion. In 1994 Gagner and Pomp first described laparoscopic pancreatoduodenectomy (LPD) [6].

Robotic technology, thanks to HD-3D vision and Endowrist instruments, makes minimally invasive pancreatic surgery easier and safer compared to conventional laparoscopy, overcoming many of its limits, in particular during the complex reconstructive phase.

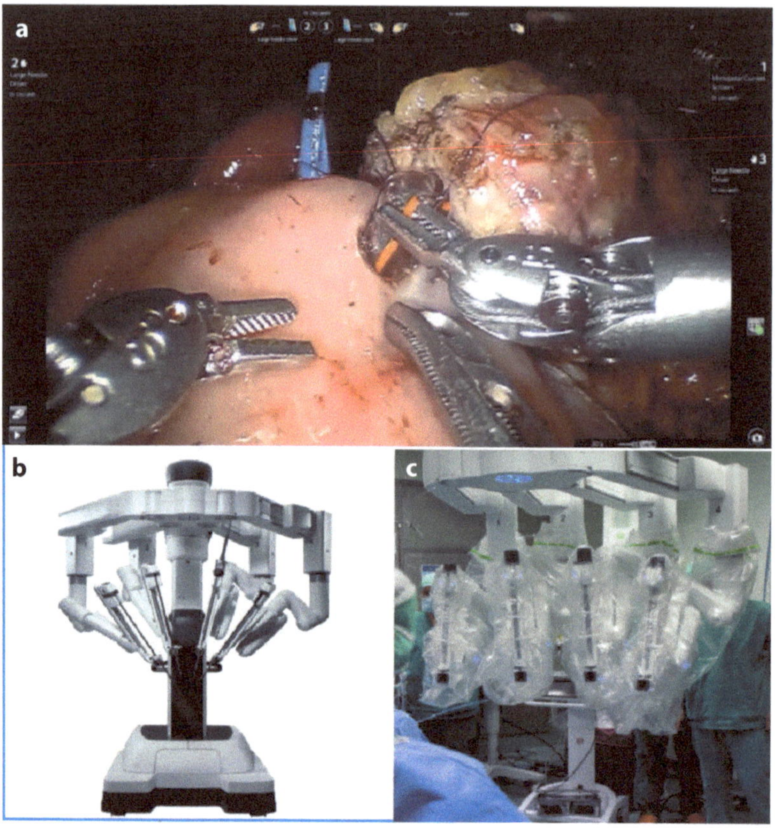

Fig. 2.2 **a** Robot-assisted duct-to-mucosa pancreatojejunostomy during pancreatoduodenectomy. **b** da Vinci Xi (Intuitive Surgical Inc.) patient cart. **c** Robotic arms with steri-drapes in operating room

Since the year 2000, when the da Vinci robot (Intuitive Surgical Inc., Sunnyvale, CA, USA) received its first FDA approval, the robot has undergone several updates, with important upgrades of the prior version. After the first-generation da Vinci Standard system came the S and Si versions. Recently, the latest upgrade, the da Vinci Xi has been introduced.

The latest generation of the da Vinci robot, the Xi surgical system (Fig. 2.2) is optimized for complex multiquadrant surgery. Yuh et al. describe 112 robotic operations using the Xi robot; 8 of them were hepatobiliary procedures and 5 were gastrointestinal interventions. In the paper they show how the new platform is a radical change from the past Si model. There are new skillsets, which can be applied, and new software is ready to communicate with new technologies. The possibility of moving the camera from one trocar to another may improve versatility and movement from one zone to another. Fighting of instruments is reduced due to the alignment of arms [7].

In response to a letter to the editor, Yuh adds that the instruments are longer, the camera is compatible with the Firefly fluorescence imaging system (while the Si needs a dedicated system), delivery of the instruments from the back tables and positioning of the surgical assistant is easier [8].

Memeo et al. published in 2016 a review about the state of the art in pancreatic robotic surgery. Advantages of robotic surgery consist of better vessel identification, easier anastomosis performance, reduction of blood loss; disadvantages are linked to the learning curve of surgeons whereas the robot docking time loss may be overcome by the use of Xi [9].

2.4 Intraoperative Ultrasonography

Intraoperative ultrasonography (IOUS) is an essential technique for diagnosis and surgical guidance in both liver and pancreatic resections, in both open and minimally invasive procedures. Particularly in pancreatic surgery, it allows evaluation of regional metastases and infiltration of vessels or surrounding organs, and identification of very small endocrine tumors. It is mostly useful for distinguishing pancreatitis from a neoplasm, driving biopsy, duct cannulation, and drainage of abscesses or cysts. Doppler and color flow may be useful for identifying vessels. Sometimes information from IOUS is so relevant as to modify the preoperative surgical strategy [10–12].

Laparoscopic IOUS is performed using a special linear flexible laparoscopic probe, generally 7.5-MHz and 10 mm in diameter. IOUS uses a linear side-view, T-shaped or microconvex probe, with a flexible tip. They can also be used for tumor staging in order to evaluate the surgical resection avoiding unnecessary laparotomy in many cases [13, 14].

A recent series of minimally invasive probes for laparoscopic and robotic surgery were made available a few years ago by BK Ultrasound (BK Medical ApS, Mileparken, Denmark). In particular, the X12C4 drop-in transducer (Fig. 2.3a) 12–3.5 MHz is a small and compact linear curved-array transducer enabling a wider field of view for faster kidney and liver navigation. The probe cable for robotic surgery is flexible, allowing studying of lesions in every abdominal space. The specially designed probe can be grasped by the articulated robotic instrument and handled by the robotic arm directly by the console, ensuring maximum control and organ contact. This means that the surgeon can control the probe directly from the console and, thanks to the so-called TilePro system, he or she can simultaneously see the operative field and the high-resolution real-time US images. (Fig. 2.3b). The color Doppler mode (Fig. 2.3c) allows identifying arterial and venous blood supply to organs (Fig. 2.3d), especially when selective clamping is needed. In addition, 3D image reconstruction is possible, thanks to special software, allowing verification of tumor location, margins and depth, enabling easier identification of key anatomical landmarks and dissection planes.

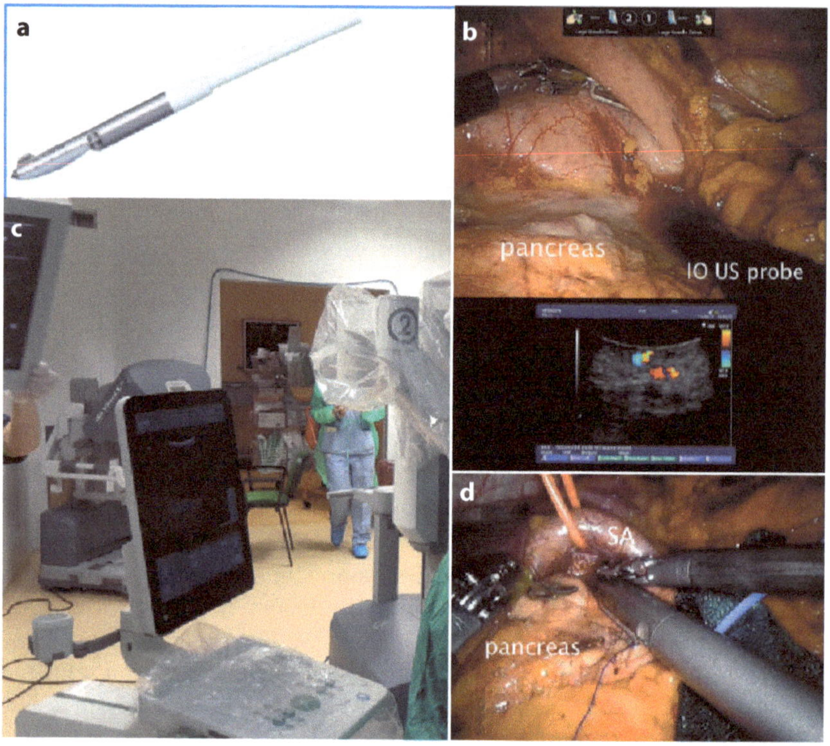

Fig. 2.3 **a** Robotic drop-in probe for intraoperative ultrasonography. **b** Real-time visualization of intraoperative field and ultrasound image. **c** Ultrasound system in the robotic operating room. **d** Robotic drop-in ultrasound transducer during pancreatic resection

2.5 Virtual Reality for Surgical Planning and Simulation

Patient-specific anatomy and pathologic lesions are currently evaluated in the preoperative setting through classical radiological studies. Despite their advancements in terms of extremely high definition at subcentimetric scale, they still have major intrinsic limits for proper surgical planning and navigation. Therefore, the analysis and understanding of the whole image series to create a precise mental model of the target anatomy remains limited to radiologists and a minority of surgeons who have specific radiological knowledge and extensive experience.

Conversely, creation of virtual reality-3D models from patients' computed tomography (CT) or magnetic resonance (MR) images may contribute to overcome these limits, offering surgeons the possibility to visualize and manipulate in a more familiar 3D fashion patient-specific anatomy and disease.

Virtual reality (VR) is a digital transposition in 3D of real objects and settings through a computer interface: it can be defined "immersive" or "non-immersive",

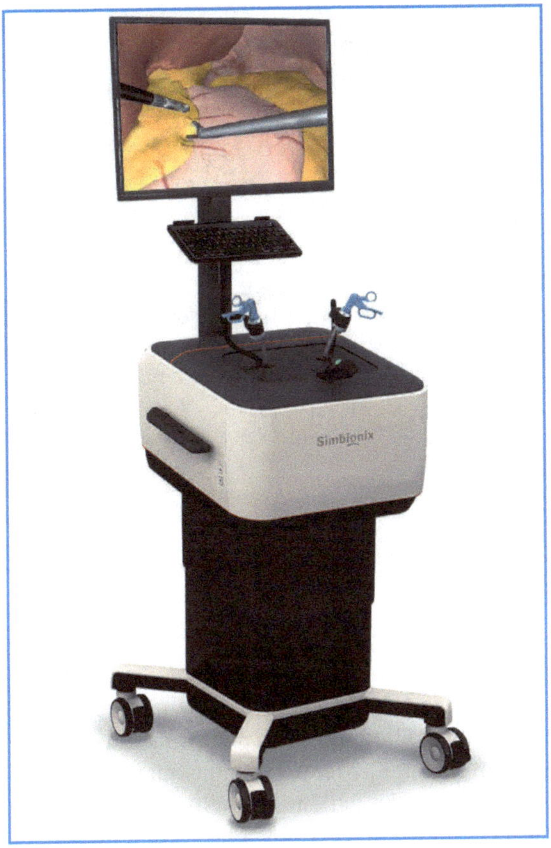

Fig. 2.4 LAP Mentor from Simbionix (Cleveland, OH, USA)

depending if you are experiencing a complete interaction with the virtual setting or not [15]. All the senses (visual and haptic) should be supported in order to get a completely immersive experience, included orientation. VR is now widely spread in other fields such as aeronautic training, video games and commercial purposes.

VR-based surgical applications can be used not only for patient-specific preoperative planning but also for preoperative training and intraoperative navigation [16]. Is well known that VR simulators (Fig. 2.4) facilitate training in young surgeons.

Indeed, simulators offer the possibility to quantify surgical performance on the basis of objective measures, which provides an unbiased assessment of surgical performance and individual progression [17]. In a review article from the Cochrane Collaboration published in 2013, Nagendran et al. evaluated the role of virtual reality for surgical trainees in laparoscopic surgery [18]. They report that virtual reality training appears to decrease the operating time and improve the operative performance of surgical trainees with limited laparoscopic experience when compared with no training or with box-trainer training.

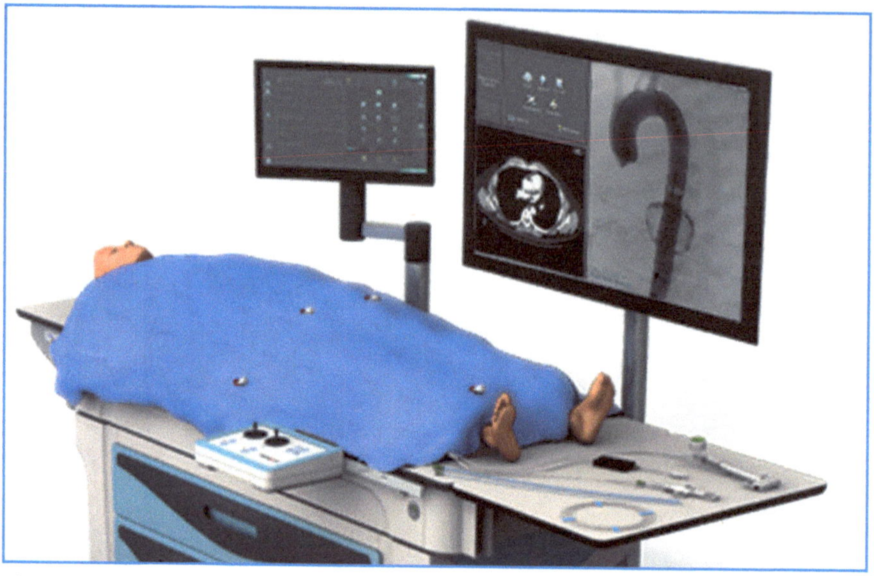

Fig. 2.5 Angio Mentor from Simbionix (Cleveland, OH, USA)

An even more promising VR training modality is represented by patient-specific VR models based on preoperative CT scan images. This promising tool has been tested on some commercially available simulating platforms and research prototype. For example, the Simbionix Angio Mentor demonstrated increased procedural training without added risks to the patient. The advantages of such VR training have been shown to be so relevant that nowadays, for surgeons in the United States to receive full board certification and authorization to practice intravascular procedures, they have to pass a VR test which is based on the Angio Mentor (Fig. 2.5) and is included in the Fundamentals of Endovascular Surgery skills testing [19].

2.6 4D Image Fusion

One special advantage of VR-based models is the possibility to produce a single 3D model of patient-specific anatomy starting from imaging examinations acquired with different technologies, different phases and even at different times: the so called 4D image fusion, the fourth dimension being the evolution over time of a given lesion. Specifically, in the case of pancreatic tumors, a VR-based model will represent at the same time the neoplasm and vascular structures based on CT images (Fig. 2.6a), while the biliary tree and pancreatic tissue will be reconstructed starting from MR acquisitions (Fig. 2.6b). The end result will be a full 3D virtual anatomical model that in one single shot will depict all the

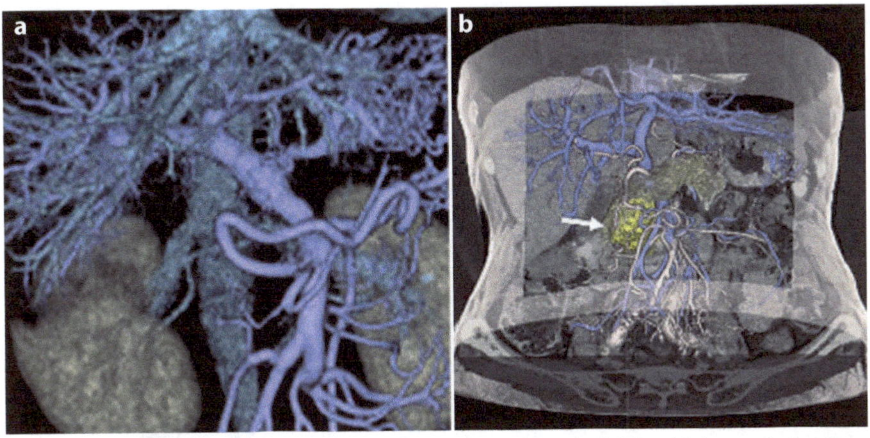

Fig. 2.6 **a** Virtual reality (VR) vascular anatomy from a CT scan. **b** VR with image fusion from CT scan and MRI

important anatomical and pathological structures with the potential to show also the evolution over time of the tumor [20]

2.7 Augmented Reality

The process of superimposing live intraoperative images with synthetic computer-generated, patient-specific preoperatively acquired, 3D reconstructed images is defined as augmented reality (AR).

AR represents an enhanced navigation tool that highlights target structures and anatomical variations through modular virtual organ transparency [21]. The process of precisely superimposing the 3D virtual model obtained from the patients' preoperative imaging anatomy onto the real patient during the operation is called "registration". Accurate registration is critical to provide correct and useful information to the surgeon. Registration is a difficult step in AR and constitutes an area of ongoing research. AR and image-guided surgery was initially applied to brain surgery and maxillofacial surgery, in which the fixed and highly contrasted structures such as bones make the virtual model highly congruent with the real patient. In abdominal surgery, especially if performed with a laparoscopic approach, AR presents several challenges (Fig. 2.7) due to respiratory motion and the deformation of soft tissues during surgical manipulation [22, 23].

The use of dedicated software, together with tools for patient-tailored training, is likely to improve clinical outcomes and patient safety. Indeed, at the present time it seems that the major obstacle to the diffusion of VR-based training and VR technologies in surgery is a cultural limitation of the surgeons themselves [24].

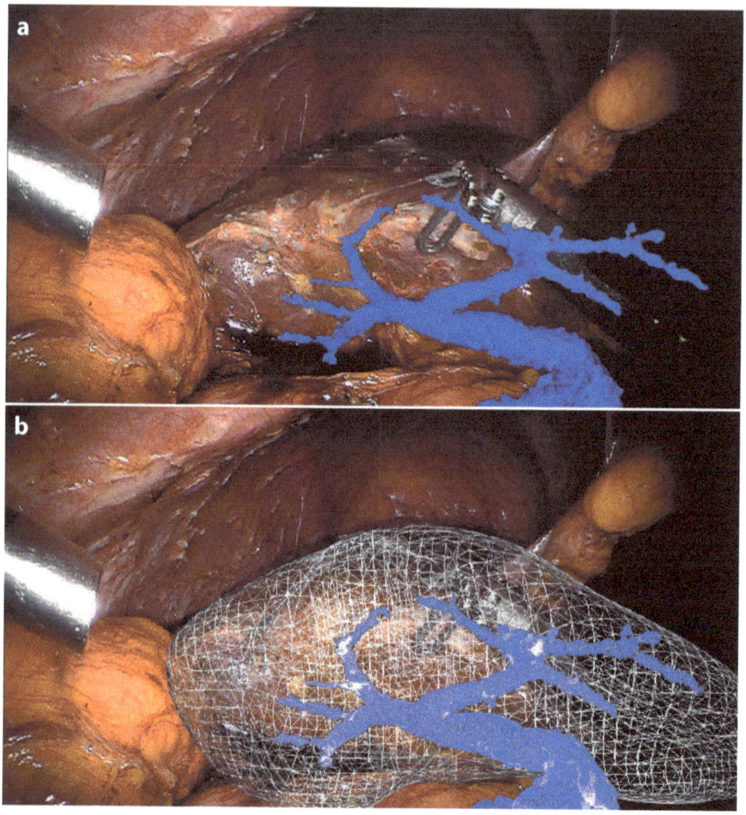

Fig. 2.7 **a** Augmented reality (AR) rigid registration. **b** AR with deformable anatomical structures

2.8 Conclusions

It is clear that technology is changing our lives in different fields. Over a few years, communications, travelling, energy production, and life sciences have all been gradually modified as a result of innovations in technology.

Surgery, and in particular pancreatic surgery, is no exception. From the first laparoscopic pancreatoduodenectomy described by Gagner and Pomp [6] in 1994, even more complex minimally invasive pancreatic procedures have been performed thanks to the improvement of technologies. A PubMed search for "laparoscopic" OR "minimally invasive" AND "pancreatic surgery" yielded more than 600 papers published in the last ten years. This spread of minimally invasive pancreatic surgery is linked to better vision and the development of sealing and cutting devices and several other tools allowing increasing numbers of surgeons to approach minimally invasive surgery.

In particular, the robotic surgery revolution boosted the development of the minimally invasive approach after the first report by Giulianotti et al. in 2003 [25]. Over the last ten years, the robotic approach has expanded, despite the flat trend in laparoscopic surgery, thanks to 3D-HD vision, Endowrist technology, new da Vinci robotic arms, optimization of IOUS robotic devices, and fluorescence integrated technology. The improvement of technologies and robotic approaches might shorten the learning curve, affording even low- and middle-volume centers the possibility to approach these challenging fields.

The introduction of virtual and augmented reality may provide new options to perform minimally invasive pancreatic surgery in a safer and more effective way.

References

1. Sørensen SM, Savran MM, Konge L, Bjerrum F (2016) Three-dimensional versus two-dimensional vision in laparoscopy: a systematic review. Surg Endosc 30(1):11–23
2. Spille J, Wenners A, von Hehn U et al (2017) 2D versus 3D in laparoscopic surgery by beginners and experts: a randomized controlled trial on a pelvitrainer in objectively graded surgical steps. J Surg Educ [Epub ahead of print] doi:10.1016/j.jsurg.2017.01.011
3. Velayutham V, Fuks D, Nomi T et al (2016) 3D visualization reduces operating time when compared to high-definition 2D in laparoscopic liver resection: a case-matched study. Surg Endosc 30(1):147–153
4. Subar D, Pietrasz D, Fuks D, Gayet B (2015) A novel technique for reducing pancreatic fistulas after pancreaticojejunostomy. J Surg Case Rep 2015(7):rjv074 doi:10.1093/jscr/rjv074
5. Kawaguchi Y, Velayutham V, Fuks D et al (2015) Usefulness of indocyanine green-fluorescence imaging for visualization of the bile duct during laparoscopic liver resection. J Am Coll Surg 221(6):e113–e117
6. Gagner M, Pomp A (1994) Laparoscopic pylorus-preserving pancreatoduodenectomy. Surg Endosc 8(5):408–410
7. Yuh B, Yu X, Raytis J et al (2016) Use of a mobile tower-based robot – The initial Xi robot experience in surgical oncology. J Surg Oncol 113(1):5–7
8. Yuh B (2016) Response to letter to the editor on "Use of a mobile tower-based robot – The initial Xi robot experience in surgical oncology". J Surg Oncol 114(8):1031
9. Memeo R, Sangiuolo F, de Blasi V et al (2016) Robotic pancreaticoduodenectomy and distal pancreatectomy: state of the art. J Visc Surg 153(5):353–359
10. Sun MR, Brennan DD, Kruskal JB, Kane RA (2010) Intraoperative ultrasonography of the pancreas. Radiographics 30(7):1935–1953
11. Piccolboni D, Ciccone F, Settembre A, Corcione F (2008) The role of echo-laparoscopy in abdominal surgery: five years' experience in a dedicated center. Surg Endosc 22(1):112–117
12. Doucas H, Sutton CD, Zimmerman A et al (2007) Assessment of pancreatic malignancy with laparoscopy and intraoperative ultrasound. Surg Endosc 21(7):1147–1152
13. Pietrabissa A, Caramella D, Di Candio G et al (1999) Laparoscopy and laparoscopic ultrasonography for staging pancreatic cancer: critical appraisal. World J Surg 23(10):998–1002
14. Zhao ZW, He JY, Tan G et al (2003) Laparoscopy and laparoscopic ultrasonography in judging the resectability of pancreatic head cancer. Hepatobiliary Pancreat Dis Int 2(4):609–611
15. Marescaux J, Clément JM, Tassetti V et al (1998) Virtual reality applied to hepatic surgery simulation: the next revolution. Ann Surg 228(5):627–634
16. Aggarwal R, Ward J, Balasundaram I et al (2007) Proving the effectiveness of virtual reality simulation for training in laparoscopic surgery. Ann Surg 246(5):771–779

17. Araujo SE, Delaney CP, Seid VE et al (2014) Short-duration virtual reality simulation training positively impacts performance during laparoscopic colectomy in animal model: results of a single-blinded randomized trial: VR warm-up for laparoscopic colectomy. Surg Endosc 28(9):2547–2554
18. Nagendran M, Gurusamy KS, Aggarwal R et al (2013) Virtual reality training for surgical trainees in laparoscopic surgery. Cochrane Database Syst Rev 8:CD006575
19. Duran C, Estrada S, O'Malley M et al (2015) The model for Fundamentals of Endovascular Surgery (FEVS) successfully defines the competent endovascular surgeon. J Vasc Surg 62(6):1660–1666
20. Uchida M (2014) Recent advances in 3D computed tomography techniques for simulation and navigation in hepatobiliary pancreatic surgery. J Hepatobiliary Pancreat Sci 21(4):239–245
21. Marescaux J, Rubino F, Arenas M et al (2004) Augmented-reality-assisted laparoscopic adrenalectomy. JAMA 292(18):2214–2215
22. Hostettler A, Nicolau SA, Rémond Y et al (2010) A real-time predictive simulation of abdominal viscera positions during quiet free breathing. Prog Biophys Mol Biol 103(2–3): 169–184
23. Pessaux P, Diana M, Soler L et al (2014) Robotic duodenopancreatectomy assisted with augmented reality and real-time fluorescence guidance. Surg Endosc 28(8):2493–2498
24. Forgione A, Guraya SY (2017) The cutting-edge training modalities and educational platforms for accredited surgical training: a systematic review. J Res Med Sci 22(1):51
25. Giulianotti PC, Coratti A, Angelini M et al (2003) Robotics in general surgery: personal experience in a large community hospital. Arch Surg 138(7):777–784

Simulation in Laparoscopy and Robotics

3

Andrea Moglia

3.1 Introduction

For more than one century surgical training has been based on the autocratic and pyramidal 'see one, do one, teach one' method developed by William Halsted at John Hopkins Hospital [1]. The advent of laparoscopy, manual first and robotically assisted later, posed new challenges on teaching the necessary technical skills a surgeon must own to operate at a safe and proficient level. These skills are different from those of traditional open surgery, and are: perceptual, visuospatial, and psychomotor (hand-eye coordination). For the assessment of perceptual and visuospatial skills, PicSOr (Pictorial Surface Orientation) and cube-comparison tests were respectively devised [2]. For the objective evaluation of psychomotor skills, virtual reality (VR) simulators have proven to be valid tools [3]. VR simulators enable users to hone their technical skills by interacting with a computer-generated environment through ad-hoc control interfaces, a physical representation of real surgical instruments. They differ from physical simulators allowing users to train on dry lab (synthetic accessories), and wet lab (animal tissues) by using actual surgical tools and viewing laparoscope images on a screen. Lastly, hybrid surgical simulators overlay virtual information on images acquired by the laparoscope and projected on the screen of the box-trainer station.

Simulation-based training is not intended to fully replace training in the operating room, but to overcome the initial learning curve. Moreover, by considering the restrictions on work hours for residents, limited to 80 hours a week in the United States and 48 hours a week in Europe, simulators enable us to educate residents in an efficient and safe way.

A. Moglia (✉)
EndoCAS – Center for Computer Assisted Surgery, University of Pisa
Pisa, Italy
e-mail: andrea.moglia@endocas.org

U. Boggi (Ed), *Minimally Invasive Surgery of the Pancreas*,
Updates in Surgery
DOI: 10.1007/978-88-470-3958-2_3, © Springer-Verlag Italia 2018

3.2 The Advent of VR Surgical Simulators

In the wake of the success of flight simulators, VR surgical simulators were pioneered by Richard Satava in early 90s within projects supported by the Defense Advanced Research Projects Agency (DARPA) [4].

VR simulators have several advantages over traditional training methods: immediate objective evaluation (summative feedback) on user performance, and automatic tracking of progress through the learning curve. Assessment is computed by considering several parameters called metrics. Good metrics are valid to distinguish optimal from suboptimal performance. Examples of metrics for assessment of psychomotor skills are time to complete, and distance covered by instruments.

VR simulators struggled before being accepted by the surgical community because of the lack of robust scientific evidence on skills transfer to the operating room [5]. Other barriers were the absence of market, and the lack of low-cost powerful computers [1]. However, things started to change once scientific evidence showed the positive effect of VR simulators for laparoscopy in skills transfer to the operating room. This proof is fundamental for the integration of simulation into surgical curricula.

3.3 VR for Laparoscopy

The expression "VR to OR" was coined by Anthony Gallagher to identify the skills transfer from VR simulators to the operating room [6]. Most of the studies addressing this aspect required a training period at VR simulators where practice was proficiency-based, repetition-based, or time-based [6]. Among these models, VR-to-OR studies coupled with the concept of reaching proficiency at a simulator twice consecutively became the benchmark. The second attempt to reach proficiency is the conventional overtraining, or additional training after initial proficiency, adopted by most authors to prove that proficiency was not reached accidentally.

A randomized control trial (RCT) conducted at Yale University showed for the first time that residents, after reaching a proficiency level on basic tasks twice consecutively at the MIST-VR simulator by Mentice (Gothenburg, Sweden), were 29% faster and made five times fewer intraoperative errors during laparoscopic cholecystectomy than the control group following conventional training [7]. Although limited to 16 residents, this study, also known as the Yale study from the center where it was conducted, demonstrated the benefits of VR training in terms of operative time and reduction of intraoperative errors. For these reasons, it became the paradigm to assess skills transfer from VR to OR. Similar results were reported in a study on 22 residents with similar design and the same VR simulator as the Yale study for the assessment of intracorporeal and suturing and knot tying [8].

Another VR-to-OR RCT on the MIST-VR simulator with 16 residents confirmed reduction of operative times and technical errors, although it was repetition-based rather than proficiency-based [9]. This last trial and the Yale study had paramount impact on training in the United States. The American College of Surgeons (ACS) published a white paper supporting VR simulators and then created a network of accredited training centers for education in surgery through simulation [10].

Since the production of the MIST-VR was discontinued, the currently available VR simulators for laparoscopy are: LapSim by Surgical Science (Gothenburg, Sweden), Mentor by 3D Systems, LAP Simbionix Products (Cleveland, OH, USA), and LapVR by CAE Healthcare (Quebec, QC, Canada). A study with 13 residents, following a similar design to the Yale RCT, showed that proficiency-based training on basic tasks with LapSim to improve psychomotor skills at a simulator reduced intraoperative errors during 10 cholecystectomies [11]. In an RCT comparing transfer of training of surgical residents from LapSim or physical simulator (box-trainer) to execution of Nissen fundoplication on real patients, there was no statistically significant difference between the two groups in time, Objective Structured Assessment of Technical Skills (OSATS) rating score, and checklist score [12].

Despite the benefits of VR-to-OR studies on improving technical performance, there is no published study assessing simulation for pancreatic surgery [13].

The cost-effectiveness of VR simulators for laparoscopy was assessed by using transfer effectiveness ratio (TER), a parameter in long-established use by the aviation industry. It is defined as the ratio between the difference in time, number of trials or errors performed by an experimental and control group until the subjects reach proficiency on the actual activity/device (safe competent flying) and time, number of trials or errors performed by experimental group until reaching proficiency on a simulator [14]. An RCT comparing different training modalities by computing TER showed that training at LapSim and box-trainer are more cost-effective than traditional training since they saved 2.31 and 1.13 hours, respectively, for each hour of conventional training [12].

3.4 VR for Robotic Surgery

Operating room costs and the availability of dedicated surgical equipment represent an even more critical issue in robotic surgery. In fact, it is estimated that the use of a da Vinci robot costs about $ 500/hour. Therefore, the purchase of one of the currently commercialized VR simulators (market price range from $ 80,000 to 150,000) for robotic surgery seems an affordable solution. The growing interest around robotic surgery and wide adoption of da Vinci surgical systems led several companies to develop VR software solutions. Today, there are different VR simulators for robotic surgery: SEP (Surgical Education Platform) by SimSurgery (Oslo, Norway), RoSS (Robotic Surgical System) by Simulated

Surgical Systems (San Jose, CA, USA), dV-Trainer by Mimic (Seattle, WA, USA), da Vinci Skills Simulator by Intuitive Surgical (Sunnyvale, CA, USA), and the recently introduced RobotiX Mentor by 3D Systems, Simbionix Products (Cleveland, OH, USA).

Many studies have been published, most of them on validity (face, content, construct, concurrent, discriminant, and predictive) [15]. Few studies addressed skills transfer from VR to inanimate models and animal tissue. However, there is no proof from any high evidence level study, such as an RCT, on VR to OR, as demonstrated for manual laparoscopy [15]. This is the main obstacle for the integration of VR simulators for robotic surgery into surgical curricula.

Evaluation on real patients was reported in only one study involving 14 subjects in the experimental group and 4 in the control group who performed supracervical hysterectomy after training on the da Vinci Skills Simulator. Aside from small numbers, this study lacked randomization [16].

A multicenter RCT involving 14 ACS-accredited training centers and aiming to validate the Fundamentals of Robotic Surgery (FRS) curriculum is currently underway. FRS is a multispecialty, proficiency-based curriculum of cognitive and technical skills (http://frsurgery.org). It was developed after reaching consensus among over 80 international robotic surgery experts, behavioral psychologists, medical educators, statisticians, and psychometricians.

The University of Pittsburgh Medical Center developed a step-wise training program for operating proficiency for complex surgical oncology procedures such as pancreatoduodenectomy. It includes VR simulation, inanimate models (bioartificial organs), and an operative curriculum [17]. A study on the first step on 17 fellows showed that they improved their performance on four tasks at the da Vinci Skills Simulator and three exercises during dry-lab with the actual da Vinci robot, after proficiency-based training at da Vinci Skills Simulator with a threshold score over 90% (with green checks in all fields) [17].

Furthermore, the cost-efficacy of VR simulators for robot-assisted surgery is not known since there is no estimate of TER. The only published study on this topic evaluated time spent on training 105 subjects at a RoSS simulator instead of a real da Vinci robot. This time was equivalent to 73 robot-assisted radical prostatectomies, realizing a saving of about 623,000 dollars [18]. However, this study did not yield an accurate estimate of cost-effectiveness since it did not use TER.

3.5 The Future of Surgical Simulators

VR simulators for laparoscopy and robotic surgery offer users a wide range of exercises to hone their technical skills in basic tasks, advanced tasks (knots and sutures), up to full procedures for different surgical specialties. The future generation of simulators might include patient-specific simulation for procedure rehearsal enabling surgeons to import radiological datasets, like computed tomography, into simulation software and rehearse the procedure before performing it on a real patient, as is currently available in VR simulators for endovascular surgery. Additionally, integration of virtual mentors will provide users with formative feedback by informing them promptly whenever an error occurs.

There is an increasing interest in the potential application of VR simulators as additional tools for objective assessment of technical skills in the selection of surgical residents. A study on innate ability for surgery among medical students by using a VR simulator for robotic surgery was conducted at the University of Pisa, Italy [19]. This study demonstrated the capability of a VR simulator to discriminate with a statistically significant difference three distinct populations: 6.6% with outstanding dexterity, 81.8% with average dexterity, and 11.6% with poor manipulative skills [19].

References

1. Gallagher AG, O'Sullivan GC (2012) Fundamentals of surgical simulation. Springer, London
2. Ritter EM, McClusky DA 3rd, Gallagher AG et al (2006) Perceptual, visuospatial, and psychomotor abilities correlate with duration of training required on a virtual-reality flexible endoscopy simulator. Am J Surg 192(3):379–384
3. Gallagher AG, Satava RM (2002) Virtual reality as a metric for the assessment of laparoscopic psychomotor skills. Learning curves and reliability measures. Surg Endosc 16(12):1746–1752
4. Satava RM (1993) Virtual reality surgical simulator: the first steps. Surg Endosc 7(3):203–205
5. Gallagher AG, Ritter EM, Champion H et al (2005) Virtual reality simulation for the operating room: proficiency-based training as a paradigm shift in surgical skills training. Ann Surg 241(2):364–372
6. Seymour NE (2008) VR to OR: a review of the evidence that virtual reality simulation improves operating room performance. World J Surg 32(2):182–188
7. Seymour NE, Gallagher AG, Roman SA et al (2002) Virtual reality training improves operating room performance: results of a randomized, double-blinded study. Ann Surg 236(4):458–463
8. Van Sickle KR, Ritter EM, Baghai M et al (2008) Prospective, randomized, double-blind trial of curriculum-based training for intracorporeal suturing and knot tying. J Am Coll Surg 207(4):560–568
9. Grantcharov TP, Kristiansen VB, Bendix J et al (2004) Randomized clinical trial of virtual reality simulation for laparoscopic skills training. Br J Surg 91(2):146–150
10. Healy GB (2002) The college should be instrumental in adapting simulators to education. Bull Am Coll Surg 87(11):10–11
11. Ahlberg G, Enochsson L, Gallagher AG et al (2007) Proficiency-based virtual reality training significantly reduces the error rate for residents during their first 10 laparoscopic cholecystectomies. Am J Surg 193(6):797–804
12. Orzech N, Palter VN, Reznick RK et al (2012) A comparison of 2 ex vivo training curricula for advanced laparoscopic skills: a randomized controlled trial. Ann Surg 255(5):833–839
13. Beyer-Berjot L, Palter V, Grantcharov T, Aggarwal R (2014) Advanced training in laparoscopic abdominal surgery: a systematic review. Surgery 156(3):676–688
14. Roscoe SN (1971) Incremental transfer effectiveness. Human Factors 13(6):561–567

15. Moglia A, Ferrari V, Morelli L et al (2016) A systematic review of virtual reality simulators for robot-assisted surgery. Eur Urol 69(6):1065–1080
16. Culligan P, Gurshumov E, Lewis C et al (2014) Predictive validity of a training protocol using a robotic surgery simulator. Female Pelvic Med Reconstr Surg 20(1):48–51
17. Hogg ME, Tam V, Zenati M et al (2016) Mastery-based virtual reality robotic simulation curriculum: the first step toward operative robotic proficiency. J Surg Educ 74(3):477–485
18. Rehman S, Raza SJ, Stegemann AP et al (2013) Simulation-based robot-assisted surgical training: a health economic evaluation. Int J Surg 11(9):841–846
19. Moglia A, Ferrari V, Morelli L et al (2014) Distribution of innate ability for surgery amongst medical students assessed by an advanced virtual reality surgical simulator. Surg Endosc 28(6):1830–1837

4 Systematic Training for Safe Implementation of Minimally Invasive Pancreatic Surgery

Sjors Klompmaker, Thijs de Rooij, Jony van Hilst,
and Marc G. Besselink

4.1 Introduction

Surgical skills are an important determinant of outcomes after abdominal surgery [1–4]. The acquisition of surgical skill over the span of a surgical career, also referred to as the "learning curve", is a well-known concept [5] that also applies to minimally invasive pancreatic surgery (MIPS), both laparoscopic [6, 7] and robot-assisted [8].

National registry [9, 10] and single center [11–15] studies on the early adoption of minimally invasive pancreatoduodenectomy (MIPD) [16–18] and distal pancreatectomy (MIDP) have revealed the presence of a learning curve. In addition, several studies have associated increased hospital case volumes and centralization of pancreatic surgery with reduced mortality and morbidity rates, as well as superior oncological outcomes [10, 19–23]. These effects can be attributed to improved acquisition of skills, experience, and practice routine by the surgeon, the operation team, and the postoperative care team. When implementing innovative surgery, the challenge is to guarantee patient safety by minimizing the impact of low case volume and lack of experience during the learning curve phase. The presence of a learning curve should also be addressed when evaluating surgical techniques, for instance within a randomized clinical trial, as the experience levels of both the surgeon and the institution can seriously confound the treatment effect [1, 24].

M.G. Besselink (✉)
Department of Surgery, Academic Medical Center
Amsterdam, The Netherlands
e-mail: m.g.besselink@amc.nl

U. Boggi (Ed), *Minimally Invasive Surgery of the Pancreas*,
Updates in Surgery
DOI: 10.1007/978-88-470-3958-2_4, © Springer-Verlag Italia 2018

4.2 Nationwide Training and Implementation

Following compelling evidence on the impact of treatment centralization on outcomes in surgery, the Dutch Society of Surgery (NVvH) has instituted a minimum annual case volume of 20 pancreatoduodenectomies. As a result, 17 out of 94 hospitals in the Netherlands (population 2017: 17 million) are currently licensed to perform pancreatic surgery. All of these centers are a member of the Dutch Pancreatic Cancer Group (DPCG), a multidisciplinary organization focusing on collaborative research and therapy improvement.

In 2014, the DPCG initiated the nationwide "Longitudinal assessment and realization of minimally invasive pancreatic surgery" (LAELAPS) program, which aimed to safely implement MIPS in the Netherlands. From January 2014 to July 2015, 32 Dutch pancreatic surgeons participated in LAELAPS-1 for MIDP training. All of the participating surgeons had multiple years of experience in open pancreatic surgery and abdominal minimally invasive surgery, but 50% had no prior experience with MIDP. In total, 14 out of 17 centers had performed <5 MIDPs prior to training [25].

LAELAPS-1 consisted of a highly detailed technique description, a video training session, and on-site proctoring by a highly experienced MIDP surgeon. During the first phase, participating surgeons learned crucial details about the minimally invasive technique, the necessary equipment, the procedural steps, and tips and tricks to prevent and solve intraoperative emergencies. After completing the first phase, surgeons were provided with operation videos, including details on critical steps and possible complications. The third phase was on-site proctoring during an MIDP, either at the surgeon's own institution or at one designated training hospital in the Netherlands. At the end of each proctoring session, the proctor would determine if the surgeon in training was ready to perform MIDPs independently. Whenever necessary, proctoring sessions were repeated [25].

As a result of LAELAPS-1, a seven-fold increase (from 9% to 47% of all DPs) was seen in the annual number of MIDPs performed in the Netherlands. After training, 12% more pancreatic adenocarcinomas were resected using MIDP ($P = 0.03$) and the conversion rate dropped from 38% to 8% ($P < 0.001$). The rates of R0 resection and pancreatic fistulae were comparable and the rate of major morbidity (Clavien-Dindo grade ≥3) was lower but not statistically significant (21% vs. 15%, $P = 0.24$). Furthermore, the median length of hospital stay decreased from 9 to 7 days ($P < 0.001$). In conclusion, LAELAPS allowed for safe introduction of MIDP with improved efficiency of treatment provision [25, 26]. After completion of the LAELAPS-1 program, a multicenter randomized controlled patient-blinded trial for open versus MIDP (LEOPARD-1) was started [27]. Results are expected by the end of 2017.

In 2015, the DPCG initiated LAELAPS-2 in order to train the Dutch pancreatic surgeons in MIPD. The curriculum was based on the LAELAPS-1 program, but now included multiple proctoring sessions, both on-site and off-site, before surgeons were allowed to perform MIPD individually. By April

2017, 14 surgeons from 6 participating centers had successfully completed all three phases of the training program and had performed 150 MIPDs combined. After completion of at least 20 MIPDs, centers were invited to participate in a multicenter randomized controlled patient-blinded trial for open versus MIPD (LEOPARD-2), of which the results are expected by the end of 2018 [28].

4.3 Mastery-Based Simulation Curriculum

Although training programs incorporating virtual reality and stepwise simulation are being applied extensively in aviation and in the military, the health care sector has been lagging behind [29]. In 2013, however, a team of hepato-pancreato-biliary surgeons at the University of Pittsburgh Medical Center (UPMC) started to implement a mastery-based simulation program to train their surgical oncology fellows in robot-assisted pancreatic surgery. The goal was to mimic and practice critical operation steps in order to minimize the risk of inferior patient outcomes during the learning curve of the surgeon. The UPMC paradigm was to embrace repetition and tailored teaching of skills during the training for minimally invasive surgery.

The curriculum consists of three phases: (1) a virtual reality training phase, (2) an inanimate training phase (using artificial biotissue, see Fig. 4.1), and (3) an operative phase. During these phases, the novices are graded using the

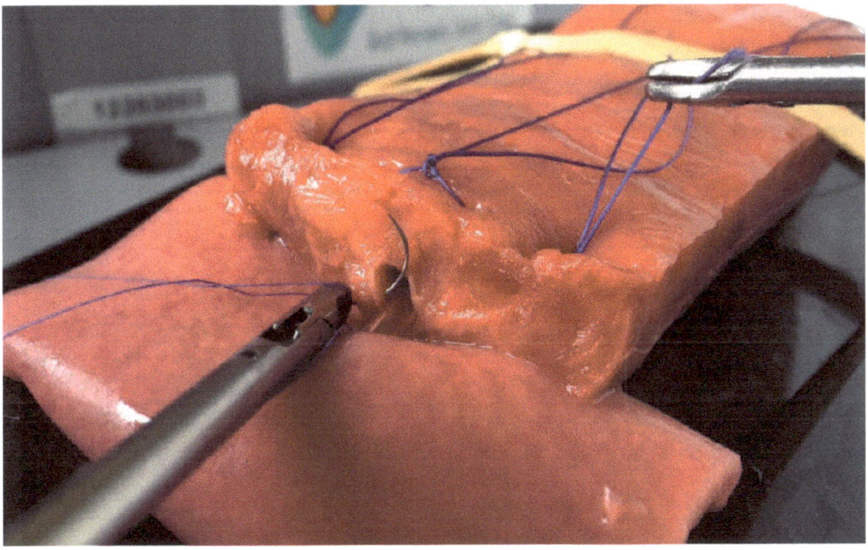

Fig. 4.1 Simulation of a laparoscopic pancreatojejunostomy using artificial biotissue (LifeLike BioTissue Inc., London, Ontario, Canada) in the Dutch LAELAPS-2 program

modified [3] Objective Structured Assessment of Technical Skills (OSATS) [2] score. The OSATS score, which has been shown to correlate to postoperative outcomes [1–4], draws on a 5-point scale (1-lowest performance, 5-highest performance) based on six domains: gentleness, time and motion, instrument handling, flow of operation, tissue exposure, and a summary score [1–2]. In an evaluative study among 17 participating surgical oncology fellows, a significant increase from pre- to post-training scores was seen and 94% of the participating fellows perceived improvement in robotic skills [30]. In a separate study, the team has confirmed that technical performance scoring independently predicts patient outcomes in pancreatic surgery [3].

4.4 Recommendations for Starting Centers

Ideally, both concepts – mastery-based simulation and nationwide training and implementation – are combined into one curriculum (Fig. 4.2). Such a program stimulates optimal exchange of knowledge and experience among surgeons with various levels of training. Each nationally or regionally initiated program would have one coordinating MIPS expert center that facilitates training and safeguards quality control. This center would need to appoint one dedicated coordinator and one or more expert proctors. Surgeons of aspiring MIPS hospitals apply to this program and matriculate through all four phases of the training. During these training phases, surgeons can use recently published decision-aid algorithms for MIPD (Fig. 4.3) and MIDP (Fig. 4.4) [31] to select cases for MIPS. Upon completion of the program, the aspiring MIPS hospitals obtain a license to

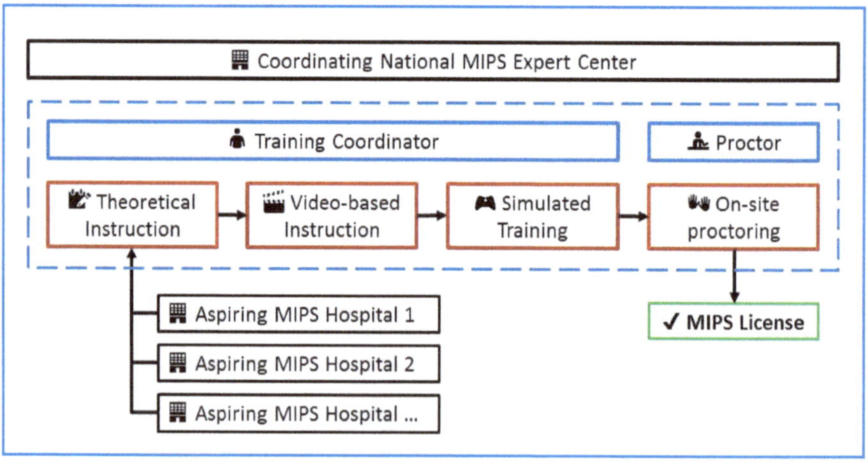

Fig. 4.2 Schematic overview of a recommended program structure for nationwide minimally invasive pancreatic surgery (MIPS) training

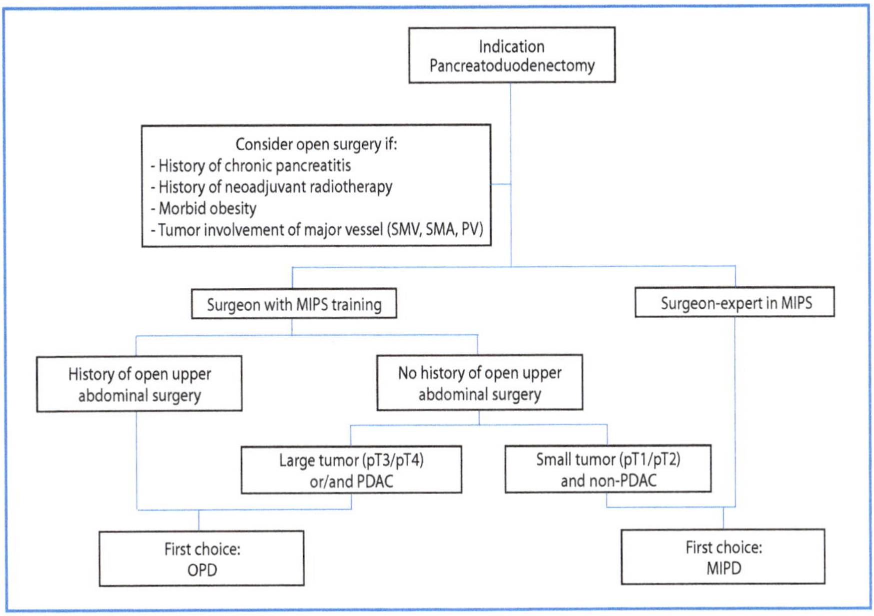

Fig. 4.3 Decision-aid algorithm for minimally invasive pancreatoduodenectomy (MIPD), based on a recent expert review [31]. *PDAC*, pancreatic ductal adenocarcinoma; *PV*, portal vein; *SMA*, superior mesenteric artery; *SMV*, superior mesenteric vein

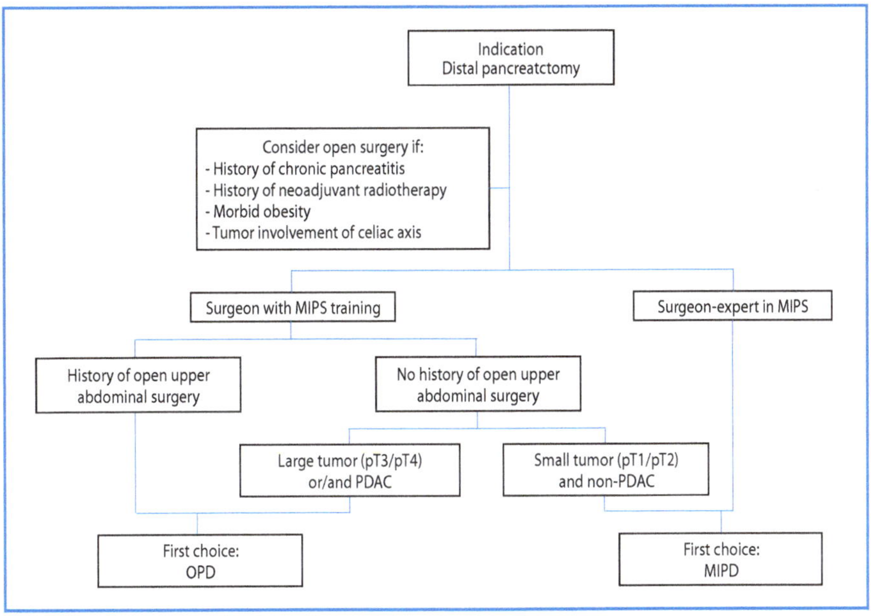

Fig. 4.4 Decision-aid algorithm for minimally invasive distal pancreatectomy (MIDP), based on a recent expert review [31]. *PDAC*, pancreatic ductal adenocarcinoma

perform MIPS independently. For such a concept to work, it is important that the coordinating center obtains a mandate from the national or regional governing body for hepato-pancreato-biliary surgery. If organized well, MIPS can be implemented on a large scale without compromising patient safety or institutional efficiency.

References

1. Birkmeyer JD, Finks JF, O'Reilly A et al (2013) Surgical skill and complication rates after bariatric surgery. N Engl J Med 369(15):1434–1442
2. Martin JA, Regehr G, Reznick R et al (1997) Objective structured assessment of technical skill (OSATS) for surgical residents. Br J Surg 84(2):273–278
3. Hogg ME, Zenati M, Novak S et al (2016) Grading of surgeon technical performance predicts postoperative pancreatic fistula for pancreaticoduodenectomy independent of patient-related variables. Ann Surg 264(3):482–491
4. Niitsu H, Hirabayashi N, Yoshimitsu M et al (2013) Using the Objective Structured Assessment of Technical Skills (OSATS) global rating scale to evaluate the skills of surgical trainees in the operating room. Surg Today 43(3):271–275
5. Tseng JF, Pisters PW, Lee JE et al (2007) The learning curve in pancreatic surgery. Surgery 141(5):694–701
6. Cuschieri A (1994) Laparoscopic surgery of the pancreas. J R Coll Surg Edinb 39(3):178–184
7. Gagner M, Pomp A (1994) Laparoscopic pylorus-preserving pancreatoduodenectomy. Surg Endosc 8(5):408–410
8. Melvin WS (2003) Minimally invasive pancreatic surgery. Am J Surg 186(3):274–278
9. Sharpe SM, Talamonti MS, Wang CE et al (2015) Early national experience with laparoscopic pancreaticoduodenectomy for ductal adenocarcinoma: a comparison of laparoscopic pancreaticoduodenectomy and open pancreaticoduodenectomy from the national cancer data base. J Am Coll Surg 221(1):175–184
10. Adam MA, Choudhury K, Dinan MA et al (2015) Minimally invasive versus open pancreaticoduodenectomy for cancer: practice patterns and short-term outcomes among 7061 patients. Ann Surg 262(2):372–377
11. Braga M, Ridolfi C, Balzano G et al (2012) Learning curve for laparoscopic distal pancreatectomy in a high-volume hospital. Updates Surg 64(3):179–183
12. Shakir M, Boone BA, Polanco PM et al (2015) The learning curve for robotic distal pancreatectomy: an analysis of outcomes of the first 100 consecutive cases at a high-volume pancreatic centre. HPB (Oxford) 17(7):580–586
13. Napoli N, Kauffmann EF, Perrone VG et al (2015) The learning curve in robotic distal pancreatectomy. Updates Surg 67(3):257–264
14. Lee SY, Allen PJ, Sadot E et al (2015) Distal pancreatectomy: a single institution's experience in open, laparoscopic, and robotic approaches. J Am Coll Surg 220(1):18–27
15. de Rooij T, Cipriani F, Rawashdeh M et al (2017) Single-surgeon learning curve in 111 laparoscopic distal pancreatectomies: does operative time tell the whole story? J Am Coll Surg 224(5):826–832
16. Speicher PJ, Nussbaum DP, White RR et al (2014) Defining the learning curve for team-based laparoscopic pancreaticoduodenectomy. Ann Surg Oncol 21(12):4014–4019
17. Kim SC, Song KB, Jung YS et al (2013) Short-term clinical outcomes for 100 consecutive cases of laparoscopic pylorus-preserving pancreatoduodenectomy: improvement with surgical experience. Surg Endosc 27(1):95–103
18. Boone BA, Zenati M, Hogg ME et al (2015) Assessment of quality outcomes for robotic pancreaticoduodenectomy: identification of the learning curve. JAMA Surg 150(5):416–422

19. Topal B, Van de Sande S, Fieuws S, Penninckx F (2007) Effect of centralization of pancreaticoduodenectomy on nationwide hospital mortality and length of stay. Br J Surg 94(11):1377–1381
20. Balzano G, Zerbi A, Capretti G et al (2008) Effect of hospital volume on outcome of pancreaticoduodenectomy in Italy. Br J Surg 95(3):357–362
21. de Wilde RF, Besselink MG, van der Tweel I et al (2012) Impact of nationwide centralization of pancreaticoduodenectomy on hospital mortality. Br J Surg 99(3):404–410
22. Onete VG, Besselink MG, Salsbach CM et al (2015) Impact of centralization of pancreatoduodenectomy on reported radical resections rates in a nationwide pathology database. HPB (Oxford) 17(8):736–742
23. van der Geest LG, van Rijssen LB, Molenaar IQ et al (2016) Volume–outcome relationships in pancreatoduodenectomy for cancer. HPB (Oxford) 18(4):317–324
24. Ergina PL, Cook JA, Blazeby JM et al (2009) Challenges in evaluating surgical innovation. Lancet 374(9695):1097–1104
25. de Rooij T, van Hilst J, Boerma D et al (2016) Impact of a nationwide training program in minimally invasive distal pancreatectomy (LAELAPS). Ann Surg 264(5):754–762
26. Hogg ME, Besselink MG, Clavien PA et al (2017) Training in minimally invasive pancreatic resections: a paradigm shift away from "See one, Do one, Teach one". HPB (Oxford) 19(3):234–245
27. de Rooij T, van Hilst J, Vogel JA et al (2017) Minimally invasive versus open distal pancreatectomy (LEOPARD): study protocol for a randomized controlled trial. Trials 18(1):166
28. LEOPARD-2 Trial – Minimally invasive versus open pancreatoduodenectomy: a multicenter randomized controlled phase 2 trial. Nederlands Trial Register, number: NTR5689. http://www.trialregister.nl/trialreg/admin/rctview.asp?TC=5689
29. Kohn KT, Corrigan JM, Donaldson MS (2000) To err is human: building a safer health system. National Academy Press, Washington DC
30. Hogg ME, Tam V, Zenati M et al (2016) Mastery-based virtual reality robotic simulation curriculum: the first step toward operative robotic proficiency. J Surg Educ 74(3):477–485
31. de Rooij T, Klompmaker S, Abu Hilal M et al (2016) Laparoscopic pancreatic surgery for benign and malignant disease. Nat Rev Gastroenterol Hepatol 13(4):227–238

Contemporary Outcome Measures in Pancreatic Surgery

5

Stefano Andrianello, Alessandro Esposito, Luca Casetti, Luca Landoni, Roberto Salvia, and Claudio Bassi

5.1 Introduction

The issue of centralizing complex procedures including major pancreatic surgery within high-volume centers has played a leading role in the debate about improving postoperative outcomes. The introduction of advanced minimally invasive techniques together with the adoption of "early recovery after surgery" (ERAS) policies and clinical care paths have led to a redefinition of pancreatic surgery since these new concepts seem to provide great results in terms of improving the quality of care for patients.

In contrast to colorectal surgery, where several indicators of quality of care and standards have been described [1], there is a lack of these in the more challenging area of pancreatic surgery. Most of the studies have mainly examined gross indicators such as case load, mortality or long-term disease-free and overall survival. However, specific indicators of effectiveness and quality of care are essential to scale the direct benefit of the minimally invasive approach for pancreatic resections.

5.2 Quality of Care in Pancreatic Surgery

Each patient who undergoes major pancreatic resection accepts the operative risk in exchange for an effective amelioration of the disease process. However, some clear goals should be accomplished every time regardless of the final

C. Bassi (✉)
General and Pancreatic Surgery – The Pancreas Institute, University of Verona Hospital Trust
Verona, Italy
e-mail: claudio.bassi@univr.it

U. Boggi (Ed), *Minimally Invasive Surgery of the Pancreas*,
Updates in Surgery
DOI: 10.1007/978-88-470-3958-2_5,

purpose. First, the surgical procedure should not endanger the patient's life and the oncological results should ensure long-term survival. It is equally important to avoid a prolonged complicated surgical course since it can be extremely challenging when several complications arise. Rather than an additive effect, their simultaneous occurrence may result in an exponential and life-threatening clinical impact. For malignant diseases, the surgical procedure should attain the correct level of oncological radicality. Following the correct indications, surgical resection should obtain complete eradication of the disease at a locoregional level. However, at the same time, it should minimize the risk of postoperative complications that might delay, or even prevent, access to adjuvant treatments. Finally, the issue of cost should be always considered. Pancreatic surgery, in fact, can be particularly expensive [2] and, as far as possible, healthcare-related costs should be contained to allow equitable access to the best level of care for every patient.

Pancreatic surgery should be considered as a unique and highly specific field of gastrointestinal surgery. The expertise gained in laparoscopic and robotic procedures applied in other gastrointestinal areas does not necessarily provide sufficient guarantees of good outcome for pancreatic surgery. In practical terms, the application of alternative surgical techniques such as laparoscopy or robotics must be preceded by the achievement of high standards in terms of structural requirements, multidisciplinary facilities, educational programs, life-long learning, surgical volume and comparative measurement of results [3–5].

5.3 Outcome Metrics in Pancreatic Surgery

Mortality is a gross indicator of quality of care in surgery, and this holds true for pancreatic surgery. Postoperative mortality must be minimized regardless of the surgical technique. A recent meta-analysis exploring the volume-outcome relationship [6] in pancreatic surgery reported a strong inverse association between hospital volume and postoperative mortality. More than 1500 Whipple procedures were performed in 2003 in some 200 Italian institutions, with an overall mortality rate of 8.1% [7]. The majority of these institutions performed fewer than five Whipple procedures per year, with a five-fold higher mortality when compared with high-volume hospitals [7]. Moreover, the probability of undergoing palliative/exploratory surgery was inversely related to volume, as reported in another survey [8].

Table 5.1 summarizes other additional metrics that need to be considered. Postoperative morbidity must be identified using updated pancreatic-specific definitions [9–11] and measured through pancreatic-specific assessment tools. Each single event influences the development and load of further complications in the postoperative course. Duration of hospital stay should no longer be considered a reliable indicator of outcome since it is dictated by healthcare policies

Table 5.1 Main indicators of quality in pancreatic surgery

Center-specific	Interventional radiology no-stop service on site
	Endoscopy no-stop service on site
	Intensive care unit on site
	Dedicated pathology
	Multidisciplinary meeting
	Nuclear medicine
	Dedicated medical and radiation oncology
	Dedicated endocrinology
	Acute and chronic pain services
	Duration of waiting list
Procedure-specific	EBL assessment
	Pancreatic stump texture assessment
	MPD size assessment
	Case load
Outcome-specific	Risk-adjusted mortality
	Pancreatic surgery-specific definitions
	ERAS protocols application
	Use of blood transfusions
	PMI assessment
	Health-care related costs reduction

EBL, estimated blood loss; *MPD*, main pancreatic duct; *ERAS*, enhanced recovery after surgery; *PMI*, postoperative morbidity index.

that vary by country and institution, quite apart from individual surgeon bias. Length of hospital stay must be minimized [12] by applying ERAS protocols for uncomplicated patients, regardless of the use of minimally invasive techniques. The planned use of a postoperative intensive care unit (ICU) is dependent on institutional policies whereas prolonged ICU stay is a viable tool to measure the impact of postoperative morbidity. This, together with the duration of hospital stay, represents a surrogate marker of the burden of the postoperative course which can be measured quantitatively using tools such as the Postoperative Morbidity Index (PMI) [13].

For pancreatoduodenectomy, for instance, high levels of intraoperative estimated blood loss (EBL) have been variably associated with an increased risk of postoperative pancreatic fistula and should be always accurately measured [14]. Equally important in predicting outcome is the assessment of pancreatic texture and main pancreatic duct size, regardless of the operative technique employed [14, 15]. Assessment of the risk of pancreatic fistula represents the only way to prevent this major complication after pancreatic resection. Goal-directed or restricted fluid administration together with a restricted use of packed red blood cell transfusion must always be pursued since liberal hydration and overuse of transfusions have been related to worse outcome [16–18].

Indicators of quality of radical resection comprise nodal retrieval and resection margin status. These can be effectively understood only after proper preoperative staging and accurate pathological examination. Accurate lymphadenectomy provides a high nodal retrieval that is associated with better disease staging and prognostic stratification [19]. Equally important is to obtain maximum clearance at the resection margins, since margin positivity has been recognized universally as a prognostic factor, in particular by applying the 1-mm clearance to define a radical resection [20].

Ultimately, costs cannot be ignored since a complicated postoperative course, can be extremely expensive [2]. Healthcare costs are an effective indicator of the proper allocation of resources and of the level of logistic organization of the institution. A network of services with expertise in pancreatic disease developed around the concept of a “Pancreas Center” can promptly handle adverse events while keeping costs low. The increased costs of minimally invasive pancreatic surgery could be justified only in the presence of significant improvement in patient outcome when compared with open surgery performed ensuring the achievement of all quality indicators.

5.4 Requirements for a Pancreatic Surgery Center

Good clinical results can only be achieved by building a system able to meet the needs resulting from the management of these complex diseases. Pancreatic surgery should be performed in referral centers able to guarantee key services including an ICU, a fully accessible digestive endoscopy group as well as diagnostic, interventional and nuclear medicine radiology, dedicated medical and radiation oncology, endocrinology, acute pain and chronic pain medicine, specialized pathology including frozen section or intraoperative consultation, expertise in rare pancreatic disease and, often, dedicated psychology. The institution should set up a specific clinical pathway for all patients such that the diagnostic and therapeutic route must be reproducible, independent of the patient’s access to the institution. These specific protocols must be underpinned by regular multidisciplinary meetings to enable discussion and decision on these most challenging cases.

Every service should have a clinical manager responsible for integration of all the professionals involved, ensuring the appropriateness of the required examination, a short waiting list, rapid diagnosis and staging as well as prompt treatment of severe symptoms such as obstructive jaundice or upper gastrointestinal tract obstruction. Radiologists should have expertise in all pancreatic imaging procedures including contrast-enhanced ultrasound, computed tomography, magnetic resonance imaging, interventional angiography and percutaneous intervention. The gastrointestinal endoscopy service should ensure both diagnostic and operative procedures. All such diagnostic and interventional services should be available at the hospital with adequate staff, to ensure rapid on-site evaluation and treatment.

The surgical waiting list should be of a maximum of 30 days (but preferably much shorter), with strict scheduling of patients based on surgical indication. Every patient should undergo an elective preoperative multidisciplinary evaluation uncovering and managing all possible factors that might decrease the surgical risk and improve outcome. Every suitable patient should be evaluated by an ERAS protocol aimed at optimizing the perioperative period. This protocol should always include preoperative nutritional counseling and interventions. All patients should undergo a fast-track protocol involving nurses, nutritionists and physiotherapists, and where the postoperative course is uneventful.

5.5 Future Prospects and the Minimally Invasive Approach

In time, more skilled laparoscopic surgeons will become available and, as a result, both distal pancreatectomy and pancreatoduodenectomy will likely be carried out routinely and safely by a minimally invasive approach. However, a technically flawless surgical procedure will be of no avail if not performed in the context of a center of excellence for pancreatic surgery where good clinical results are already ensured by high quality of care. The personal skills of each pancreatic surgeon are of utmost importance, however, a dedicated "pancreas team" plays the greater role in impacting positively on patient outcome [21, 22]. The outcomes of pancreatic surgery are independent from the skills of the single surgeon and the optimal clinical environment is by far more important even when applied to minimally invasive surgery. Future studies should be implemented in a context that guarantees the correct indication for surgery, lower mortality rates, a low burden of postoperative morbidity through early recognition of adverse events and prevention of predictable complications, high standards of oncological radicality, prompt recovery with access to adjuvant therapy as soon as possible, and reduction of healthcare-related costs.

Only once a wider application of minimally invasive pancreatic surgery integrates effectively with the outcome-improving effect of a dedicated pancreatic team, will we be able to assess more precisely the putative benefits of the minimally invasive approach.

References

1. Gooiker GA, Kolfschoten NE, Bastiaannet E et al (2013) Evaluating the validity of quality indicators for colorectal cancer care. J Surg Oncol 108(7):465–471
2. Vollmer CM (2013) The economics of pancreas surgery. Surg Clin North Am 93(3):711–728
3. Nathan H, Cameron JL, Choti MA et al (2009) The volume-outcomes effect in hepato-pancreato-biliary surgery: hospital versus surgeon contributions and specificity of the relationship. J Am Coll Surg 208(4):528–538
4. Bilimoria KY, Bentrem DJ, Lillemoe KD et al; Pancreatic Cancer Quality Indicator Development Expert Panel, American College of Surgeons (2009) Assessment of pancreatic cancer care in the United States based on formally developed quality indicators. J Natl Cancer Inst 101(12):848–859
5. Sabater L, García-Granero A, Escrig-Sos J et al (2014) Outcome quality standards in pancreatic oncologic surgery. Ann Surg Oncol 21(4):1138–1146
6. Gooiker GA, van Gijn W, Wouters MW et al (2011) Systematic review and meta-analysis of the volume-outcome relationship in pancreatic surgery. Br J Surg 98(4):485–494
7. Balzano G, Zerbi A, Capretti G et al (2008) Effect of hospital volume on outcome of pancreaticoduodenectomy in Italy. Br J Surg 95(3):357–362
8. Balzano G, Capretti G, Callea G et al (2016) Overuse of surgery in patients with pancreatic cancer. A nationwide analysis in Italy. HPB (Oxford) 18(5):470–478
9. Bassi C, Dervenis C, Butturini G et al (2005) Postoperative pancreatic fistula: an international study group (ISGPF) definition. Surgery 138(1):8–13
10. Wente MN, Bassi C, Dervenis C et al (2007) Delayed gastric emptying (DGE) after pancreatic surgery: a suggested definition by the International Study Group of Pancreatic Surgery (ISGPS). Surgery 142(5):761–768
11. Wente MN, Veit JA, Bassi C et al (2007) Postpancreatectomy hemorrhage (PPH): an International Study Group of Pancreatic Surgery (ISGPS) definition. Surgery 142(1):20–25
12. Xiong J, Szatmary P, Huang W et al (2016) Enhanced recovery after surgery program in patients undergoing pancreaticoduodenectomy: a PRISMA-compliant systematic review and meta-analysis. Medicine (Baltimore) 95(18):e3497
13. Miller BC, Christein JD, Behrman SW et al (2013) Assessing the impact of a fistula after a pancreaticoduodenectomy using the Post-operative Morbidity Index. HPB (Oxford) 15(10):781–788
14. Callery MP, Pratt WB, Kent TS et al (2013) A prospectively validated clinical risk score accurately predicts pancreatic fistula after pancreatoduodenectomy. J Am Coll Surg 216(1):1–14
15. Shubert CR, Wagie AE, Farnell MB et al (2015) Clinical risk score to predict pancreatic fistula after pancreatoduodenectomy: independent external validation for open and laparoscopic approaches. J Am Coll Surg 221(3):689–698
16. Mavros MN, Xu L, Maqsood H et al (2015) Perioperative blood transfusion and the prognosis of pancreatic cancer surgery: systematic review and meta-analysis. Ann Surg Oncol 22(13):4382–4391
17. Eng OS, Goswami J, Moore D et al (2013) Intraoperative fluid administration is associated with perioperative outcomes in pancreaticoduodenectomy: a single center retrospective analysis. J Surg Oncol 108(4):242–247
18. Grant F, Brennan MF, Allen PJ et al (2016) Prospective randomized controlled trial of liberal vs restricted perioperative fluid management in patients undergoing pancreatectomy. Ann Surg 264(4):591–598
19. Showalter TN, Winter KA, Berger AC et al (2011) The influence of total nodes examined, number of positive nodes, and lymph node ratio on survival after surgical resection and adjuvant chemoradiation for pancreatic cancer: a secondary analysis of RTOG 9704. Int J Radiat Oncol Biol Phys 81(5):1328–1335
20. Konstantinidis IT, Warshaw AL, Allen JN et al (2013) Pancreatic ductal adenocarcinoma: is there a survival difference for R1 resections versus locally advanced unresectable tumors? What is a "true" R0 resection? Ann Surg 257(4):731–736

21. Ghaferi AA, Birkmeyer JD, Dimick JB (2009) Complications, failure to rescue, and mortality with major inpatient surgery in Medicare patients. Ann Surg 250(6):1029–1034
22. Ghaferi AA, Birkmeyer JD, Dimick JB (2009) Variation in hospital mortality associated with inpatient surgery. N Engl J Med 361(14):1368–1375

6 Preoperative Evaluation and Anesthesia in Minimally Invasive Surgery of the Pancreas

Gabriella Amorese

6.1 Introduction

Pancreatic surgery has long remained a stronghold of open surgery because of a combination of technical, anatomic, and oncologic factors. An additional limiting issue was the training of most pancreatic surgeons that, until very recently, did not include advanced laparoscopic techniques [1]. Centralization of pancreatic surgery to high-volume centers [2] reinforced this surgical enclave, further slowing the diffusion of minimally invasive pancreatic resection (MIPR). Lack of enthusiasm and support from well-respected surgeons possibly prevented younger colleagues from embarking upon the serious undertaking of initiating a program for MIPR, especially for pancreatoduodenectomy [3]. MIPR was eventually accepted as an alternative approach to open surgery in selected patients [4, 5]. A standardized approach to anesthesia is therefore required to enhance the value of MIPR.

As compared with surgeons, anesthetists were probably more prepared to face the challenges of laparoscopy, because they are not usually focused on an organ or apparatus and they had the opportunity to practice with laparoscopy in other subspecialties. On the other hand, modern anesthesia for pancreatic surgery, and in particular for pancreatoduodenectomy, requires specific knowledge and cultural dedication, as evidence is emerging that the occurrence of several complications could be reduced by the implementation of newer strategies of pre-, intra-, and early postoperative treatment [6–10]. The establishment of these new and quite revolutionary concepts, made it crucial for anesthetists to become more deeply involved in the care of patients undergoing pancreatic surgery, either open or minimally invasive. As a consequence, also anesthetists had to go through

G. Amorese (✉)
Division of Anesthesia and Intensive Care, Azienda Ospedaliero-Universitaria Pisana
Pisa, Italy
e-mail: g.amorese@ao-pisa.toscana.it

U. Boggi (Ed), *Minimally Invasive Surgery of the Pancreas*,
Updates in Surgery
DOI: 10.1007/978-88-470-3958-2_6, © Springer-Verlag Italia 2018

a learning curve, because MIPR created some counterintuitive circumstances, such as the need to find a balance between the reduction in cardiac output, caused by pneumoperitoneum and reverse Trendelenburg position, and the need to limit the volume of infused fluids, despite a long and complex procedure with inherent risk of bleeding [11–13].

6.2 Preoperative Evaluation

The decision to resect a pancreatic tumor is a complex and multidisciplinary process balancing the risks of surgery against the benefits of resection.

There are basically two scenarios: symptomatic patients, with either a benign or malignant tumor, and asymptomatic patients, with premalignant or malignant tumors. In either instance, the contribution of the anesthetist to the multidisciplinary evaluation is to remove barriers to surgery, optimize preoperative conditions, define the type of anesthesia, anticipate the need for intensive postoperative care, and plan for postoperative analgesia. In rare circumstances the anesthetist will define a prohibitive operative risk profile making surgery contraindicated. In symptomatic patients an alternative treatment strategy will be necessary, typically in the form of a less invasive operation or an interventional procedure. Anesthesia will be required in either instance. In patients with malignant pancreatic tumors, the prognostic weight of a negative anesthesiologic evaluation, contraindicating resection, has obvious implications. In the absence of alternative therapies aiming at the cure of patients with pancreatic tumors, surgery should rarely be withheld on the basis of age and comorbidity alone [14].

The initial evaluation of patients candidate for MIPR follows the same path usually employed in patients undergoing open pancreatic resections (Table 6.1), eventually resulting in grading of the surgical risk according to the classification of physical health of the American Society of Anesthesiologists (ASA). The ASA score is considered an imperfect tool to assess the surgical risk, mostly because of subjective assessment of patients' overall health [15]. Other scores were indeed developed [16–20] but, although usually more sophisticated and reliable than the ASA classification, they are not used routinely. Therefore, using the ASA score, and accepting a degree of variability in anesthetists' evaluation, no major problems related to the patients' physical health are anticipated in the majority of persons classified in class I or II, because a correlation between ASA score and postoperative course is evident only for classes III and IV [15, 20]. ASA class I and II patients can therefore undergo all types of pancreatic resections and, if otherwise indicated, a MIPR can be offered. ASA grades III and IV include a large proportion of patients requiring a pancreatic resection. Some ASA III patients are not really sicker than ASA II patients, and pose no additional problems when considered for MIPR. Other patients, instead, may

Table 6.1. Evaluation of patients candidate for pancreatic resections

1. History	• Family history • Past medical history • Past anesthesiologic history • Past surgical history • Smoking habit • Daily alcohol intake • Use of drugs • Pharmacologic history/allergies • Current medical/surgical history
2. Physical examination	• General physical examination • Assessment of heart rate and rhythm (radial artery palpation) • Measurement of arterial blood pressure • Assessment of relative ease of endotracheal intubation • Determination of height and weight
3. Basic tests/consultations	• ECG, with a written diagnosis from a cardiologist. • Chest X-Ray • Blood typing (group, Rh) • Complete blood count, coagulation studies, and biochemical tests • Urinalysis • Serological markers of infectious diseases (upon written informed consent from the patient)
4. Additional tests/consultations	• Cardiologic consultation[a] • Pneumological consultation[b] • Neurologic consultation[c] • Hematologic consultation[d] • Infectious disease consultation[e] • Other consultations (as indicated)

[a] **Cardiologic consultation** if: 1. History, symptoms, or signs of cardiac disease; 2. Abnormal findings in the ECG; 3. History of diabetes; 4. Severe hypertension; 5. Obesity; 6. Non cardiac symptoms (e.g. unexplained dyspnea) or signs (e.g. edema of the lower extremities) possibly indicating heart problems; 7. History of syncope or sudden loss of consciousness; 8. History of alcohol or drug abuse; 9. Chronic respiratory disease; 10. Congenital disorders and abnormalities; 11. Patients with connective tissue disorders; 12. Patients with serious infections; 14. Patients treated with cardiotoxic medications; 15. Transplant recipients.

[b] **Pneumological consultation** if: 1. History, symptoms, or signs of respiratory disease; 2. Age > 80 years; 3. Smoking ≥20 cigarettes per day; 4. Obesity; 5. Sleep apnea syndrome; 6. Abnormal Chest X-Ray; 7. Occupational exposure to potentially toxic substances.

[c] **Neurological consultation** if: 1. History, symptoms, or signs of acute or chronic neurologic disease; 2. Treatment with neurologic drugs; 3. History of serious and prolonged headache; 4. Abnormal findings in a CT, MRI scan or the EEG.

[d] **Hematologic consultation** if: 1. History, symptoms, or signs of hematologic disease; 2. History of thrombo-embolic episodes; 3. Spontaneous bleeding; 4. Abnormal blood count or coagulation studies.

[e] **Infectious disease consultation** if: 1. History, symptoms, or signs of infectious disease; 2. Preoperative biliary drainage.

be at higher surgical risk so that the preoperative multidisciplinary assessment of physiologic resectability of the tumor could involve also the type of surgical approach, namely open or laparoscopic. In general, MIPR is associated with more complicated intraoperative management, but also with smoother postoperative recovery as compared with open surgery. On practical grounds, the sicker the patient the greater the benefit of a minimally invasive approach; however, the challenges associated with anesthesia are also greater. A decision algorithm to help the anesthetist to decide between open and MIPR is proposed in Fig. 6.1.

In the "grey" area including ASA III and IV patients, an individualized approach should be adopted. This approach brings the anesthetist much more in the context of clinical management of patients with pancreatic tumors, rather than relegating him or her solely to the role of a consulting physician. Some of the parameters to be considered regard patient frailty, while other variables regard the complexity of the procedure. Some parameters can be modified with proper planning of the procedure, such as the nutritional status or the level of ability of the operating surgeon. Other parameters, instead, are static, such as the type of tumor or the patient's age. The combination of all these variables produces quite a complex scenario with no absolute certainties. For instance, a frail ASA IV patient requiring a straightforward enucleation of a "small and superficial" pancreatic tumor could be safely operated upon, and would benefit greatly from MIPR. On the other hand, a relatively fit ASA III patient requiring pancreatoduodenectomy for a borderline-resectable pancreatic cancer, after neoadjuvant chemoradiation, could be best managed by an open procedure.

It is worth noting the role that the surgeon's ability plays in the decision algorithm. It is commonplace that surgical talent, experience and proficiency are keys to the success of any surgical procedure. This popular belief was so well founded that it eventually became a science with clear definitions and high levels of evidence [21]. Measuring surgical ability is currently receiving even greater attention because the diffusion of minimally invasive techniques made the issue of surgical training, credentialing and quality assessment stringent [22]. The anesthetist's non-technical and technical skills are expected to play a similar role but, for the moment, have not received the same degree of attention [23, 24]. Overall, professional factors play a major role in the treatment outcome of pancreatic tumors and should be taken into serious account when planning for major surgical procedures such as MIPR.

Finally, a common problem in clinical practice, which has to be solved in the preoperative workup, is whether or not patients should discontinue oral aspirin and/or other antiplatelet therapies. This question pertains only to patients receiving single-agent antiaggregation for "prophylactic" purposes, because persons undergoing dual antiplatelet therapy to ensure patency of endovascular stents are a different category. In these patients, according to the cardiologist's evaluation, a personalized approach can be defined, but one of the two antiplatelet therapies has to be maintained [25]. As regards patients taking only aspirin, no specific evidence is currently available for aspirin withdrawal/

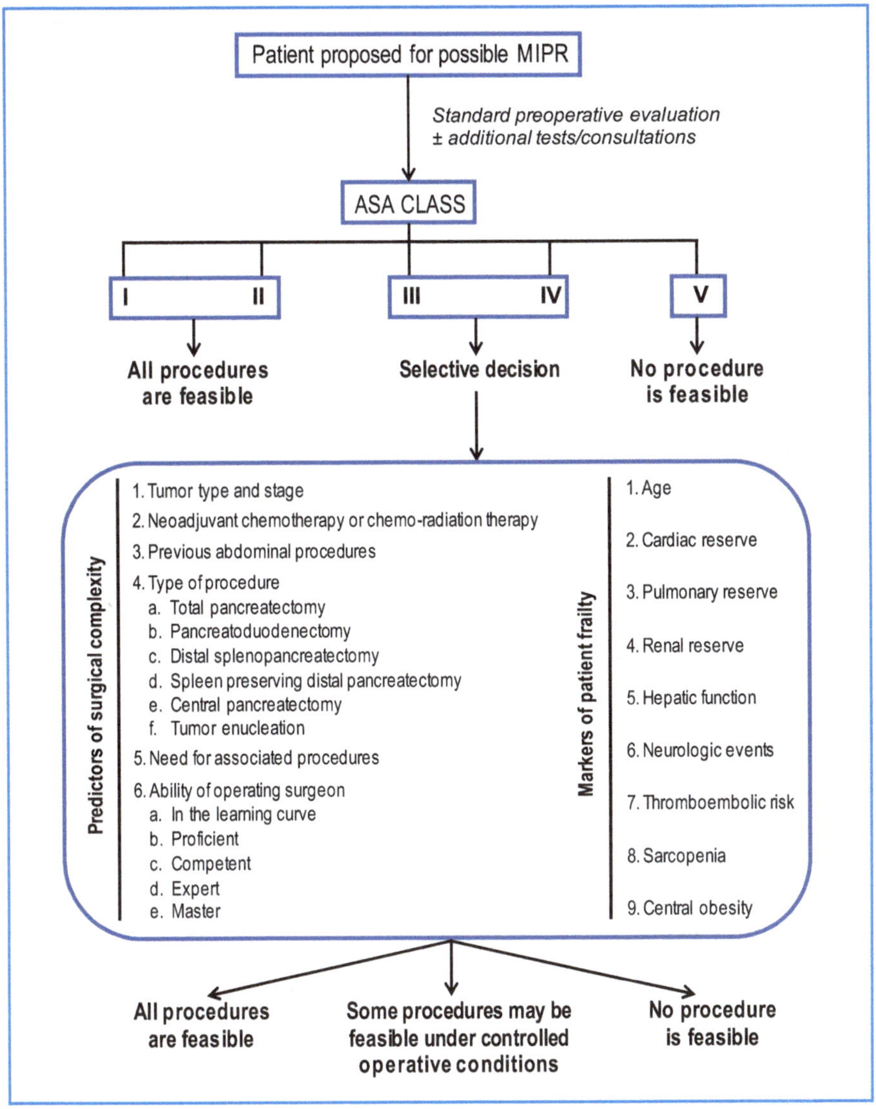

Fig. 6.1 Decision algorithm for anesthesiologic evaluation of patient candidate for minimally invasive pancreatic resection (MIPR). *ASA*, American Society of Anesthesiologists

maintenance before MIPR, and data from open surgery are quite conflicting [26, 27]. In open surgery, Wolf et al. showed that aspirin was safely maintained [26], while Mita et al. reported a higher incidence of postpancreatectomy hemorrhage [27]. Experience with other non-pancreatic procedures [28] demonstrates that antiplatelet therapy should not be discontinued. Our approach is permissive in MIPR, especially when there are specific risk factors for vascular thrombosis and the patient requires a distal pancreatectomy. A more restrictive approached is used for pancreatoduodenectomy, especially in patients with jaundice.

6.3 The Case of Robotic Surgery

At the time of writing, the term robotic surgery, at least in abdominal surgery, corresponds to da Vinci surgery. The da Vinci surgical system (dVss) (Intuitive Surgical, Sunnyvale, California, USA) was indeed the only system available on the market from 1998 to 2015. Recently, the TELELAP ALF-X has been launched (SOFAR S.p.A., ALF-X Surgical Robotics Department, Trezzano Rosa, Milan, Italy) [29], and other systems are awaited in the future.

Robotic surgery is a variant of laparoscopic surgery that employs a complex device, the dVss, to enhance surgical dexterity. Contrary to the common meaning of the word "robot", which indicates a machine capable of programmed, or autonomous, actions, the dVss is a telemanipulator that transfers the movements of the hands of a remote surgeon to the tips of miniaturized intracorporeal instruments. As compared with conventional laparoscopy, robotic surgery offers a high-definition, stereoscopic, steady, and immersive view (vs. bidimensional view), the use of surgical instruments with seven degrees of freedom (vs. four degrees of freedom), and optimal ergonomy (vs. static, and often awkward, working postures).

Four different models of dVss have been marketed since 1998: the dVss Standard, the dVss S, the dVss Si, and the dVss Xi. The basic components of all systems are similar: the surgeon console, the patient side cart (PSC), and the vision cart. From an anesthesiologist's perspective, the component of the dVss that makes most of the difference in intraoperative management (vs. conventional laparoscopy) is the PSC.

The PSC is a bulky tower, weighing between 550 and 820 kg depending on the model, with three or four operative arms holding the camera and the robotic instruments. Because of the design of the robotic system, the PSC of all systems but the Xi has to come from the side opposite to the target anatomy. In MIPR, the PSC is placed immediately over the head of the patient, thus largely preventing accessibility to airways and infusion lines. The dVss Xi has partially solved this problem, because the newer design of the PSC offers 270° accessibility around the patient. In MIPR, the PSC of the dVss is placed at one side of the patient, leaving the access to the head and the neck of the patient quite unobstructed. Although accessibility to airways and infusion lines is improved, the bulk of the system and its "rigidity" still restrict the ability of the anesthesia team to freely intervene on the endotracheal tube and infusion lines. Additionally, it is accepted that conventional laparoscopy requires deep neuromuscular blockade to ensure optimal working space [30], with reduced pneumoperitoneum pressures, and to avoid accidental visceral piercing by a laparoscopic instrument in case of unplanned reversal of blockade with contraction of abdominal muscles. In robotic surgery, a smaller working space is required, allowing the use of lower pneumoperitoneum pressures [31, 32]. Despite this, deep neuromuscular blockade is still required, because the absolute fixation of ports and instruments to robotic arms can have catastrophic consequences, in terms of visceral and/or vascular injuries, in the case of sudden reversal of neuromuscular blockade.

As a matter of fact, if robotic surgery means "remote surgery", because the surgeon is sitting far from the patient, robotic surgery also means "remote anesthesia", because the anesthetist cannot freely manipulate the endotracheal tube, the infusion lines, and the arterial line. Anesthesia in robotic surgery requires more accurate planning and stronger team coordination as compared with all other types of surgery [33]. The systematic and overprotective approach required by anesthesia in robotic surgery improves the approach to standard laparoscopic procedures, where patient accessibility and manpower are also reduced as compared with open surgery.

6.4 Hemodynamic and Respiratory Changes in MIPR

Hemodynamic and respiratory alterations in laparoscopic surgery result from the higher intra-abdominal pressure created by pneumoperitoneum, the absorption of CO_2 into the blood, and the position of the patient. Interestingly enough, the level of the peritoneum and patient position have the same purpose: providing working space and improving exposure. As a consequence, surgeons may be willing to increase pneumoperitoneum pressure and place patients in steep positions. Extreme "head-up" postures result in reduced venous return, facilitating hypotension and potentially leading to myocardial and cerebral ischemia. Elderly patients, hypovolemic patients, and those with pre-existing ischemic heart disease or cerebrovascular disease are particularly vulnerable to posture-related hemodynamic changes.

Pneumoperitoneum increases abdominal pressure, raises the diaphragm, decreases perfusion of abdominal viscera, and increases both systemic vascular resistances and pulmonary vascular resistances [34, 35]. As a consequence, central venous pressure increases, and heart rate accelerates. Most of these changes are well tolerated by ASA I and II patients and by most fit ASA III patients. The lower cardiac output is compensated by increased heart rate and arterial pressure, resulting in a stable hemodynamic state. It is, however, important to note that this equilibrium is quite unsteady and may easily turn into overt hemodynamic instability if an acute hemorrhage occurs.

In ASA III and IV patients, with more relevant cardiac disease, the increase of vascular resistance associated with pneumoperitoneum [36], which is affected by patient position being aggravated by the reverse Trendelenburg position [37], may lead to a relevant reduction in cardiac output.

As mentioned earlier, absorption of CO_2 leads to a tendency to hypercapnia. If CO_2 is not eliminated efficiently with pulmonary ventilation, hypercapnia arises, followed by acidosis. Acidosis can depress myocardial function and predispose to arrhythmia and cardiovascular collapse. CO_2 has also direct effects on the heart [38].

The increased intra-abdominal pressure has also respiratory implications. The reverse Trendelenburg position alleviates these changes. If pneumoperitoneum pressure is maintained over 15 mmHg, airway and intrathoracic pressures increase, leading to compression of the great and small vessels with associated hemodynamic consequences [39].

In ASA I and II patients, capnography and pulse oximetry provide reliable monitoring of $PaCO_2$ and arterial oxygen saturation [40]. In ASA III and IV patients, and in particular in persons with impaired CO_2 excretion capacity, there is a less reliable correlation between $PaCO_2$ and end-tidal carbon dioxide tension. In these patients arterial blood sampling is recommended [40, 41].

Before proceeding with surgery, all pressure points must be padded and the patient has to be secured to the operating table using wide bandings.

6.5 Monitoring and Preparation for Anesthesia

All patients undergoing MIPR must be monitored for ECG, arterial pressure, capnography, pulse oximetry, and urinary volumes. Verification of ventilatory parameters is also essential (volumes, inspiratory pressure, oxygen concentration). Measurement of arterial pressure by radial artery cannulation is required in sicker patients but is advised in all patients because of anticipated long duration of MIPR and for better assessment of pH and electrolyte balance.

As maintenance of thermal homeostasis is key, body temperature should also be monitored, and a fluid warming device has to be available. The use of thermic blankets is also important.

At least one large-bore (14 or 16 G) intravenous cannula must be placed in either arm to ensure the possibility of fluid infusion at all times. In patients with limited possibility of peripheral venous cannulation a central venous line may be placed. Stockings, connected to a sequential compression device, are placed on the legs to reduce blood pooling and lessen the risk of deep venous thrombosis. A nasogastric tube is inserted after induction of anesthesia. The tube may be removed at the end of the procedure, at the discretion of the operating surgeon.

In ASA III and IV patients, invasive measurement of arterial pressure is mandatory and the placement of a central venous line may be helpful in maintaining more physiologic levels of cardiac preload. Although it is known that stroke volume variation is a better predictor of fluid responsiveness as compared with central venous pressure [42], changes in central venous pressure after the first infusion bolus predict later variations in stroke volume [43].

6.6 Neuromuscular Blockade and Ventilatory Strategy

Deep neuromuscular blockade is key in all laparoscopic procedures to allow the surgeon to work with low pneumoperitoneum pressures [44]. Rocuronium bromide provides optimal neuromuscular blockade but the dose has to be reduced to 0.075–0.1 mg/kg, because of the known interactions with volatile anesthetics resulting in augmentation of the intensity of neuromuscular blockade [45]. The level of blockade is measured using the TOF-watch, a device that gives an electrical stimulus to the ulnar nerve and measures the contraction in the adductor pollicis muscle. To define a deep level of neuromuscular blockage, the post-tetanic count has to be assessed by giving several stimuli and measuring the number of contractions. A post-tetanic count of 1–2 corresponds to a deep level of neuromuscular blockade, but could still not reflect complete paralysis of the diaphragm and lateral abdominal muscles, which are instead the true endpoint of neuromuscular blockade [30]. These muscles can indeed still demonstrate contractions when the adductor pollicis muscle is completely paralyzed because they are more resistant to the action of rocuronium bromide [46, 47]. While providing deeper neuromuscular blockade is not a problem during the procedure it could become an issue towards the end of the procedure. Availability of sugammadex, which fully reverses the neuromuscular blockade within few minutes, can be of help in this regard [48].

A tidal volume of 6–8 mL/kg of ideal body weight reduces the degree of lung injury caused by either stress or strain and may have a positive impact on the development of postoperative pulmonary complications. Applying a positive end-expiratory pressure (PEEP) is effective in improving dynamic intratidal compliance, with beneficial effects on damage from alveolar opening-closing. PEEP reduces the incidence of atelectasis, restores fractional reserve capacity and improves respiratory mechanics, with consequent positive effects on applied pressure and gas exchange [49].

Although volume-controlled and pressure-controlled ventilation can be both employed, we prefer pressure-controlled ventilation because of better respiratory data [50]. On practical grounds, we establish the baseline ventilation parameters with volume-controlled ventilation, with constant flow, a tidal volume of 6–8 mL/kg, and 12 breaths per minute. We switch to pressure-controlled ventilation after creation of the pneumoperitoneum. Since it is known that pressure-controlled ventilation does not guarantee the tidal volume, we adjust the pressure limit to obtain a tidal volume as close as possible to the one previously settled in volume-controlled ventilation. The initial respiratory rate of 12 breaths per minute is adjusted to maintain an end-tidal CO_2 of 35–40 mmHg. An inspiratory/expiratory ratio of 1:2 is used with an end-inspiratory pause of 10% of the inspiration time, and the lowest PEEP value that reaches satisfactory ventilatory parameters. A mathematical model to quickly and safely switch from volume-controlled to pressure-controlled ventilation was proposed by Agrò et al. [51].

We prefer to switch to pressure-controlled ventilation because this modality achieves higher instantaneous flow peaks, minimizing peak pressures, and it improves alveolar recruitment and oxygenation. Additionally, the use of titrated levels of PEEP can be employed to reduce alveolar de-recruitment. The increase of PEEP, however, must be very prudent since high levels are expected to potentiate the negative effects of pneumoperitoneum on cardiac output.

Anesthesia is maintained with sevoflurane in 50% oxygen/air.

6.7 Anesthesia

A synopsis of our pharmacologic protocol during anesthesia for MIPR is provided in Table 6.2.

Regarding the type of anesthesia (volatile vs. intravenous) we prefer inhaled drugs [52]. Although there is no striking evidence favoring either volatile or intravenous anesthesia in MIPR, the use of propofol is known to reduce cardiac parasympathetic tone leading to lower hemodynamic stability [53, 54]. Insecure hemodynamic stability may become a problem at the time of sudden bleeding, and/or may accentuate the challenges associated with maintenance of optimal tissue perfusion because of the cardiopulmonary implications of pneumoperitoneum. Additionally, intravenous anesthesia promotes intestinal peristalsis thereby complicating intestinal reconstruction during some procedures, such as pancreatoduodenectomy.

The bronchodilator response to the use of sevoflurane, observed both in animals [55] and in humans [56], is an additional factor that justifies our preference for volatile anesthesia.

Table 6.2 Pharmacologic protocol and fluids infusions during volatile anesthesia for MIPR

Premedication	Midazolam 0.07–0.1 mg/kg i.v. bolus * Atropine 0.1–0.2 mg/kg i.v. bolus
Induction and neuromuscular blockade	Fentanyl 1 μg/kg i.v. bolus Propofol 1% 1,5–2,5 mg/kg i.v. bolus Rocuronium bromide 0.6 mg/kg i.v. bolus
Maintenance	Fentanyl 0.35–1.4 μg/kg (25–100 μg) i.v. bolus Sevorane target minimum alveolar concentration based on patient age Rocuronium bromide 0.15 mg/kg i.v. infusion
Fluid replacement	(4–6 mL/kg/h) Ringer lactate (40%) Succinylated gelatin 4% (60%)

*Final dose adjusted in small boluses (1–2 mg each) based on patient response.

6.8 Practical Considerations

Intraoperative transfusions increase the risk of serious postoperative infections [57] and the rate of 30-day readmissions [58] and worsen oncologic prognosis [59]. However, it also known that postoperative morbidity and mortality increase for each gram of decrement when the hemoglobin concentration is <7.0 mg/dL [60], and patients with cardiovascular disease are more vulnerable to the effects of anemia [61, 62]. Although the postoperative incidence of complications is reduced when fresh blood is transfused (i.e., blood stored for <35 days) [63], proper management of blood transfusions is among the major treatment objectives of anesthesia during pancreatic resections.

In the modern era of pancreatic surgery, and in MIPR in particular, the amount of intraoperative bleeding is usually limited. However, intraoperative blood transfusions are still required in 9% to 78% of the patients undergoing pancreatoduodenectomy [64, 65]. Rarely, patients may experience massive bleeding as a consequence of surgical misadventure [13].

Although patients with very low hemoglobin levels (<7.0 mg/dL) are likely to benefit from transfusion of packed red blood cells, we prefer to rely more on delta hemoglobin (ΔHb) to decide when transfusions are needed [66]. ΔHb is defined as the difference between first intraoperative Hb level, determined immediately after anesthesia induction and nadir intraoperative Hb level. Although personalized decisions are required, in ASA I and II patients we prefer to avoid transfusions if ΔHb is ≤50%, and Hb is >7.0 mg/dL. In ASA III and IV patients we accept a ΔHb ≤30%, but transfusions may be given even when Hb >7.0 mg/dL, if the patient is at high cardiovascular risk and/or the procedure is complex and further bleeding is anticipated.

Recent data suggest that patients at high risk for pancreatic fistula may benefit from intravenous hydrocortisone treatment. The first bolus of steroids is given at the induction of anesthesia. A total of eight doses are suggested given every 8 hours in the postoperative period [67].

Although given quite often, somatostatin analogs may decrease the incidence of pancreas-related postoperative complications but do not reduce perioperative mortality [68]. A recent multi-institutional study showed that perioperative use of octreotide was associated with a three-fold increase in the risk of postoperative pancreatic fistula [69]. The prophylactic use of somatostatin analogs is questionable.

Elevated intrabdominal pressure, caused by pneumoperitoneum, increases intrathoracic and intracranial pressures. Higher thoracoabdominal pressure reduces venous drainage from the brain. Elevated intracranial pressure increases cerebral blood volume because of the vasodilatory effect of CO_2. Changes in intracranial pressure and in blood supply to the brain may affect cerebral perfusion and eventually cerebral oxygenation, leading to a longer recovery and impaired cognition. To prevent, or reduce, these phenomena we provide intraoperative mannitol infusion in association with albumin drip [70]. The combination of mannitol and dopamine is also useful to preserve renal function [71]. Vasopressors may also be used, as required, to maintain optimal blood pressure. Attention is also paid to maintain electrolyte balance.

Optimal management of postoperative pain is also key to the success of complex abdominal operations, such as MIPR. The use of opioids should be reduced as much as possible in order to prevent their side-effects on intestinal motility [52]. Pain management is a main component in modern protocols for enhanced recovery [72].

6.9 Conclusions

Modern management of anesthesia during pancreatic resections in general, and during MIPR in particular, requires dedication and commitment. While the role of the anesthetist, in many circumstances, is still relegated to delivering anesthesia to enable surgery, in MIPR anesthetists have to be fully embedded in the multidisciplinary team caring for these patients.

References

1. van Hilst J, de Rooij T, Abu Hilal M et al (2017) Worldwide survey on opinions and use of minimally invasive pancreatic resection. HPB (Oxford) 19(3):190–204
2. Gooiker GA, van Gijn W, Wouters MW et al (2011) Systematic review and meta-analysis of the volume-outcome relationship in pancreatic surgery. Br J Surg 98(4):485–494
3. Kendrick ML, van Hilst J, Boggi U et al (2017) Minimally invasive pancreatoduodenectomy. HPB (Oxford) 19(3):215–224
4. Vollmer CM, Asbun HJ, Barkun J et al (2017) Proceedings of the first international state-of-the-art conference on minimally-invasive pancreatic resection (MIPR). HPB (Oxford) 19(3):171–177
5. Huang Y, Chua TC, Gill AJ, Samra JS (2017) Impact of perioperative fluid administration on early outcomes after pancreatoduodenectomy: a meta-analysis. Pancreatology 17(3):334–341
6. Bruns H, Kortendieck V, Raab HR, Antolovic D (2016) Intraoperative fluid excess is a risk factor for pancreatic fistula after partial pancreaticoduodenectomy. HPB Surg 2016:1601340 doi:10.1155/2016/1601340
7. Grant F, Brennan MF, Allen PJ et al (2016) Prospective randomized controlled trial of liberal vs restricted perioperative fluid management in patients undergoing pancreatectomy. Ann Surg 264(4):591–598
8. Xiong J, Szatmary P, Huang W et al (2016) Enhanced recovery after surgery program in patients undergoing pancreaticoduodenectomy: a PRISMA-compliant systematic review and meta-analysis. Medicine (Baltimore) 95(18):e3497
9. Joliat GR, Labgaa I, Petermann D et al (2015) Cost-benefit analysis of an enhanced recovery protocol for pancreaticoduodenectomy. Br J Surg 102(13):1676–1683
10. Hamza N, Darwish A, O'Reilly DA et al (2015) Perioperative enteral immunonutrition modulates systemic and mucosal immunity and the inflammatory response in patients with periampullary cancer scheduled for pancreaticoduodenectomy: a randomized clinical trial. Pancreas 44(1):41–52

11. Ross A, Mohammed S, Vanburen G et al (2013) An assessment of the necessity of transfusion during pancreatoduodenectomy. Surgery 154(3):504–511
12. Boggi U, Napoli N, Costa F et al (2016) Robotic-assisted pancreatic resections. World J Surg 40(10):2497–2506
13. Chalikonda S, Aguilar-Saavedra JR, Walsh RM (2012) Laparoscopic robotic-assisted pancreaticoduodenectomy: a case-matched comparison with open resection. Surg Endosc 26(9):2397–2402
14. Petrowsky H, Clavien PA (2005) Should we deny surgery for malignant hepato-pancreatico-biliary tumors to elderly patients? World J Surg 29(9):1093–1100
15. Mak PH, Campbell RC, Irwin MG; American Society of Anesthesiologists (2002) The ASA Physical Status Classification: inter-observer consistency. American Society of Anesthesiologists. Anaesth Intensive Care 30(5):633–640
16. Tamijmarane A, Bhati CS, Mirza DF et al (2008) Application of Portsmouth modification of physiological and operative severity scoring system for enumeration of morbidity and mortality (P-POSSUM) in pancreatic surgery. World J Surg Oncol 6:39
17. Ouellette JR, Small DG, Termuhlen PM (2004) Evaluation of Charlson-Age Comorbidity Index as predictor of morbidity and mortality in patients with colorectal carcinoma. J Gastrointest Surg 8(8):1061–1067
18. de Castro SM, Biere SS, Lagarde SM et al (2009) Validation of a nomogram for predicting survival after resection for adenocarcinoma of the pancreas. Br J Surg 96(4):417–423
19. Gulbinas A, Barauskas G, Pundzius J (2004) Preoperative stratification of pancreas-related morbidity after the Whipple procedure. Int Surg 89(1):39–45
20. Mogal H, Vermilion SA, Dodson R et al (2017) Modified frailty index predicts morbidity and mortality after pancreaticoduodenectomy. Ann Surg Oncol 24(6):1714–1721
21. Satava RM, Gallagher AG, Pellegrini CA (2003) Surgical competence and surgical proficiency: definitions, taxonomy, and metrics. J Am Coll Surg 196(6):933–937
22. Hogg ME, Besselink MG, Clavien PA et al (2017) Training in minimally invasive pancreatic resections: a paradigm shift away from "See one, Do one, Teach one". HPB (Oxford) 19(3): 234–245
23. Jepsen RM, Dieckmann P, Spanager L et al (2016) Evaluating structured assessment of anaesthesiologists' non-technical skills. Acta Anaesthesiol Scand 60(6):756–766
24. Gjeraa K, Jepsen RM, Rewers M et al (2016) Exploring the relationship between anaesthesiologists' non-technical and technical skills. Acta Anaesthesiol Scand 60(1):36–47
25. Savonitto S, Caracciolo M, Cattaneo M, De Servi S (2011) Management of patients with recently implanted coronary stents on dual antiplatelet therapy who need to undergo major surgery. J Thromb Haemost 9(11):2133–2142
26. Wolf AM, Pucci MJ, Gabale SD et al (2014) Safety of perioperative aspirin therapy in pancreatic operations. Surgery 155(1):39–46
27. Mita K, Ito H, Takahashi K et al (2016) Postpancreatectomy hemorrhage after pancreatic surgery in patients receiving anticoagulation or antiplatelet agents. Surg Innov 23(3): 284–290
28. Fujikawa T, Tanaka A, Abe T et al (2013) Does antiplatelet therapy affect outcomes of patients receiving abdominal laparoscopic surgery? Lessons from more than 1,000 laparoscopic operations in a single tertiary referral hospital. J Am Coll Surg 217(6):1044–1053
29. Stark M, Pomati S, D'Ambrosio A et al (2015) A new telesurgical platform – preliminary clinical results. Minim Invasive Ther Allied Technol 24(1):31–36
30. Rosenberg J, Fuchs-Buder T (2016) Why surgeons need to know about anaesthesia. Surg Endosc 30(9):3661–3664
31. Christensen CR, Maatman TK, Maatman TJ, Tran TT (2016) Examining clinical outcomes utilizing low-pressure pneumoperitoneum during robotic-assisted radical prostatectomy. J Robot Surg 10(3):215–219
32. Angioli R, Terranova C, Plotti F et al (2015) Influence of pneumoperitoneum pressure on surgical field during robotic and laparoscopic surgery: a comparative study. Arch Gynecol Obstet 291(4):865–868

33. Gill A, Randell R (2016) Robotic surgery and its impact on teamwork in the operating theatre. J Perioper Pract 26(3):42–45
34. Demyttenaere SV, Taqi A, Polyhronopoulos GN et al (2007) Targeting individual hemodynamics to maintain renal perfusion during pneumoperitoneum in a porcine model. Surgery 142(3):350–356
35. Yavuz Y, Rønning K, Lyng O et al (2001) Effect of increased intraabdominal pressure on cardiac output and tissue blood flow assessed by color-labeled microspheres in the pig. Surg Endosc 15(2):149–155
36. Galizia G, Prizio G, Lieto E et al (2001) Hemodynamic and pulmonary changes during open, carbon dioxide pneumoperitoneum and abdominal wall-lifting cholecystectomy. A prospective, randomized study. Surg Endosc 15(5):477–483
37. Odeberg S, Ljungqvist O, Svenberg T et al (1994) Haemodynamic effects of pneumoperitoneum and the influence of posture during anaesthesia for laparoscopic surgery. Acta Anaesthesiol Scand 38(3):276–283
38. Crystal GJ (2015) Carbon dioxide and the heart: physiology and clinical implications. Anesth Analg 121(3):610–623
39. Rauh R, Hemmerling TM, Rist M, Jacobi KE (2001) Influence of pneumoperitoneum and patient positioning on respiratory system compliance. J Clin Anesth 13(5):361–365
40. Bures E, Fusciardi J, Lanquetot H et al (1996) Ventilatory effects of laparoscopic cholecystectomy. Acta Anaesthesiol Scand 40(5):566–573
41. Lebowitz P, Yedlin A, Hakimi AA et al (2015) Respiratory gas exchange during robotic-assisted laparoscopic radical prostatectomy. J Clin Anesth 27(6):470–475
42. Marik PE, Cavallazzi R (2013) Does the central venous pressure predict fluid responsiveness? An updated meta-analysis and a plea for some common sense. Crit Care Med 41(7):1774–1781
43. Hahn RG, He R, Li Y (2016) Central venous pressure as an adjunct to flow-guided volume optimisation after induction of general anaesthesia. Anaesthesiol Intensive Ther 48(2):110–115
44. Neudecker J, Sauerland S, Neugebauer E et al (2002) The European Association for Endoscopic Surgery clinical practice guideline on the pneumoperitoneum for laparoscopic surgery. Surg Endosc 16(7):1121–1143
45. Wulf H, Ledowski T, Linstedt U et al (1998) Neuromuscular blocking effects of rocuronium during desflurane, isoflurane, and sevoflurane anaesthesia. Can J Anaesth 45(6):526–532
46. Cantineau JP, Porte F, d'Honneur G, Duvaldestin P (1994) Neuromuscular effects of rocuronium on the diaphragm and adductor pollicis muscles in anesthetized patients. Anesthesiology 81(3):585–590
47. Kirov K, Motamed C, Combes X et al (2000) Sensitivity to atracurium in the lateral abdominal muscles. Ann Fr Anesth Reanim 19(10):734–738 [Article in French]
48. Jones RK, Caldwell JE, Brull SJ, Soto RG (2008) Reversal of profound rocuronium-induced blockade with sugammadex: a randomized comparison with neostigmine. Anesthesiology 109(5):816–824
49. Güldner A, Kiss T, Serpa Neto A et al (2015) Intraoperative protective mechanical ventilation for prevention of postoperative pulmonary complications: a comprehensive review of the role of tidal volume, positive end-expiratory pressure, and lung recruitment maneuvers. Anesthesiology 123(3):692–713
50. Wang JP, Wang HB, Liu YJ et al (2015) Comparison of pressure- and volume-controlled ventilation in laparoscopic surgery: a meta-analysis of randomized controlled trial. Clin Invest Med 38(3):E119–E141
51. Agrò FE, Cappa P, Sciuto SA, Silvestri S (2006) Linear model and algorithm to automatically estimate the pressure limit of pressure controlled ventilation for delivering a target tidal volume. J Clin Monit Comput 20(1):1–10
52. De Pietri L, Montalti R, Begliomini B (2014) Anaesthetic perioperative management of patients with pancreatic cancer. World J Gastroenterol 20(9):2304–2320
53. Husedzinović I, Tonković D, Barisin S et al (2003) Hemodynamic differences in sevoflurane versus propofol anesthesia. Coll Antropol 27(1):205–212

54. Kanaya N, Hirata N, Kurosawa S et al (2003) Differential effects of propofol and sevoflurane on heart rate variability. Anesthesiology 98(1):34–40
55. Lele E, Petak F, Fontao F et al (2006) Protective effects of volatile agents against acetylcholine-induced bronchoconstriction in isolated perfused rat lungs. Acta Anaesthesiol Scand 50(9):1145–1151
56. Goff MJ, Arain SR, Ficke DJ et al (2000) Absence of bronchodilation during desflurane anesthesia: a comparison to sevoflurane and thiopental. Anesthesiology 93(2):404–408
57. Zhang L, Liao Q, Zhang T et al (2016) Blood transfusion is an independent risk factor for postoperative serious infectious complications after pancreaticoduodenectomy. World J Surg 40(10):2507–2512
58. Fisher AV, Fernandes-Taylor S, Campbell-Flohr SA et al (2017) 30-day readmission after pancreatic resection: a systematic review of the literature and meta-analysis. Ann Surg [Epub ahead of print] doi:10.1097/SLA.0000000000002230
59. Sutton JM, Kooby DA, Wilson GC et al (2014) Perioperative blood transfusion is associated with decreased survival in patients undergoing pancreaticoduodenectomy for pancreatic adenocarcinoma: a multi-institutional study. J Gastrointest Surg 18(9):1575–1587
60. Carson JL, Noveck H, Berlin JA, Gould SA (2002) Mortality and morbidity in patients with very low postoperative Hb levels who decline blood transfusion. Transfusion 42(7):812–818
61. Carson JL, Duff A, Poses RM et al (1996) Effect of anaemia and cardiovascular disease on surgical mortality and morbidity. Lancet 348(9034):1055–1060
62. Nair D, Shlipak MG, Angeja B et al (2005) Association of anemia with diastolic dysfunction among patients with coronary artery disease in the Heart and Soul Study. Am J Cardiol 95(3):332–336
63. Kim Y, Amini N, Gani F et al (2017) Age of transfused blood impacts perioperative outcomes among patients who undergo major gastrointestinal surgery. Ann Surg 265(1):103–110
64. Barreto SG, Singh A, Perwaiz A et al (2017) Maximum surgical blood order schedule for pancreatoduodenectomy: a long way from uniform applicability! Future Oncol 13(9): 799–807
65. Di Giorgio A, Alfieri S, Rotondi F et al (2005) Pancreatoduodenectomy for tumors of Vater's ampulla: report on 94 consecutive patients. World J Surg 29(4):513–518
66. Spolverato G, Bagante F, Weiss M et al (2016) Impact of delta hemoglobin on provider transfusion practices and post-operative morbidity among patients undergoing liver and pancreatic surgery. J Gastrointest Surg 20(12):2010–2020
67. Laaninen M, Sand J, Nordback I et al (2016) Perioperative hydrocortisone reduces major complications after pancreaticoduodenectomy: a randomized controlled trial. Ann Surg 264(5):696–702
68. Gurusamy KS, Koti R, Fusai G, Davidson BR (2013) Somatostatin analogues for pancreatic surgery. Cochrane Database Syst Rev 30:CD008370
69. McMillan MT, Soi S, Asbun HJ et al (2016) Risk-adjusted outcomes of clinically relevant pancreatic fistula following pancreatoduodenectomy: a model for performance evaluation. Ann Surg 264(2):344–352
70. Zhou X, Wu MC, Wang YL et al (2013) Mannitol improves cerebral oxygen content and postoperative recovery after prolonged retroperitoneal laparoscopy. Surg Endosc 27(4):1166–1171
71. Bolte SL, Chin LT, Moon TD et al (2006) Maintaining urine production and early allograft function during laparoscopic donor nephrectomy. Urology 68(4):747–750
72. Morgan KA, Lancaster WP, Walters ML et al (2016) Enhanced recovery after surgery protocols are valuable in pancreas surgery patients. J Am Coll Surg 222(4):658–664

7 Contribution of Radiology as an Enabling Medical Specialty

Davide Caramella, Carla Cappelli, Rosa Cervelli, and Greg Strowig

7.1 Introduction

Radiology has changed dramatically in the last few decades. From the old paradigm of a diagnostic specialty reacting to a referring doctor's request by performing a given imaging study for a given clinical situation, in recent years radiologists have been proactively taking part in clinical management by acquiring and integrating multimodality information obtained from different equipment able to generate mono- as well as multiparametric image datasets. Furthermore, hybrid acquisition makes it possible to fuse radiology and nuclear medicine images, and quantitative imaging is emerging with the aim of obtaining useful imaging biomarkers [1, 2].

All these developments have been increasingly applied in patient candidates for pancreatic surgery with the aim of predicting the risk of postoperative complications, by adding in the diagnostic workup dynamic contrast-enhanced magnetic resonance imaging (DCE-MRI) and diffusion-weighted imaging (DWI) together with the intravoxel incoherent motion model. DCE-MRI has been recently applied in patients with pancreatic adenocarcinomas also to quantify pharmacokinetic parameters such as K^{trans} and k_{ep} values [3], which can be considered prognostic indicators of clinical outcome (in terms of both tumor response and patient survival). Fat quantification and DWI, with the intravoxel incoherent motion model, are used to evaluate several pancreatic glandular factors [4], such as soft-tissue texture, pancreatic steatosis, absence of fibrosis, and small pancreatic duct size, which are associated with an increased rate of postoperative pancreatic complications [5, 6]. Finally, the introduction of advanced 3D reconstruction [7] has proved useful in assisting surgeons to better

D. Caramella (✉)
Diagnostic and Interventional Radiology, Department of Translational Research and New Technologies in Medicine and Surgery, University of Pisa
Pisa, Italy
e-mail: davide.caramella@med.unipi.it

U. Boggi (Ed), *Minimally Invasive Surgery of the Pancreas*, Updates in Surgery
DOI: 10.1007/978-88-470-3958-2_7,

appreciate complex anatomy whose knowledge is of paramount importance in planning pancreatic interventions [8, 9].

In addition to that, a series of recent disruptive innovations are paving the way towards new hi-tech applications aimed at helping the surgeon during the laparoscopic or robotic operation by augmented reality [10, 11].

This exponential and multifaceted technological development resulted in a hyper-growth of digital information that has to be processed and stored for each patient to manage newly emerging health problems as well as to monitor the evolution of chronic conditions over time. We are effectively entering an era in which radiology is no longer required to produce and distribute just diagnostic images, since its role has evolved into the hospital-wide enabler of the technical and clinical integration of all medical data (diagnostic images being still the largest portion of them) at the point of care and beyond.

7.2 Radiology as a Diagnostic Medical Discipline

If we go back in time to the old days of film, diagnostic images were organized, indexed, and stored in the hospital's film room. Couriers went back and forth between the film room and the various departments that needed to see these images. Simple, and sometimes sophisticated, light box systems were found throughout the hospital where film could be displayed. As all of this digitization of medical imaging occurred, it became necessary to put procedures in place to manage all of this data. It was out of this need that the Picture Archiving and Communications System (PACS) was born. These systems were produced by major healthcare technology vendors, film manufacturers, and a host of upstart companies who stepped in to fill the need for image management technology (Fig. 7.1).

However, PACS was conceived as filling just the departmental needs of radiology. There was no view of PACS serving beyond this department or specialties. PACS was good at storing data created in that specific department and retrieving and displaying the data created in that department. If you were a clinician outside that department and wished to see the images, the solution was to walk to the department and view them on the very expensive PACS workstations that the radiologists were using. Or, if your hospital was well equipped, you might be able to walk over to a PACS workstation that had been installed in your department or somewhere on the hospital floor. And, if the data were needed for a patient referral outside of the hospital, the images were printed on film and given to the patients to carry with them.

As PACS evolved in the first decade of this century, it was not uncommon for these systems to be replaced every three years. And, when this replacement happened, all of the data from the outgoing PACS needed to be moved to the incoming PACS. In the early days, this wasn't a big problem as there was not

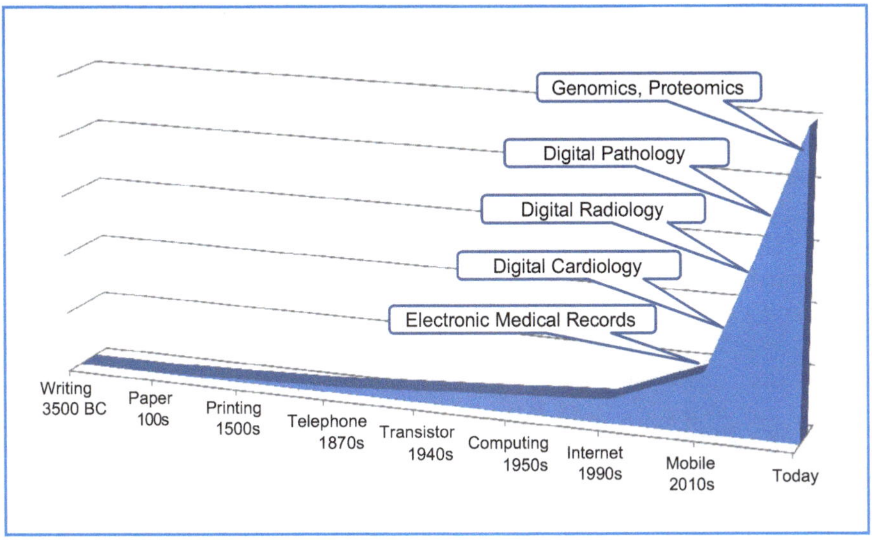

Fig. 7.1 Historic data growth

that much data to move. However, as more and more data were generated each year, the migration of these data became a very time-consuming and challenging effort. Often, part of the data would be problematic to move. Either the data were irretrievable due to storage technology issues, such as tape corruption, or they were not stored in a compatible format for the new system to use. Further, despite standards being established to facilitate the flow and storage of medical images such as Digital Image and Communication in Medicine (DICOM), modality and PACS manufacturers often did not fully implement the standards. Some PACS manufacturers retained data such as text overlays, annotations, and other necessary data in their systems database so they could be displayed properly on their own workstations. However, if the data were migrated or otherwise sent to another brand of workstation, often these data were missing as they were "stuck" in the original system's database and not passed along with the image.

Data migrations would also often be required simply when there was no change in PACS software vendor. This would happen when the same vendor would upgrade their storage system from one version to the next. New technologies either developed in-house or from a recently purchased company, would replace the old technology. If a hospital wanted to simply upgrade from PACS version one to PACS version two, a storage upgrade was in the offering.

With all of these data migrations, a further complication of cost was involved. It was like having to move the hospital's film room across the hall and back, just to paint the room. Further complicating the issue of cost when transitioning from one vendor to another, outgoing vendors had little incentive to assist in migrating data out of their system, which was being shut down. So they would begrudgingly help, but at an even greater cost to the hospital.

Lastly, during the 1990s and 2000s, it was very common that PACS vendors resold storage technology (plenty of disks) with their solution. Hospitals were required to purchase this infrastructure, and continue to upgrade it as the PACS vendor evolved their solution. However, these storage technologies came at a premium price from the PACS vendors who were marking up the solution from storage vendors like EMC, HP, IBM, Dell, etc. And, by decree of the PACS vendors, these storage technologies could only be used with the PACS and nothing else. This often infuriated the information technology professionals in the hospital as they knew storage could be purchased at a lower cost, direct from the manufacturer, and they also wanted to buy something that could provide enterprise-wide data storage, not just for radiology images.

However, in 1998 and 2001, two startup companies took a different approach to managing medical images. Emageon, Inc. was started in 1998 as a research project at the University of Alabama at Birmingham before being formed as a venture capital-backed company. Similarly, TeraMedica, Inc. was formed in late 2001 out of an idea that the Mayo Clinic had for managing medical images. Both of these companies were founded out of an idea to separate the archival and data management of these medical images from the ever-changing workstation and workflow technologies. Further, their new technology would service medical images from more than just one specialty as PACS focused on. Additionally, with TeraMedica, their product was purely software, with hospitals providing their own servers and storage as they desired. Emageon went on to purchase a radiology workstation company and refocus itself as a PACS vendor. Then, it merged with several other companies and was eventually acquired by Merge Healthcare, a division of IBM. TeraMedica remained focused on the image management and archival marketspace and is now a division of Fujifilm.

These two companies were the start of a new healthcare information technology product category that, sometime around 2008, became known as vendor-neutral archives (VNAs). By this time, a few other startup vendors had joined this product category with VNAs of their own. Later, the large, global healthcare information technology vendors also promoted their own VNAs. As a product category name, it is not very descriptive of what these systems do. Certainly, all of these systems are created by vendors, so what is the meaning of “vendor-neutral”? Furthermore, these systems offer much more than archiving of information; rather, they provide storage, retrieval, sharing, and universal access to all patient-related clinical content – images or otherwise.

The idea behind calling these systems “vendor-neutral” was because they were independent and agnostic as to what systems they were connecting to. VNA was indeed produced by a vendor, but it did not matter if the customer wished to connect different vendors’ PACS, modalities, 3D workstations, or other technology. This independence allowed the VNAs to focus on the interoperability of their solution rather than tight integration with another product manufactured by that same company. “True VNAs” were often built from the ground up by vendors who did not sell PACS. Later, PACS vendors started selling variants

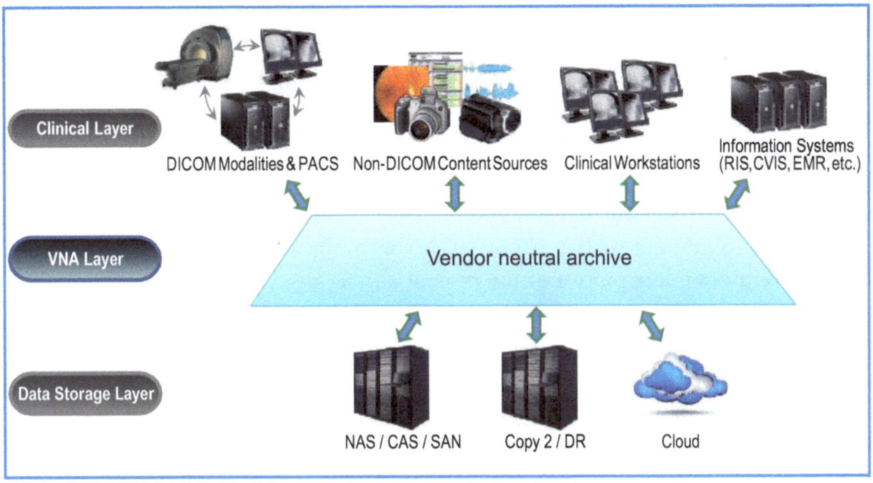

Fig. 7.2 Typical role for a vendor-neutral archive (*DR*, disaster recovery)

of their PACS or their PACS archive product as a VNA. However, often, these systems were optimized to work with that vendor's PACS and not with a myriad of other vendors' products.

A VNA was often implemented as the last stop for images as they made their way through the radiology workflow. For instance, diagnostic images would be generated at the modality, sent to the PACS for quality control checks and adjustment, read by the radiologist, and stored in the VNA. No longer was it required to have vast amounts of storage attached to the PACS. When the PACS needs the imaging study for prior comparison again, it is retrieved from the VNA to the PACS. It was now the VNA whose storage infrastructure was going to grow and grow (Fig. 7.2).

As hospital systems across the world began implementing VNAs, the PACS vendors took notice. Suddenly, the sales of storage hardware with their PACS declined sharply. Furthermore, the virtual grip that PACS vendors had on hospital systems was loosened. Hospitals were able to upgrade systems much more easily. They were also able to replace a PACS vendor much more easily. No longer were they beholden to the concern that they would have to pay significant money and expend hundreds or thousands of hours, just to migrate their own patient data. Now, these data were resident in the VNA, which could remain in place while the information technology world around it changed. Furthermore, VNAs often included software functionality to migrate data between various storage infrastructures that it had stored data on, thus making technology upgrades easier on a hospital system. "Vendor-neutral" was the benefit of being able to change systems easily, without being concerned about what would happen to the data.

VNAs started out with their focus on DICOM radiological images. These images are generated by the various modalities in radiology and are created, routed, and stored in the DICOM standard format. Often, especially until around 2010, there might be several PACS in a single hospital – one PACS for general radiology, one PACS for cardiology, one PACS for endoscopy, another PACS for radiotherapy planning, and so on. To see a complete view of the patient's imaging, clinicians would need to navigate to several PACS, often having to physically go to a different workstation. There was no hope of seeing images in different PACS side by side. And, of course, each system had its own idiosyncrasies in how users would need to interact with it. So often, it was more trouble than it was worth to try and see a complete record of the patient's imaging.

However, as VNAs came into vogue, data from all of these source PACS and modalities were now being stored centrally. Around this same time, implementation of electronic medical record (EMR) systems became the dominant focus of healthcare information technology in the United States. These systems, analogous in many ways to VNAs, were centralized repositories of large amounts of patient clinical data. Things such as patient history and physical results, laboratory results, clinical notes, oncologic treatments, etc. were all kept in this centralized EMR. And, in the VNA industry, it made perfect sense to integrate the centralized VNA with the centralized EMR. VNAs were good at storing and managing clinical images while EMRs were good at storing and managing clinical text. Thus, this created another new healthcare information technology software product category, enterprise image viewers, sometimes called universal image viewers.

Enterprise image viewers were developed by a myriad of companies, including VNA manufacturers. These viewers focused on being able to integrate with the EMR, display the image content in the VNA regardless of its original source, and deliver simple viewing tools to the masses using standard desktop technologies. No longer were medical images just the domain of those who had access to expensive PACS workstations; rather, images were now accessible to any authorized practitioner in the hospital. And, because they provided simple viewing tools, the deployment of these systems required little, if any, training of the users.

VNAs also offered hospital information technology staff a way to manage the content that was being amassed in the VNA. TeraMedica patented their technology to understand the contents of the DICOM medical images and to classify them into various storage retention policies. For instance, imaging studies with no pathology could be stored on a slow and inexpensive storage system as it was unlikely they would be retrieved again. However, imaging studies for a cancer patient showing pathology could be stored on a fast and expensive storage system for quick and frequent retrieval. Further, mammography images or pediatric studies can be stored longer than other types of studies, as most legal image retention laws dictate. And, finally, VNAs often provided for the eventual deletion of studies after this legal retention period had expired (Fig. 7.3).

These storage, or information lifecycle, management abilities were thought to be desirable in the early days of VNAs. Storage costs were growing exponentially

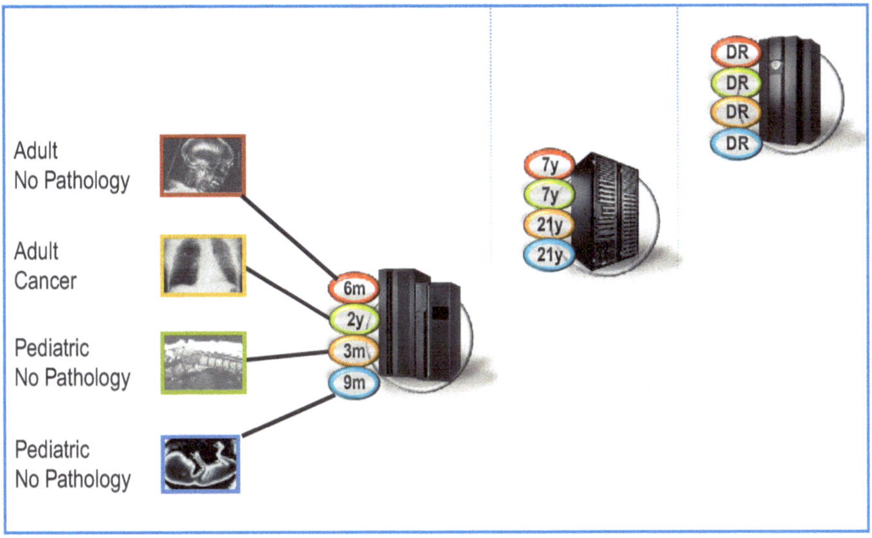

Fig. 7.3 Vendor-neutral archive: clinical information lifecycle management (*DR*, disaster recovery)

for hospitals, PACS had no facility to differentiate the storage of imaging studies, and PACS could not delete studies after a configured retention period. However, in practice, VNA vendors found that storage costs per terabyte were dropping quickly and that the storing of studies across many different tiers of storage was just too complicated for hospitals to manage. Further, with the advent of enterprise image viewers and the evolution of users' expectations, it was no longer acceptable to store an imaging study on a slow media where it would take a long time to retrieve. EMR users who clicked on a six-year-old imaging study wanted to see images immediately, just as they had become accustomed to using the Internet or video streaming services at home. With PACS, it was more predictable as to what imaging studies the radiologist might want to see from the VNA. However, EMR users were not predictable and their desire was to have immediate access to everything.

Moreover, while the idea of being able to delete studies at the end of their legal retention period was a good one, VNA vendors found out that most hospitals had not yet come to terms with this in the digital world. In the days of the film room, clerks would have no problem periodically culling through the old film and sending it to the silver recycler. But, once everything became digital, then people's expectations changed. Physicians demanded that images be retained forever as they might have clinical value. Hospital administrators couldn't figure out what the right retention policies were. PACS were still not able to delete references to imaging studies in their database. Thus, the PACS might continue to reference studies in the VNA that had been purged by the VNA. For these and other reasons, VNA's ability to delete images did not get utilized as much as originally envisioned.

VNAs originally focused on the world of medical images, namely those created by radiology and cardiology devices and stored in the DICOM format. However, VNAs soon found themselves in the position of being the centralized repository for all types of clinical content, both in the DICOM format and in non-DICOM formats. Images from endoscopy, anesthesiology data, genetic data and data of other specialties needed to be stored and managed in the hospital. Videos from surgery among others, were soon finding their way into the VNA. Scanned documents, EKG and EEG wave forms, anesthesiology monitoring strips, and other types of content that could be output digitally from all over the hospital were sent to the VNA for permanent keeping and distribution through the enterprise viewing solution. Even proprietary files, such as radiation treatment plans, that could only be viewed or used on the same type of device that created the file were stored in the VNA. Often, this was to facilitate hospital-to-hospital sharing of the file or to ensure that the data was professionally stored, backed up, available during a disaster, and secured.

Interestingly, in Europe, hospitals did not follow the same path to management of all of this clinical content. PACS continued to have a strong foothold in the management of radiology data. A unique concept called PACS2 grew in Europe, which basically meant a system to manage all non-DICOM clinical content. Thus, hospitals would have both a PACS and a PACS2. But, because they did not move the storage management of all the PACS data to a separate system, such as a VNA, they did not reap the control and financial benefits. Thus, when PACS was replaced, they had to endure the painful and costly PACS-to-PACS migration. Only in the past few years have European hospitals started down the path of combining the data management of their PACS with their PACS2 solutions into a VNA system. Europe also was much quicker than the rest of the world to adopt the Cross-Document Sharing (XDS) framework for sharing content between hospital facilities.

Today's VNAs are generally accepted to perform the following functions:

- Storage of DICOM and non-DICOM clinical content;
- Connectivity through an embedded or third-party enterprise viewing solution;
- Information lifecycle management of the data over its medical and legal lifetime, including deletion of the data at the end of its use;
- Sharing of clinical content to other hospitals and clinics;
- Integration and interoperability between modalities, workstations, and information.

7.3 Radiology as an Enabling Medical Specialty

As VNAs become more and more prevalent in the world, there will be greater demands placed on these systems by their users. The content within VNAs continues to grow, with data flowing into them from a myriad of specialties across the hospital. Physicians are finding that the ability to look at more data in the course of diagnosing and treating a patient is opening new doors to better information, better diagnosis, and greater clinician collaboration. For example, radiologists who previously did not have access to radiation treatment plans for cancer patients, but suddenly have this at their fingertips, are now able to make more informed diagnoses and meaningful reports. And, in the near future, it will not be uncommon for genomic and proteomic data to be stored within the VNA, all ready for access and correlation.

Large pools of data, such as that which resides in a VNA, are perfect for correlating with the EMR to bring the complete picture of each patient to life. By combining patient history and physical information, pharmaceutical information, diagnosis, treatment paths, and outcomes, these new systems will be able to derive new insights from all of this data into better patient care at lower costs.

However, as this information grows, so too does the difficulty that humans have in processing large amounts of data. Further, when cost and resource constraints are prevalent in a hospital, there is little time for searching, reading, viewing, and correlating these data. Thus, with the benefits that a VNA and EMR provide, there are difficulties in using all of this information, especially if it is not filtered, interpreted, and presented in the right context at the right time. This is where the next wave of information technology will move VNAs and EMRs. With big data, analytics, machine learning, and artificial intelligence, these technologies will help sift through the data and present relevant information to the clinician.

Further, as these technologies evolve, and as privacy concerns can be assured, the massive amounts of data that exist across many hospital VNAs and EMRs can be combined into research cohort studies that look across geographies and country borders. Through artificial intelligence, patient care paths will be recommended by systems capable of processing and associating large amounts of data in real time. Machine learning and deep learning will be informed by patient outcomes to improve this intelligence over time.

All these developments are transforming the role of radiology, from a diagnostic medical discipline to an enabling medical specialty whose key role is to provide increasingly complex image datasets to the clinical community, helping to integrate them with laboratory and pathology results, quantitative imaging biomarkers, and anesthesiological as well as surgical information, thus enabling the creation of a shared archive from which a huge amount of multidisciplinary data can be easily retrieved with the possibility to select and compare all of them by artificial intelligence, creating a new scenario for personalized patient care [12].

References

1. Hoffman JM, Gambhir SS (2007) Molecular imaging: the vision and opportunity for radiology in the future. Radiology 244(1):39–47
2. Sorensen AG (2006) Magnetic resonance as a cancer imaging biomarker. J Clin Oncol 24(20):3274–3281

3. Kim H, Arnoletti PJ, Martin JC et al (2014) Pancreatic adenocarcinoma: a pilot study of quantitative perfusion and diffusion-weighted breath-hold magnetic resonance imaging. Abdom Imaging 39(4):744–752
4. Yoon JH, Lee JM, Lee KB et al (2016) Pancreatic steatosis and fibrosis: quantitative assessment with preoperative multiparametric MR imaging. Radiology 279(1):140–150
5. Kirihara Y, Takahashi N, Hashimoto Y et al (2013) Prediction of pancreatic anastomotic failure after pancreatoduodenectomy: the use of preoperative, quantitative computed tomography to measure remnant pancreatic volume and body composition. Ann Surg 257(3):512–519
6. Mathur A, Pitt HA, Marine M et al (2007) Fatty pancreas: a factor in postoperative pancreatic fistula. Ann Surg 246(6):1058–1064
7. Yang J, Fang CH, Fan YF et al (2014) To assess the benefits of medical image three-dimensional visualization system assisted pancreaticoduodenectomy for patients with hepatic artery variance. Int J Med Robot 10(4):410–417
8. Butturini G, Damoli I, Crepaz L et al (2015) A prospective non-randomised single-center study comparing laparoscopic and robotic distal pancreatectomy. Surg Endosc 29(11):3163–3170
9. Joyce D, Morris-Stiff G, Falk GA et al (2014) Robotic surgery of the pancreas. World J Gastroenterol 20(40):14726–14732
10. Volonté F, Pugin F, Bucher P et al (2011) Augmented reality and image overlay navigation with OsiriX in laparoscopic and robotic surgery: not only a matter of fashion. J Hepatobiliary Pancreat Sci 18(4):506–509
11. Volonté F, Buchs NC, Pugin F et al (2013) Augmented reality to the rescue of the minimally invasive surgeon. The usefulness of the interposition of stereoscopic images in the Da Vinci robotic console. Int J Med Robot 9(3):e34–e38
12. Brink JA, Arenson RL, Grist TM et al (2017) Bits and bytes: the future of radiology lies in informatics and information technology. Eur Radiol [Epub ahead of print] doi:10.1007/s00330-016-4688-5

8 Laparoscopic Staging for Pancreatic Cancer

Robert Memba, Donal B. O'Connor, and Kevin C. Conlon

8.1 Introduction

Pancreatic cancer is the one of leading causes of cancer mortality in developed countries. The most common type is pancreatic ductal carcinoma (PDC), which accounts for approximately 85% of cases. The incidence of PDC has been increasing worldwide but it varies greatly across regions and populations. In Western Europe and North America, the incidence ranges between 7.3 and 7.4 per 100,000 people; 55.5% of the new cases of PDC are registered in more developed regions. PDC is the seventh most common cancer in men and the fourteenth in women but, more importantly, it is among the five most frequent causes of cancer-related mortality in North America and Europe. Certain risk factors have been identified, such as cigarette smoking, positive family history and genetics, diabetes mellitus, obesity, dietary factors, alcohol use and physical inactivity [1, 2].

PDC is a devastating disease associated with a poor prognosis for the majority of patients. The main reasons for the low survival of PDC patients are aggressive biology, the resistance to conventional and targeted therapeutic agents, the lack of biomarkers for early detection and the fact that most patients present with advanced disease. At presentation, approximately 50–55% of patients have metastatic disease and a further 20–25% have locally advanced disease. Only 20% of patients with PDC undergo potentially curative resection [3, 4]. The 5-year survival is only 10% following resection with curative intent and median survival after resection ranges from 12 to 24 months [5, 6]. The most common disease factors precluding resection are due to locoregional growth, leading to invasion of surrounding vessels, and the early systemic spread of ductal adenocarcinoma leading to disseminated disease, most commonly involving the liver. Diagnostic imaging is not sufficiently accurate to detect the presence

R. Memba (✉)
Professorial Surgical Unit, Surgery Department, Tallaght Hospital, Trinity College Dublin
Dublin, Ireland
e-mail: membar@tcd.ie

U. Boggi (Ed), *Minimally Invasive Surgery of the Pancreas*,
Updates in Surgery
DOI: 10.1007/978-88-470-3958-2_8,

Table 8.1 TNM classification for pancreatic ductal carcinoma

TX	Primary tumor cannot be assessed
T0	No evidence of primary tumor
Tis	Carcinoma in situ
T1	Tumor limited to the pancreas, 2 cm or less in greatest dimension
T2	Tumor limited to the pancreas, more than 2 cm in greatest dimension
T3	Tumor extends beyond the pancreas but without involvement of the celiac axis or the superior mesenteric artery
T4	Tumor involves the celiac axis or the superior mesenteric artery (unresectable primary tumor)
NX	Regional lymph nodes cannot be assessed
N0	No regional lymph node metastasis
N1	Regional lymph node metastasis
M0	No distant metastasis
M1	Distant metastasis

Table 8.2 Anatomic stage/prognostic groups for pancreatic ductal carcinoma

Stage 0	Tis N0 M0
Stage IA	T1 N0 M0
Stage IB	T2 N0 M0
Stage IIA	T3 N0 M0
Stage IIB	T1 N1 M0 T2 N1 M0 T3 N1 M0
Stage III	T4 Any N M0
Stage IV	Any T Any N M1

of all metastatic disease or vessel invasion. Accurate staging is essential for treatment planning and to avoid non-resectional laparotomies [3]. Laparoscopic staging (LS) has a role in detecting small peritoneal metastases and features of local vessel invasion when combined with laparoscopic ultrasonography (LUS) and has demonstrated upstaging of approximately 20% of patients deemed resectable after conventional imaging staging [7]. However, routine use of LS is not universally applied and its yield may be lower in the era of more advanced non-invasive imaging. The American Joint Committee on Cancer (AJCC) TNM classification [8] is used to describe the stages of PDC (Table 8.1) and prognosis groups (Table 8.2).

Several risk factors have been identified to be associated with an increased risk of non-resectability at laparotomy. The presence of these factors could be used to more accurately select patients who would benefit from LS.

Tumor size is one of the most important staging criteria and prognostic indicator in PDC, and primary larger tumor size is associated with metastases not identified on preoperative CT. According to some authors, tumor size ranging between 3 cm and 4.8 cm predicts unresectability and can be used in addition to imaging studies to consider the indication of LS [9–14].

Regarding tumor localization, PDC of the body and tail are associated with a worse prognosis, presumably because of the advanced stage of disease at diagnosis, compared with pancreatic head cancers which present earlier with signs of obstructive jaundice [15, 16]. However, if resectable they have a similar oncological outcome when compared to patients with resectable tumors in the pancreatic head [17].

Concerning tumor markers, carcinoembryonic antigen (CEA) and carbohydrate antigen 19-9 (CA 19-9) are serum tumor markers used in the management of PDC. Both tumor markers have limitations with respect to specificity, being elevated in other cancers and benign diseases. Several researchers [18–22] have demonstrated a correlation between a combination of high CEA and CA 19-9 levels and advanced disease, concluding that preoperative tumor marker levels can be independently used for the prediction of resectability (R0 resection) in patients with PDC. Ca 19-9 is the most commonly used for PDC. The cut-off value used to predict unresectability ranges between 92.77 and 353.15 IU/mL. However, CA 19-9 is also increased in the presence of hyperbilirubinemia, which makes interpretation in the presence of obstructive jaundice difficult [5]. It is also undetectable in 4–15% of the population with Lewis negative (a-b-) phenotype. Some authors have adjusted tumor marker levels to account for obstructive jaundice by dividing the serum tumor marker level by the bilirubin levels [22].

Resectable PDC (Fig. 8.1) includes tumors with the following criteria: absence of distant metastases, lack of evidence of tumor involvement of superior mesenteric artery (SMA) or hepatic artery (HA), and in cases of venous invasion, a suitable segment of portal vein (PV) above and superior mesenteric vein (SMV) below the site of venous involvement to allow for venous reconstruction; providing that adequate inflow and outflow veins are present and a R0/R1 resection is reasonably expected [23, 24].

Borderline resectable (BLR) PDC (Fig. 8.2) comprise an imprecise entity between resectable and unresectable disease on the initial radiological evaluation, which due to vessel involvement predicts a challenge in achieving a resection with negative surgical margins [25, 26]. There is no universally accepted definition of BLR PDC. Consensus statements from the American Hepato-Pancreato-Biliary Association (AHPBA), the Society for Surgery of the Alimentary Tract (SSAT) and the Society of Surgical Oncology (SSO) have been adopted by the National Comprehensive Cancer Network (NCCN) and define BLR PDC as the presence of venous involvement of the SMV/PV demonstrating tumor abutment, encasement, or short segment venous occlusion, but with suitable vessel proximal and distal

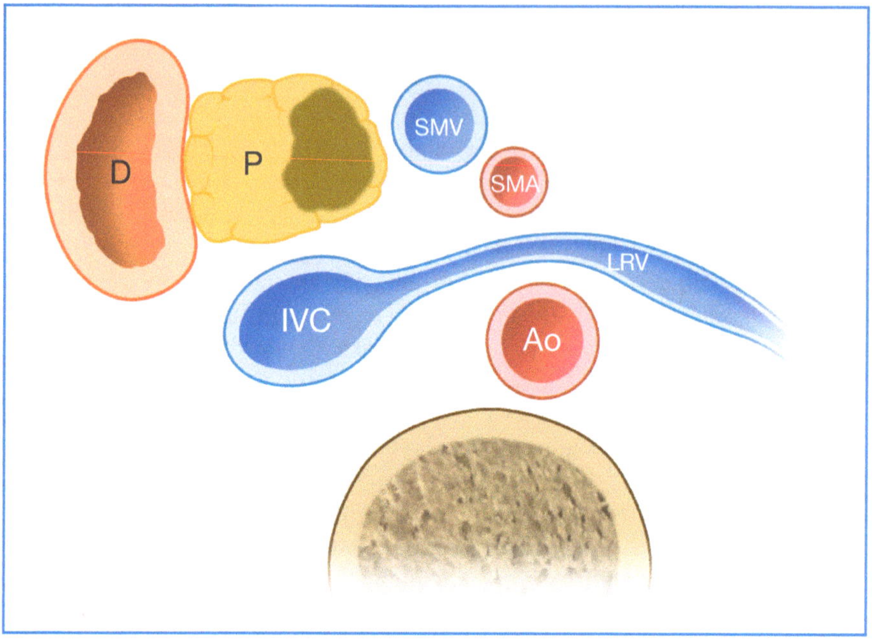

Fig. 8.1 Diagram showing resectable pancreatic ductal carcinoma

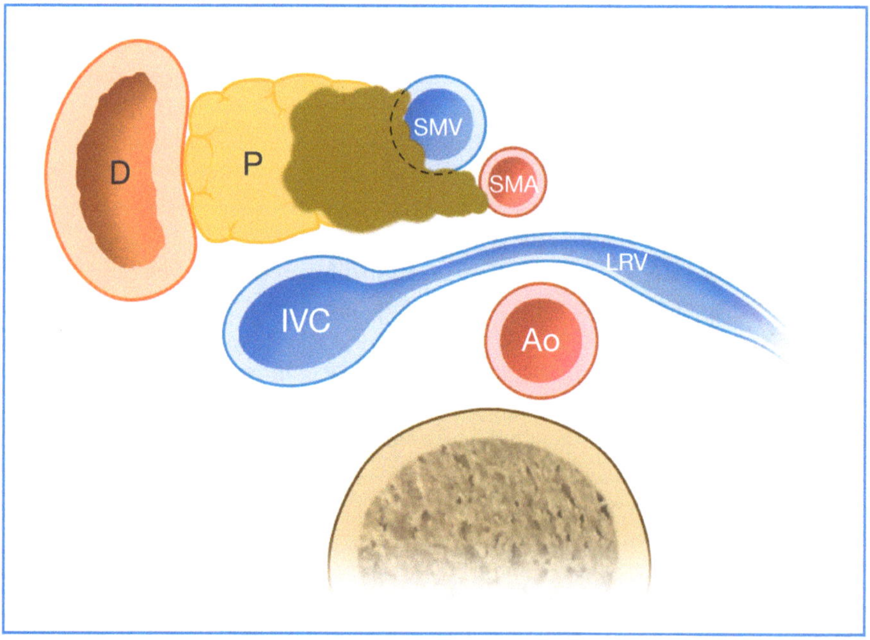

Fig. 8.2 Diagram showing borderline resectable pancreatic ductal carcinoma

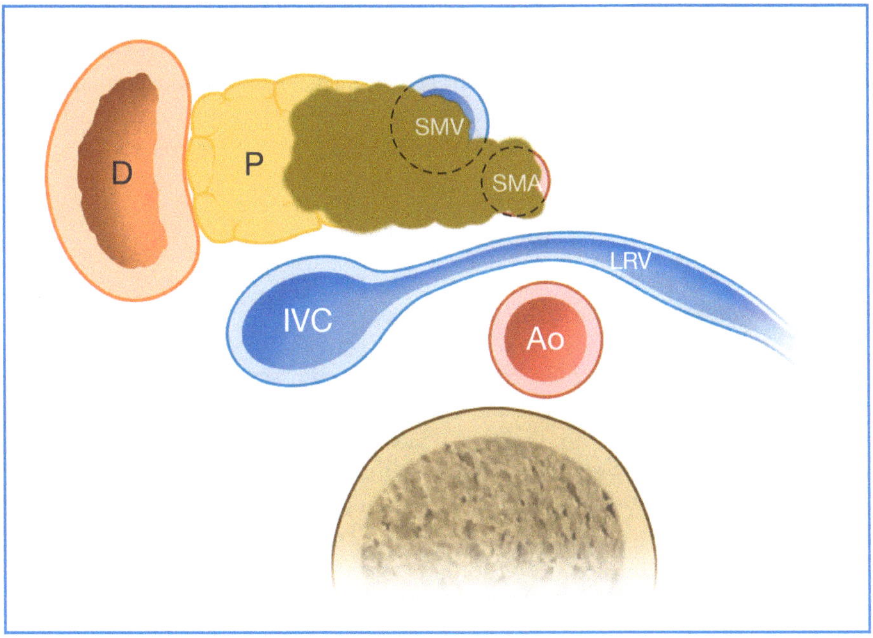

Fig. 8.3 Diagram showing locally advanced pancreatic ductal carcinoma

to the area of vessel involvement, allowing for safe resection and reconstruction; gastroduodenal artery encasement up to the HA and short segment encasement/direct tumor abutment of the HA with no extension to the celiac axis; or tumor-SMA involvement <180 degrees [27]. However, the American Joint Committee on Cancer (AJCC) defines all venous occlusion as a feature of local unresectability [28]. The recent consensus from the International Study Group for Pancreatic Surgery (ISGPS) supports the NCCN definition [29]. Due to the lack of an accepted definition, all patients with potential BLR PDC should be discussed by multidisciplinary teams in high volume centers. BLR PDC may benefit from resection after restaging when preceded by neoadjuvant therapy, based on chemotherapeutic combinations of gemcitabine or 5-fluorouracil and radiation therapy [26, 27, 30, 31]. The purpose of neoadjuvant therapy is downstaging, providing an opportunity for a R0 resection and increasing long-term survival [32]. Given the higher risk of occult metastases in BLR PDC, many centers advocate LS prior to initiation of neoadjuvant therapy in order to improve the reliability of initial staging [26, 30, 33].

Unresectable PDC (Fig. 8.3) includes patients with locally advanced disease or those with distant metastases. The unequivocal radiographic findings for locally advanced disease are circumferential encasement of the SMA or celiac axis or proximal HA, as defined by >180 degrees of the circumference of the vessel; and major venous thrombosis of the PV or SMV extending for several centimeters, without the possibility for venous reconstruction [27, 34].

8.2 Staging Modalities in Pancreatic Cancer

Accurate staging is essential for optimal patient care. All staging algorithms include computed tomography (CT) scan. Other tests such as magnetic resonance imaging (MRI), endoscopic ultrasound (EUS), positron emission tomography (PET) scanning or LS may be used in addition to CT scanning to further assess resectability [3].

8.2.1 Computed Tomography Scan

Conventional CT was replaced by dynamic thin-section CT, spiral CT, multidetector CT (MDCT), and three-dimensional reconstruction, increasing its reliability (Fig. 8.4). Current MDCT have improved their ability to predict resectability in patients with PDC with a sensitivity of up to 90% for detection and an accuracy of 80–90% for staging [35]. However, limitations remain including the sensitivity of CT to detect tumors less than 1 cm in diameter, thus limiting the detection of small liver metastases and peritoneal micrometastases. In addition, CT scanning usually cannot distinguish between reactive lymphadenopathy and malignant deposits [36].

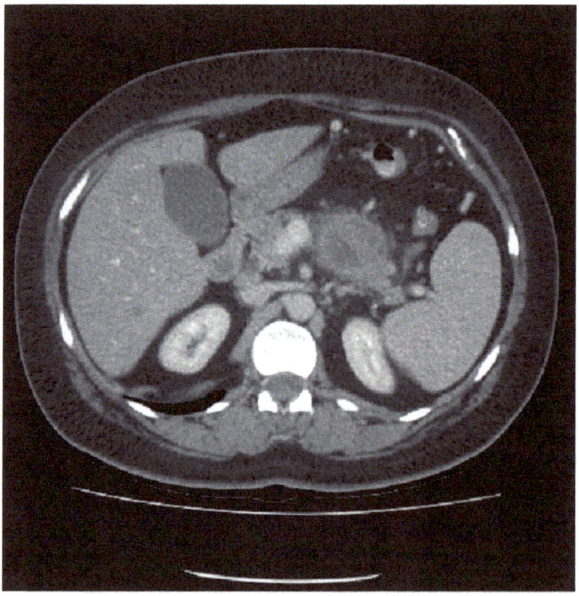

Fig. 8.4 CT abdomen showing liver metastases in patient with distal pancreatic ductal carcinoma

8.2.2 Magnetic Resonance Imaging

MRI liver and magnetic resonance cholangiopancreatography (MRCP) are rapidly evolving, becoming more sophisticated and improving in imaging quality, therefore in diagnostic accuracy. Regarding PDC, MRI currently provides essentially similar information to CT scanning, so in most of patients, it may not be needed. However, it may be superior to CT scan in specific circumstances such as small tumors, hypertrophied pancreatic head, isoattenuating PDC, and focal fatty infiltration of the parenchyma [35–37].

8.2.3 Endoscopic Ultrasound

EUS is commonly used to detect small pancreatic masses when there is a high suspicion for pancreatic cancer but no mass is clearly identified by CT scan. EUS is considered one of the most accurate methods for the detection of pancreatic focal lesions and EUS-guided fine-needle aspiration (EUS-FNA) has replaced endoscopic retrograde cholangiopancreatography (ERCP) with brush cytology as the endoscopic test of choice for tissue acquisition due to its higher efficacy and lower rate of complications. The most common complication after EUS are bleeding or pancreatitis, which are mostly mild and self-limited. With regard to staging, EUS is also a sensitive test for portal vein invasion and it is superior to CT in determining tumor size, extent, and lymph node status. Where available, EUS should be performed supplementary to CT scanning and may provide better assessment of T staging and certain types of vascular invasion. Thus, EUS plays a major role to further evaluate borderline patients with non-metastatic disease that appears resectable on initial imaging. However, EUS is limited by the experience and expertise of the ultrasonographer [35, 36, 38].

8.2.4 Positron Emission Tomography

It is a well-established imaging modality, combining the anatomical information of a helical CT with the functional information of a PET scanner using metabolic detection of fluorine 18-fluorodeoxyglucose (FDG), a glucose analogue. On the one hand, it has a utility in some situations as for the differential diagnosis of PDC and mass-forming chronic pancreatitis. On the other hand, as a whole body exam, PET/CT possesses a unique advantage for M staging, therefore it has also shown a role detecting metastatic lesions that were not identified by CT scan, especially peritoneal metastasis. Finally, PET/CT is also able to detect early recurrences during the follow-up. However, PET/CT false positive results can be seen in various inflammatory conditions such as pancreatitis and false negative results in hyperglycemic states like in diabetic patients, due to competition of endogenous glucose with FDG. It is not performed routinely in PDC staging, however it has a significant role in the follow-up, to differentiate between recurrence and postoperative changes [35, 39, 40].

8.2.5 Laparoscopic Staging

The main reason, however, to consider diagnostic laparoscopy for PDC is the considerable proportion of patients who undergo unnecessary laparotomy because of underestimation of the extent of the cancer on CT scanning [3, 5, 41]. LS for PDC was initially described by Bernheim [42] of Johns Hopkins University in 1911 and was reintroduced by Cuscheri [43, 44] from the University of Dundee in 1978, and by Warshaw from the Harvard Medical School in 1986 [45]. However, laparoscopic inspection allows only two-dimensional inspection of the surface of the liver and the peritoneal cavity and a lack of tactile sensation may limit the identification of small intraparenchymal hepatic metastases and make it difficult to evaluate the critical retroperitoneal tumor-vessel relationships. Therefore, John et al. [46], of The Royal Infirmary, introduced LUS in 1995. The development of LUS, also reported by Minnard et al. [47], improved the yield by allowing the surgeon to examine the liver, the porta hepatis, and the PV and SMA predicting resectability up to as high as 98% [36, 48–50].

LS appears to be a safe and cost-effective way of directing appropriate therapy and avoiding unnecessary exploration not only in PDC, but also in other upper gastrointestinal malignancies like hepatobiliary, esophageal or gastric cancers [48]. In fact, LS reduces morbidity, postoperative pain, operating costs, hospitalization and gives a higher likelihood of receiving systemic therapy in patients with unresectable pancreatic cancer compared to exploratory laparotomy and surgical palliation [5]. Laparoscopy allows internal visualization of the abdomen and can detect peritoneal spread of the cancer or the involvement of adjacent structures. In addition, biopsy and histopathological examination of any suspicious liver or peritoneal lesions and washings for cytology can easily be performed during the procedure [3]. Conlon, at the Memorial Sloan-Kettering Cancer Center, developed a multiport technique to stage and assess resectability of peripancreatic malignancy, mimicking the surgical assessment of resectability performed at open operation [7], and making it a routine procedure in PDC evaluation. Regarding cytology, where results are not available at the time of surgery, information obtained can only be utilized in clinical decision-making afterwards [36]. Therefore, LS can either be performed as a separate procedure, or immediately prior to major laparotomy as part of a scheduled pancreatectomy. The main advantages of performing diagnostic laparoscopy immediately prior to planned resective surgery are that the patient needs only one hospital admission and one general anesthetic. However, if the patient is diagnosed as having unresectable disease at laparoscopy and the subsequent laparotomy is then cancelled, it means that operation theatre time is wasted [3]. Despite its apparent benefits, the value of staging laparoscopy is not universally accepted. Opinions range from recommending its routine use for all patients before laparotomy to not performing laparoscopy in any circumstance [27]. Recently, some authors argued against using LS routinely in all PDC, as the proportion of patients found to have metastatic disease at laparoscopy is decreasing due to the increased sensitivity of CT [5]. Critics argue that if today's highest quality imaging is properly used, only a minority of patients would actually benefit from LS. A Cochrane review and meta-analysis recently conducted by Allen et al. included fifteen studies with a total of 1015 patients, in order to assess the diagnostic accuracy of LS performed after CT staging in pancreatic and periampullary cancers [41]. This review demonstrated that the addition of LS to CT scanning decreases the probability of unresectable disease from 41.4% to 20%. They concluded that LS with biopsy and histopathological confirmation of suspicious lesions prior to laparotomy would avoid 21 unnecessary laparotomies per 100 patients in whom resection of cancer with curative intent is planned [3, 41].

8.3 Surgical Technique of Laparoscopic Staging

The aim of LS is identifying or ruling out regional extension of the primary tumor and/or metastatic disease. The operative time in experienced hands should be between 20 and 40 minutes. LS is performed under general anesthesia with the patient in the supine position. It can be carried out as an ambulatory/outpatient procedure with excellent patient satisfaction.

8.3.1 Trocar Placement

The periumbilical region is the most used site for initial access. A periumbilical skin incision and open Hasson technique is performed, placing a 10-mm blunt port. Pneumoperitoneum is kept at low levels (8–12 mmHg). Additional (5 mm) trocars are used at the discretion of the surgeon as needed for exposure and for potential biopsies, ultrasound or intervention. These secondary ports should be placed in the line of the planned skin incision for laparotomy.

8.3.2 Intra-Abdominal Examination

A 30-degree angled scope is used at the periumbilical trocar site for inspection of the intra-abdominal organs, including the surface of the liver, gallbladder, stomach, intestine, pelvic organs, and visible retroperitoneal surfaces along with

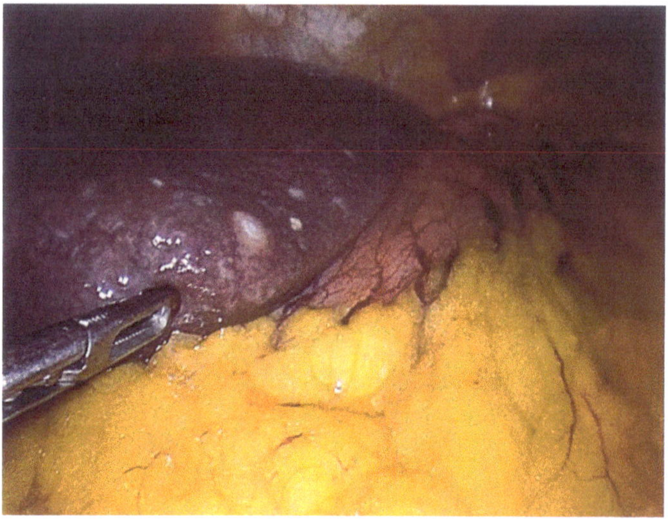

Fig. 8.5 Liver surface evaluation performed during laparoscopic staging showing malignant suspicious lesions

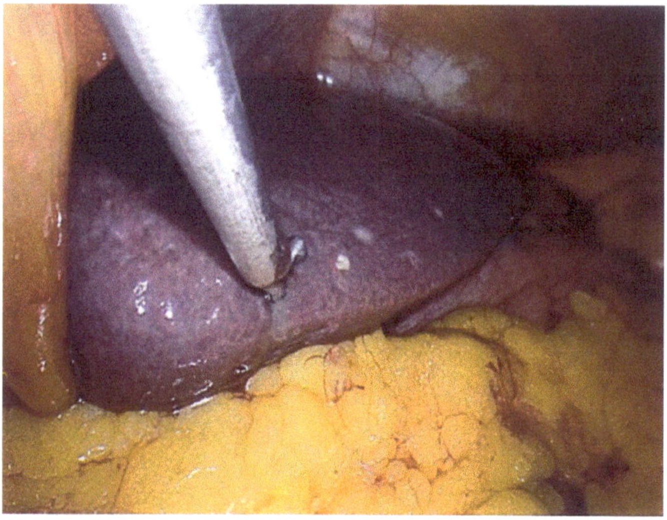

Fig. 8.6 Laparoscopic biopsy forceps used for cup biopsy to confirm liver metastases

examination of free intraperitoneal fluid (Fig. 8.5). Intraperitoneal adhesions, if present, are divided. If present, initial aspiration of ascites for cytology is performed. Peritoneal washings for cytology are also collected after instilling between 200 and 400 cc of saline into both upper quadrants and pelvis prior to any manipulation of the tumor. Systematic examination of peritoneum, FNA cytology or biopsies of any suspicious serosal findings are performed (Fig. 8.6).

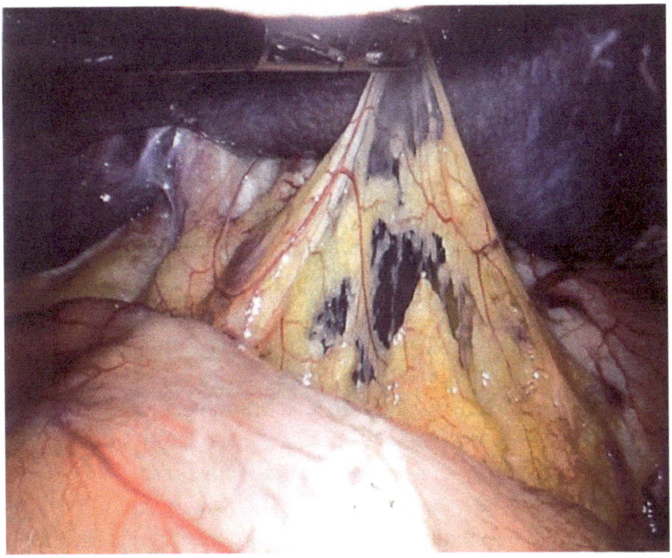

Fig. 8.7 Lesser sac exposure to access tumor

Extent, size and mobility of the primary tumor is assessed. Systematic inspection of the liver and diaphragmatic surface after positioning the patient in a 20-degree reverse Trendelenburg is carried out. Incision of the gastrohepatic omentum, exposing the caudate lobe, celiac axis and inferior vena cava is performed. HA is visualized and biopsies of portal, perigastric and celiac lymph nodes, if enlarged, are carried out. The lesser sac is entered with the camera via the right upper quadrant port for evaluation of the tumor (Fig. 8.7). The patient is positioned at 10 degrees Trendelenburg and the omentum is placed in the left upper quadrant. The transverse colon is lifted to visualize the ligament of Treitz, transverse mesocolon, middle colic vein and surrounding lymph nodes.

8.3.3 Laparoscopic Ultrasonography

Laparoscopic ultrasound (LUS) is performed to evaluate potential small intraparenchymal hepatic lesions, invasion of PV, SMA or SMV, as well as peripancreatic extension of the tumor and local and regional lymph nodes. A 6 to 10 MHz T-shaped linear or curvilinear-array transducer is placed. In addition, Doppler allows vessel identification and assessment of tumor-vessel surface. LUS can also facilitate biopsies and needle aspirations of suspicious lesions.

The signs of unresectability are: histological confirmation of hepatic, serosal, peritoneal or omental metastasis; peripancreatic tumor extension, celiac or portal positive lymph nodes; high PV involvement by tumor or invasion and/or encasement of the celiac trunk, HA or SMA [51–54].

8.4 Algorithm

In summary, selective use of staging laparoscopy may be of benefit to avoid a non-therapeutic laparotomy in patients deemed initially resectable after conventional imaging in PDC. The addition of LUS during laparoscopic staging enhances the ability of laparoscopy to determine resectability. In order to select patients for LS, based on the available data, the most reliable surrogate markers to predict unresectability in patients with CT-defined resectable PDC are CA 19-9 and tumor size. Therefore, LS and LUS might be indicated in the following situations (Fig. 8.8):

1. Tumors larger than 3 cm and markedly elevated CA 19-9;
2. If high-quality imaging is in any way suggestive of indeterminate metastatic disease (equivocal peritoneal/liver metastases, low-volume ascites);
3. In preoperative staging of BLR PDC, in order to more accurately select patients for neoadjuvant protocols.

Further prospective investigations are needed to validate these statements. Although some other studies suggest a role for tumor location (body and tail of the pancreas), CEA levels, weight loss or jaundice, there is not enough evidence currently to support their inclusion into an algorithm to select patients for LS [5, 27, 33, 36].

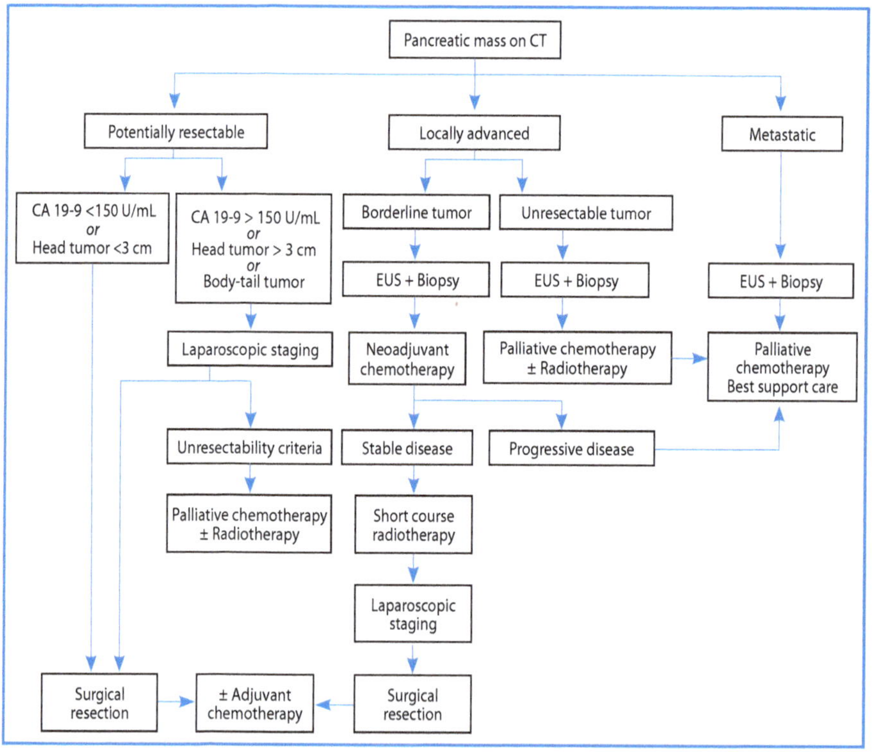

Fig. 8.8 Suggested algorithm for management of patients with pancreatic ductal carcinoma. *CT*, computed tomography; *CA 19-9*, carbohydrate antigen 19-9; *EUS*, endoscopic ultrasound

References

1. Ilic M, Ilic I (2016) Epidemiology of pancreatic cancer. World J Gastroenterol 22(44):9694–9705
2. Zhang Q, Zeng L, Chen Y et al (2016) Pancreatic cancer epidemiology, detection, and management. Gastroenterol Res Pract 2016:8962321
3. Allen VB, Gurusamy KS, Takwoingi Y et al (2013) Diagnostic accuracy of laparoscopy following computed tomography (CT) scanning for assessing the resectability with curative intent in pancreatic and periampullary cancer. Cochrane Database Syst Rev 2013(11):CD009323
4. Hariharan D, Saied A, Kocher HM (2008) Analysis of mortality rates for pancreatic cancer across the world. HPB (Oxford) 10(1):58–62
5. De Rosa A, Cameron IC, Gomez D (2016) Indications for staging laparoscopy in pancreatic cancer. HPB (Oxford) 18(1):13–20
6. Wolfgang CL, Herman JM, Laheru DA et al (2013) Recent progress in pancreatic cancer. CA Cancer J Clin 63(5):318–348
7. Conlon KC, Dougherty E, Klimstra DS et al (1996) The value of minimal access surgery in the staging of patients with potentially resectable peripancreatic malignancy. Ann Surg 223(2):134–140
8. National Comprehensive Cancer Network (2013) NCCN Clinical practice guidelines in oncology (NCCN Guidelines): Pancreatic adenocarcinoma (Version 1.2013). https://www.nccn.org/professionals/physician_gls/f_guidelines.asp
9. De Jong MC, Li F, Cameron JL et al (2011) Re-evaluating the impact of tumor size on survival following pancreaticoduodenectomy for pancreatic adenocarcinoma. J Surg Oncol 103(7):656–662
10. Agarwal B, Correa AM, Ho L (2008) Survival in pancreatic carcinoma based on tumor size. Pancreas 36(1):e15–e20
11. Shimada K, Sakamoto Y, Sano T et al (2006) Reappraisal of the clinical significance of tumor size in patients with pancreatic ductal carcinoma. Pancreas 33(3):233–239
12. Chiang KC, Yeh CN, Lee WC et al (2009) Prognostic analysis of patients with pancreatic head adenocarcinoma less than 2 cm undergoing resection. World J Gastroenterol 15(34):4305–4310
13. Fortner JG, Klimstra DS, Senie RT, Maclean BJ (1996) Tumor size is the primary prognosticator for pancreatic cancer after regional pancreatectomy. Ann Surg 223(2):147–153
14. Chiang KC, Lee CH, Yeh CN et al (2014) A novel role of the tumor size in pancreatic cancer as an ancillary factor for predicting resectability. J Cancer Res Ther 10(1):142–146
15. Fujioka S, Misawa T, Okamoto T et al (2007) Preoperative serum carcinoembryonic antigen and carbohydrate antigen 19-9 levels for the evaluation of curability and resectability in patients with pancreatic adenocarcinoma. J Hepatobiliary Pancreat Surg 14(6):539–544
16. Contreras CM, Stanelle EJ, Mansour J et al (2009) Staging laparoscopy enhances the detection of occult metastases in patients with pancreatic adenocarcinoma. J Surg Oncol 100(8):663–669
17. Ruess DA, Makowiec F, Chikhladze S et al (2015) The prognostic influence of intrapancreatic tumor location on survival after resection of pancreatic ductal adenocarcinoma. BMC Surg 15:123
18. Ong SL, Garcea G, Thomasset SC et al (2008) Surrogate markers of resectability in patients undergoing exploration of potentially resectable pancreatic adenocarcinoma. J Gastrointest Surg 12(6):1068–1073
19. Kilic M, Gocmen E, Tez M et al (2006) Value of preoperative serum CA 19-9 levels in predicting resectability for pancreatic cancer. Can J Surg 49(4):241–244
20. Mehta J, Prabhu R, Eshpuniyani P (2010) Evaluating the efficacy of tumor markers CA 19-9 and CEA to predict operability and survival in pancreatic malignancies. Trop Gastroenterol 31(3):190–194

21. Karachristos A, Scarmeas N, Hoffman JP (2005) CA 19-9 levels predict results of staging laparoscopy in pancreatic cancer. J Gastrointest Surg 9(9):1286–1292
22. Kim YC, Kim HJ, Park JH et al (2009) Can preoperative CA19-9 and CEA levels predict the resectability of patients with pancreatic adenocarcinoma? J Gastroenterol Hepatol 24(12):1869–1875
23. Evans DB, Farnell MB, Lillemoe KD et al (2009) Surgical treatment of resectable and borderline resectable pancreas cancer: expert consensus statement. Ann Surg Oncol 16(7):1736–1744
24. Wong JC, Raman S (2010) Surgical resectability of pancreatic adenocarcinoma: CTA. Abdom Imaging 35(4):471–480
25. Okada K, Kawai M, Tani M et al (2014) Predicting factors for unresectability in patients with pancreatic ductal adenocarcinoma. J Hepatobiliary Pancreat Sci 21(9):648–653
26. Mahipal A, Frakes J, Hoffe S, Kim R (2015) Management of borderline resectable pancreatic cancer. World J Gastrointest Oncol 7(10):241–249
27. Callery MP, Chang KJ, Fishman EK et al (2009) Pretreatment assessment of resectable and borderline resectable pancreatic cancer: expert consensus statement. Ann Surg Oncol 16(7):1727–1733
28. Edge SB, Compton CC (2010) The American Joint Committee on Cancer: the 7th edition of the AJCC cancer staging manual and the future of TNM. Ann Surg Oncol 17(6):1471–1474
29. Bockhorn M, Uzunoglu FG, Adham M et al (2014) Borderline resectable pancreatic cancer: a consensus statement by the International Study Group of Pancreatic Surgery (ISGPS). Surgery 155(6):977–988
30. Varadhachary GR, Tamm EP, Abbruzzese JL et al (2006) Borderline resectable pancreatic cancer: definitions, management, and role of preoperative therapy. Ann Surg Oncol 13(8): 1035–1046
31. Lopez NE, Prendergast C, Lowy AM (2014) Borderline resectable pancreatic cancer: definitions and management. World J Gastroenterol 20(31):10740–10751
32. Laurence JM, Tran PD, Morarji K et al (2011) A systematic review and meta-analysis of survival and surgical outcomes following neoadjuvant chemoradiotherapy for pancreatic cancer. J Gastrointest Surg 15(11):2059–2069
33. O'Connor DB, Ta R, Sulistijo A et al (2016) The utility of staging laparoscopy for potentially resectable pancreatic cancer: a systematic review. Pancreatology 16(3):S104
34. Fathi A, Christians KK, George B et al (2015) Neoadjuvant therapy for localized pancreatic cancer: guiding principles. J Gastrointest Oncol 6(4):418–429
35. Lee ES, Lee JM (2014) Imaging diagnosis of pancreatic cancer: a state-of-the-art review. World J Gastroenterol 20(24):7864–7877
36. Camacho D, Reichenbach D, Duerr GD (2005) Value of laparoscopy in the staging of pancreatic cancer. JOP 6(6):552–561
37. Tapper E, Kalb B, Martin DR et al (2011) Staging laparoscopy for proximal pancreatic cancer in a magnetic resonance imaging-driven practice: what's it worth? HPB (Oxford) 13(10):732–737
38. Iglesias García J, Lariño Noia J, Domínguez Muñoz JE (2009) Endoscopic ultrasound in the diagnosis and staging of pancreatic cancer. Rev Esp Enferm Dig 101(9):631–638
39. Wang XY, Yang F, Jin C, Fu DL (2014) Utility of PET/CT in diagnosis, staging, assessment of resectability and metabolic response of pancreatic cancer. World J Gastroenterol 20(42):15580–15589
40. Michl P, Pauls S, Gress TM (2006) Evidence-based diagnosis and staging of pancreatic cancer. Best Pract Res Clin Gastroenterol 20(2):227–251
41. Allen VB, Gurusamy KS, Takwoingi Y et al (2016) Diagnostic accuracy of laparoscopy following computed tomography (CT) scanning for assessing the resectability with curative intent in pancreatic and periampullary cancer. Cochrane Database Syst Rev 2016(7):CD009323
42. Bernheim BM (1911) IV Organoscopy: cystoscopy of the abdominal cavity. Ann Surg 53(6):764–767

43. Cuschieri A (1988) Laparoscopy for pancreatic cancer: does it benefit the patient? Eur J Surg Oncol 14(1):41–44
44. Cuschieri A, Hall AW, Clark J (1978) Value of laparoscopy in the diagnosis and management of pancreatic carcinoma. Gut 19(7):672–677
45. Warshaw AL, Tepper JE, Shipley WU (1986) Laparoscopy in the staging and planning of therapy for pancreatic cancer. Am J Surg 151(1):76–80
46. John TG, Greig JD, Carter DC, Garden OJ (1995) Carcinoma of the pancreatic head and periampullary region. Tumor staging with laparoscopy and laparoscopic ultrasonography. Ann Surg 221(2):156–164
47. Minnard EA, Conlon KC, Hoos A et al (1998) Laparoscopic ultrasound enhances standard laparoscopy in the staging of pancreatic cancer. Ann Surg 228(2):182–187
48. Conlon KC, Minnard EA (1997) The value of laparoscopic staging in upper gastrointestinal malignancy. Oncologist 2(1):10–17
49. Hann LE, Conlon KC, Dougherty EC et al (1997) Laparoscopic sonography of peripancreatic tumors: preliminary experience. AJR Am J Roentgenol 169(5):1257–1262
50. de Werra C, Quarto G, Aloia S et al (2015) The use of intraoperative ultrasound for diagnosis and stadiation in pancreatic head neoformations. Int J Surg 21(Suppl 1):S55–S58
51. Doyle MBM, Pratt WB (2012) Intraoperative diagnostic techniques. In: Jarnagin WR (ed) Blumgart's surgery of the liver, biliary tract and pancreas, 5th edn. Elsevier, Philadelphia, PA, vol 1, pp 369–375
52. Conlon KC, Gallagher TK (2013) Laparoscopic staging and approaches to cancer. In: Zinner MJ, Ashley SW (eds) Maingot's abdominal operations,12th edn. McGraw-Hill, New York. pp 75–95
53. Ganta SV, Conlon KC (2001) Laparoscopic staging for pancreatic carcinoma. In: Greene FL, Heniford BT (eds) Minimally invasive cancer management. Springer, New York, pp 123–130
54. Conlon KC, Johnston SM (2007) Laparoscopic staging of periampullary neoplasms. In: Clavien P-A, Sarr MG, Fong Y, Georgiev P (eds) Atlas of upper gastrointestinal and hepato-pancreato-biliary surgery. Springer, New York, pp 917–927

Thoracoscopic Splanchnicectomy for the Treatment of Severe Pancreatic Pain

9

Luigi Pugliese, Andrea Peri, Emma Cavazzi, and Andrea Pietrabissa

9.1 Introduction

The alleviation of severe chronic pain is often required in patients with unresectable pancreatic ductal adenocarcinoma (PDAC) and chronic pancreatitis (CP) [1, 2]. Failure in pain control with standard analgesia, usually employed as a first step, is common; also, addiction to narcotics and their burdensome side effects limit long-term usage [3]. Invasive treatments have been proposed over time with the aim of suppressing the transmission of pain impulse from the celiac region along the splanchnic nerves. Celiac plexus neurolysis by alcohol injection in the celiac ganglia has been widely adopted by percutaneous approach and, more recently, under endoscopic ultrasound guidance [4]. Although effective for pain relief, the limited duration of pain response with no clear benefit in opiate consumption and the occurrence of major complications account for the shareable criticism [4–6]. Thoracoscopic splanchnicectomy (TS) has gained popularity as a less invasive alternative to the open transhiatal or transthoracic approach, whose related morbidity exceeded the benefit of denervation [3]. Its safety and effectiveness in relieving intractable pain with satisfactory outcomes on quality of life have been widely attested [4]. If compared to chemical neurolysis, TS allows for higher precision in nerve fiber interruption and prevents erosive complications related to alcohol injection in the celiac region [7].

9.2 Anatomical Overview

Three splanchnic nerves originate from the lower eight ganglia of the sympathetic thoracic chain: the greater splanchnic nerve (GSN) from T5-T9,

A. Pietrabissa (✉)
Department of Surgery, Fondazione IRCCS Policlinico San Matteo
Pavia, Italy
e-mail: a.pietrabissa@smatteo.pv.it

U. Boggi (Ed), *Minimally Invasive Surgery of the Pancreas*,
Updates in Surgery
DOI: 10.1007/978-88-470-3958-2_9,

the lesser splanchnic nerve from T10-T11, the least splanchnic nerve from T12 [8–9]. They contain both efferent and afferent visceral fibers, the latter conducting pain impulse from prevertebral ganglia such as the celiac ones. While the lesser and least splanchnic nerves are inconstant, the GSN after perforating the diaphragm runs cephalad in the posterior mediastinum along the thoracic aorta on the left side and the azygos vein on the right side. Anatomical studies on cadavers have shown the presence of multiple communicating collateral nerve branches both between the GSN and the lesser splanchnic nerve (when the latter is present) and between these trunks and the sympathetic chain [8–9].

9.3 Technical Considerations

From the anatomo-surgical point of view, two different TS techniques have been described: one implies cutting of the main nerve trunks right above the diaphragm; the other consists in the division of every single root forming the splanchnic nerves from the sympathetic chain [10]. Since intercommunicating collateral nerve fibers may exist, a segmental resection of the GSN has been proposed in order to increase the likelihood of TS effectiveness [8]. These fibers may provide an alternative neural pathway responsible for pain recurrence after TS [9]. However, this has never been demonstrated on living subjects.

According to the available literature, TS application encompasses different technical variants in terms of patient decubitus (lateral or prone), side of denervation (left or right), extent (unilateral or bilateral) and timing of the procedure relative to pain onset (early vs. late phase). The prone position has been proposed for simultaneous bilateral TS, given the optimal visual exposure of the thoracic anatomy offered by the posterior route with no need for single lung ventilation or intraoperative changes in patient positioning [11]. However, bilateral TS has not proved to be necessarily recommended as a first-step operation; in fact, the unilateral procedure has been largely preferred among the published series resulting in immediate pain relief that lasts for months in the majority of cases [3].

Contralateral TS can be proposed in non-responders or for recurrent pain [3, 7]. At any rate, considering the short life expectancy of PDAC patients, the need for a second intervention may never occur [7]. Here, pain relapse weeks or months after TS might be ascribable to many factors independent from nerve transmission along the splanchnic trunks: cancer spread beyond the afferent fibers from celiac ganglia; diffusion to the peritoneal surface triggering somatic pain; development of bone metastasis. In all these situations, a contralateral TS would be ineffective [8, 12].

Some authors support bilateral TS considering the frequent need for a contralateral procedure in CP patients [13]; however, pain in CP has multifactorial etiology and complex mechanisms which are absent in PDAC [2]. Moreover, transient orthostatic hypotension and diarrhea are observed after bilateral TS, but not after single-side TS [7, 8].

The lateral approach, which we favor, can equally be performed without selective lung intubation thanks to a low-pressure (8 mmHg) CO_2 insufflation allowing an adequate working space. The benefit of this positive pressure inside the pleural cavity is to increase the downward displacement of the diaphragm, which enables the surgeon to transect the GSN trunk below the merging of the most distal nerve roots; this is expected to increase the extent of denervation and consequently pain control. In a previous report, we have shown the safety of low-pressure CO_2 pneumothorax which made a two-trocars procedure feasible in some patients (Fig. 9.1), the lung being sufficiently collapsed to obviate retraction through an auxiliary port [12]. Short median operative times and hospital stay were made possible by this approach [12].

No definitive consensus has been reached on which side should be treated to maximize pain relief [9]. Based on current knowledge, left TS should be adopted for left-sided or central pain and also for bilateral pain, while right TS for predominant right pain [4, 8, 9, 12].

Results from several series of patients show the efficacy of TS as a salvage therapy for intractable pain resistant to high dose medications.

The perception of pain relief might be limited by further tumor spread/retroperitoneal inflammation and by the poor general conditions worsened by the heavy side effects of opiates. Hence, invasive management via TS performed early after or even before the onset of pain has been advocated as a sound option for patients with PDAC end-stage disease or CP refractory to medical therapy [12, 14, 15]. Early surgical treatment may be more successful by avoiding the side effects of medical therapy; it might offer higher, long-lasting efficacy with improved quality of life despite the progression of cancer or chronic inflammation [14, 15].

Dense pleural adhesions represent the only real contraindication to TS, which can be mostly anticipated based on known previous thoracic disease or surgery and on chest X-ray [12].

As adverse effects, transient intercostal neuralgia might develop in the early postoperative course for a few days or weeks [8, 12]. Bleeding from intercostal vessels is rare and it is especially related to multiple port positioning and trocar size (>5 mm) [13]; the risk for major vessel injuries is theoretical and should be considered when extended division of all the GSN roots is planned [8]. Transient pleural effusion or residual pneumothorax requiring chest-tube placement after surgery may occur [7, 8, 12]. Postoperative chylothorax has occasionally been reported after either unilateral or bilateral TS; care should be taken in nerve dissection, especially if performed at the upper level of the GSN on the left side, to prevent injury of the thoracic duct or of small collateral lymphatic branches [8, 16].

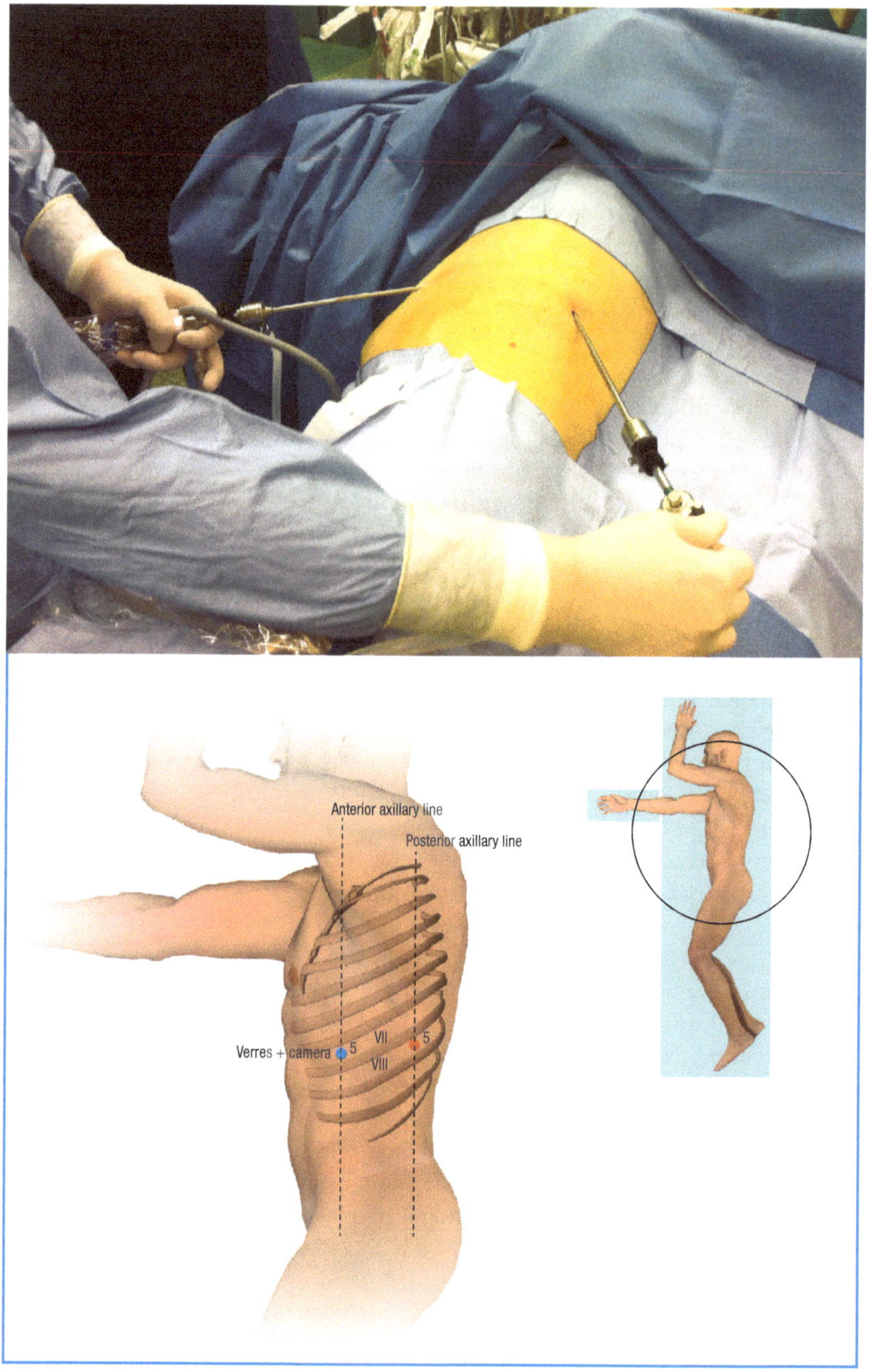

Fig. 9.1 Intraoperative setting for left thoracoscopic splanchnicectomy using the two-trocars technique

9.4 Operative Technique

We herein describe our current technique for truncal unilateral TS which can be performed by a single surgeon with no need for further assistance. The patient is placed in lateral decubitus lying on the opposite flank relative to the side of the scheduled intervention. Double-lung ventilation is provided via conventional endotracheal tube. Partial pneumothorax up to 8 mmHg of working pressure is obtained by inflating CO_2 through a Veress needle inserted in the 7th intercostal space at the anterior axillary line, while the endotracheal tube is temporarily disconnected from ventilation. A 5-mm trocar accommodating a 5-mm 30° optic is inserted replacing the Veress needle, while another 5-mm trocar is placed in the 8th intercostal space at the posterior axillary line. Three-millimeter ports, camera and instruments can be used instead of 5 mm if available. The pleura is opened by a horizontal 2–3-cm incision at the posterior costophrenic reflection just above the diaphragm, lateral to the descending aorta for a left TS and to the azygos vein for a right TS. The GSN and the lesser and/or least splanchnic nerve when present are identified, isolated with blunt dissection and then sectioned with cold scissors as distally as possible (Fig. 9.2). Clips are not essential before section since almost no bleeding arises from the nerve transection. Complete suction of CO_2 along with full lung reinflation ends the procedure. A chest tube is not routinely left in place unless injuries to the visceral pleura are suspected.

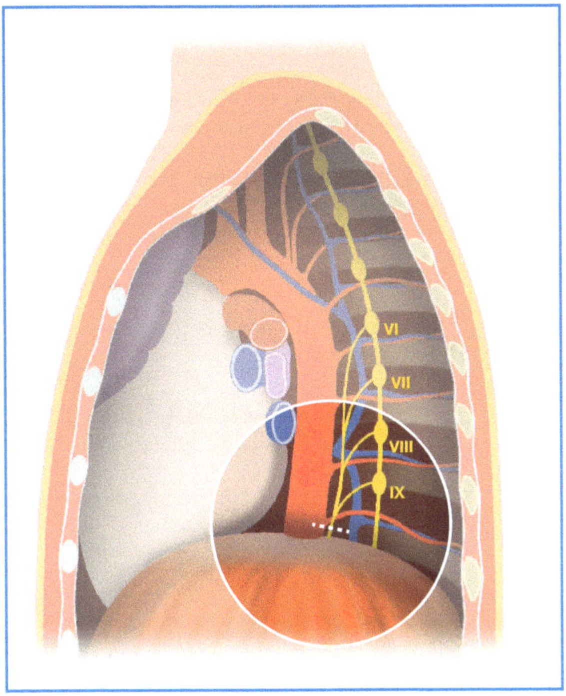

Fig. 9.2 Anatomical illustration of a greater splanchnic nerve (GSN) transection. The nerve trunk is divided just above the diaphragm, below the merging of the most distal roots

References

1. Siegel R, Ma J, Zou Z, Jemal A (2014) Cancer statistics, 2014. CA Cancer J Clin 64(1):9–29
2. Malec-Milewska MB, Tarnowski W, Ciesielski AE et al (2013) Prospective evaluation of pain control and quality of life in patients with chronic pancreatitis following bilateral thoracoscopic splanchnicectomy. Surg Endosc 27(10):3639–3645
3. Masuda T, Kuramoto M, Shimada S et al (2014) Splanchnicectomy for pancreatic cancer pain. Biomed Res Int 2014:941726
4. Nagels W, Pease N, Bekkering G et al (2013) Celiac plexus neurolysis for abdominal cancer pain: a systematic review. Pain Med 14(8):1140–1163
5. Luz LP, Al-Haddad MA, DeWitt JA (2014) EUS-guided celiac plexus interventions in pancreatic cancer pain: an update and controversies for the endosonographer. Endosc Ultrasound 3(4):213–220
6. Yasuda I, Wang HP (2017) Endoscopic ultrasound-guided celiac plexus block and neurolysis. Dig Endosc 29(4):455–462
7. Katri KM, Ramadan BA, Mohamed FS (2008) Thoracoscopic splanchnicectomy for pain control in irresectable pancreatic cancer. J Laparoendosc Adv Surg Tech A 18(2):199–203
8. Kang CM, Lee HY, Yang HJ et al (2007) Bilateral thoracoscopic splanchnicectomy with sympathectomy for managing abdominal pain in cancer patients. Am J Surg 194(1):23–29
9. Naidoo N, Partab P, Pather N et al (2001) Thoracic splanchnic nerves: implications for splanchnic denervation. J Anat 199(Pt 5):585–590
10. Worsey J, Ferson PF, Keenan RJ et al (1993) Thoracoscopic pancreatic denervation for pain control in irresectable pancreatic cancer. Br J Surg 80(8):1051–1052
11. Cuschieri A, Shimi SM, Crosthwaite G, Joypaul V (1994) Bilateral endoscopic splanchnicectomy through a posterior thoracoscopic approach. J R Coll Surg Edinb 39(1):44–47
12. Pietrabissa A, Vistoli F, Carobbi A et al (2000) Thoracoscopic splanchnicectomy for pain relief in unresectable pancreatic cancer. Arch Surg 135(3):332–335
13. Ihse I, Zoucas E, Gyllstedt E et al (1999) Bilateral thoracoscopic splanchnicectomy: effects on pancreatic pain and function. Ann Surg 230(6):785–790; discussion 790–791
14. Dobosz L, Stefaniak T, Dobrzycka M et al (2016) Invasive treatment of pain associated with pancreatic cancer on different levels of WHO analgesic ladder. BMC Surg 16:20
15. Issa Y, Ahmed Ali U, Bouwense SA et al (2014) Preoperative opioid use and the outcome of thoracoscopic splanchnicectomy in chronic pancreatitis: a systematic review. Surg Endosc 28(2):405–412
16. Selzer DJ, Howard TJ, Kesler KA (1999) Management of chylothorax after thoracoscopic splanchnicectomy. J Laparoendosc Adv Surg Tech A 9(3):273–276

10 Minimally Invasive Biliary Bypass

Stefano Berti, Andrea Gennai, and Elisa Francone

10.1 Introduction

Pancreatic cancer is deemed unresectable in up to 85% of affected patients, with 5-year survival rates lower than 5%. Therefore, the proposable treatment for the majority of patients is palliative care. Obstructive jaundice is the most common presenting symptom of pancreatic head cancer, affecting 70% of patients. Severe, persistent abdominal pain and itch are other symptoms that may require palliation [1].

The ideal palliative treatment for unresectable cancer causing biliary obstruction must provide a low treatment-related mortality and a long-term resolution of jaundice with minimal need for reintervention, with the ultimate intent of delivering optimum preservation and restoration of quality of life with minimal physical trauma, rapid recovery and a high rate of success in symptom relief [2]. Biliary decompression can be obtained either with interventional procedures (endoscopic stenting and percutaneous treatment) or with surgery, associated with reduced early and late complications, respectively. The decision to perform biliary stenting or surgical bypass depends on several factors including life expectancy, safety, and the patient's preference. It is fundamental that a multidisciplinary team reviews the patient's clinical data in order to determine the best approach for each patient, also considering the site of the obstruction, the risk factors and the expertise of the surgical team.

A proposed paradigm to decide on surgical bypass versus stenting could be the following: patients with impaired performance status or advanced disease may be better served with "definitive" endobiliary stenting, which minimizes inpatient length of stay and costs of care; conversely, carefully selected patients with low surgical risk, good performance status, and non-metastatic cancer who

E. Francone (✉)
Department of Surgery, S. Andrea Hospital, POLL-ASL5
La Spezia, Italy
e-mail: elisafrancone@gmail.com

U. Boggi (Ed), *Minimally Invasive Surgery of the Pancreas*,
Updates in Surgery
DOI: 10.1007/978-88-470-3958-2_10,

are projected to have a reasonable survival rate, should be considered for surgical bypass [3, 4].

Patients who are reasonable candidates for conservative or surgical techniques may experience fewer subsequent invasive procedures if early surgical biliary bypass is offered, reducing overall costs and hospitalization. Since the same principles adopted during open surgery are applied, minimally invasive surgical (MIS) biliary bypass combines the best of both surgical and conservative approaches: lower morbidity and faster recovery with reduced risk of recurrent jaundice. In this setting, MIS biliary-enteric bypass can be performed in the same session as the staging laparoscopy, once the tumor is deemed unresectable and a frozen section confirmation (if necessary) is obtained, as already proposed by some authors. Alternatively, laparoscopic palliation of malignant distal biliary obstruction can be performed in patients in whom endoscopic and percutaneous approaches failed [2, 4].

The addition of prophylactic gastric bypass to the palliative biliary bypass does not seem to increase operative morbidity or mortality whether the surgery is carried out by an open or an MIS approach [5].

10.2 Minimally Invasive Surgical Biliary Bypass

10.2.1 General Considerations

Regardless of the surgical approach adopted, if a biliary bypass is planned, adequate exposure is essential to safely access the porta hepatis. Accordingly, the liver has to be retracted, the lesser omentum should be opened and the duodenal-pancreatic block may have to be lowered. Structures in the hepatoduodenal ligament are usually recognizable by inspection and palpation, especially if a biliary stent has been positioned. However, if in doubt, intraoperative ultrasound may be helpful. The bile duct should be prepared taking care to avoid excessive dissection of the surrounding tissue in order to preserve blood supply to the duct.

Some fundamental rules should be followed to perform a trophic and patent biliary anastomosis, including preservation of adequate blood supply, avoidance of tension, mucosa-to-mucosa apposition, widely patent caliber, and accurate placement of sutures [6, 7]. Sutures should be a single layer of a thin monofilament absorbable material (e.g., 4-0/5-0 for normal ducts and 3-0/4-0 for thickened ducts), to prevent choledocholithiasis possibly related to non-absorbable sutures. Extensive placement of stitches should be avoided to preserve blood supply. Interrupted or double-running sutures can be both safely performed, in accordance with the exposure and the bile duct caliber.

10.2.2 Preoperative Patient Preparation

Routine prophylactic broad-spectrum antibiotic therapy is administered intravenously during anesthesia and is possibly continued for several days. Low-molecular weight heparin is routinely administered during the postoperative phase. Intermittent pneumatic compression of the lower limbs is also used intraoperatively.

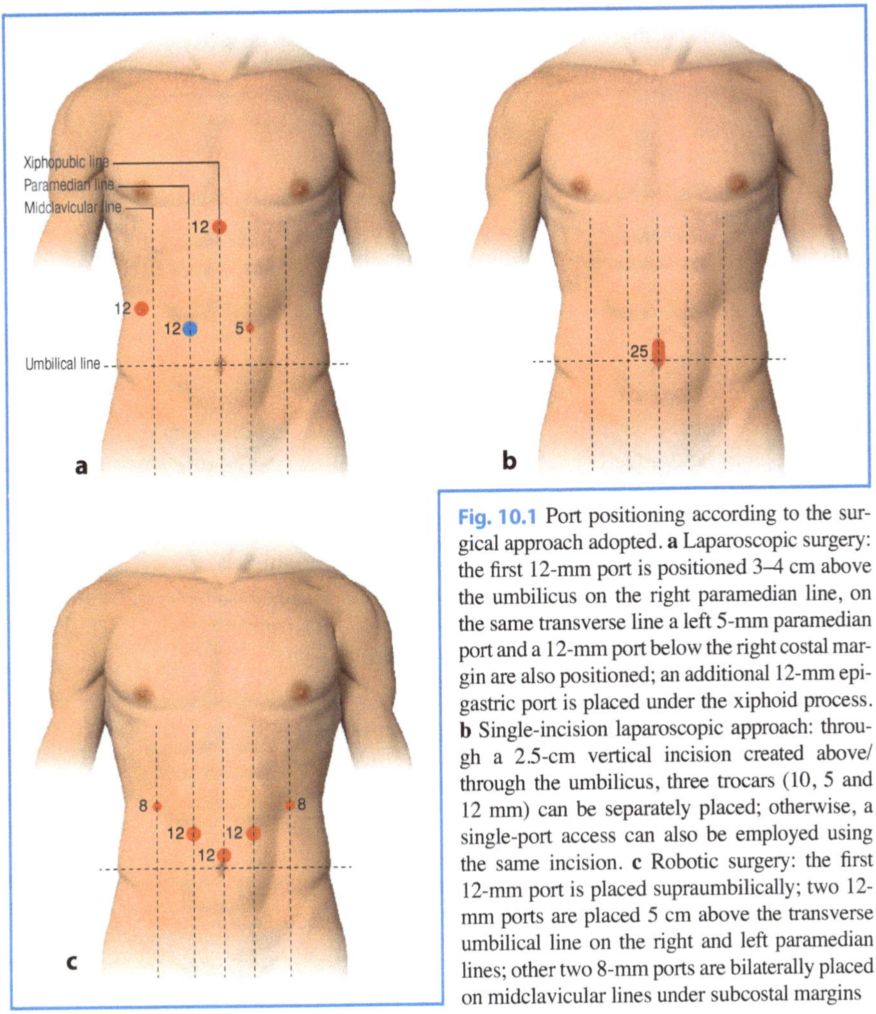

Fig. 10.1 Port positioning according to the surgical approach adopted. **a** Laparoscopic surgery: the first 12-mm port is positioned 3–4 cm above the umbilicus on the right paramedian line, on the same transverse line a left 5-mm paramedian port and a 12-mm port below the right costal margin are also positioned; an additional 12-mm epigastric port is placed under the xiphoid process. **b** Single-incision laparoscopic approach: through a 2.5-cm vertical incision created above/through the umbilicus, three trocars (10, 5 and 12 mm) can be separately placed; otherwise, a single-port access can also be employed using the same incision. **c** Robotic surgery: the first 12-mm port is placed supraumbilically; two 12-mm ports are placed 5 cm above the transverse umbilical line on the right and left paramedian lines; other two 8-mm ports are bilaterally placed on midclavicular lines under subcostal margins

10.2.3 Patient and Port Positioning

10.2.3.1 Laparoscopic Surgery

The patient is supine with head-up position, on a deflectable sandbag and with arms and legs spread apart. The surgeon stands between the patient's legs. The procedure can be approached with a four- or five-port technique (Fig. 10.1a). Pneumoperitoneum is established at a mean pressure of 12 mmHg.

10.2.3.2 Single-incision Laparoscopic Approach

Single-incision laparoscopic biliary bypass has seldom been reported in the literature, partly attributed to technical challenges [8]. The patient's and surgeon's position does not differ from the above described laparoscopic approach with multiple ports. An umbilical incision can be used for trocar accesses (Fig. 10.1b).

10.2.3.3 Robotic Surgery

The patient is positioned in a 20° reverse Trendelenburg position. The laparoscopic surgeon stands between the patient's legs, while the robotic surgeon operates from the console. A five-port technique is usually employed (Fig. 10.1c).

10.2.4 Procedures

10.2.4.1 Choledochoduodenostomy

In order to perform a choledochoduodenostomy, adequate duodenal mobilization should be achieved and Kocher and Cattell maneuvers may be required in order to avoid any tension at the anastomosis. The setting for side-to-side or end-to-side choledochoduodenostomy varies depending on bile duct size; nevertheless, an effort should be made to prevent strictures and cholangitis.

In cases of dilated common bile duct (CBD), the choledochoduodenal anastomosis can be performed by single-layer double-running sutures. The ideal length of the stitches for a continuous suture should be 15 cm to allow the surgeon a way to accomplish the final knot [9]; however, special threads equipped with absorbable clips can also be safely used, to avoid knot-tying maneuvers and reduce operative times. We usually use the PDS II Suture Endo-Clip 3.0 with Absolok Plus (Ethicon, Somerville, NJ, USA) with great outcomes.

For smaller CBD, instead, interrupted sutures should be preferred. In this case, 10 cm should be the adequate length of stitches [9]. Stay sutures can be usefully placed on the opposite sides of the bile duct cut. This expedient will improve traction, exposure and orientation of the anastomosis.

In both cases with running or separate stiches, the anastomosis begins from the posterior row. In interrupted suture, the stitches are all individually placed from inside the lumen, tied in order and cut. Once the posterior row has been fashioned, the duodenum is longitudinally incised at approximately 3 mm from the previous suture and the anterior row of the anastomosis is performed, with either continuous or interrupted sutures.

10.2.4.2 Choledochojejunostomy

Choledochojejunostomy is probably the most performed biliary bypass procedure, and it is ideal for malignant distal bile duct strictures due to periampullary cancer or advanced cancer of the head of the pancreas.

As previously described for choledochoduodenostomy, the setting for a side-to-side or end-to-side choledochojejunostomy varies depending on the size of the bile duct, and the same principles have to be followed in order to construct a patent and trophic anastomosis. In an end-to-side anastomosis, if the CBD is small, an anterior longitudinal incision in the duct wall can be made to enlarge the caliber. On the other hand, a wall shared between the CBD and the cystic duct can be divided.

The jejunal loop should be cut from 15 to 20 cm distal to the Treitz ligament. The transection can be performed with a surgical endostapler. Some authors recommend retrocolic loop transposition for benign disease, and antecolic passage in the case of malignancy or in obese patients [2]. If a transmesocolic route is chosen, mesenteric structures, which can impair blood flow to the limb, should be carefully avoided. At the same time, the breach created in the mesocolon should not be extensively wide, in order to avoid formation of Petersen's hernia, a condition with a high morbidity and mortality rate.

According to the size of the duct and the extension of the cut, either side-to-side or end-to-side anastomosis can be proposed [2] (Fig. 10.2), following the same general principles discussed above. Stay sutures can be usefully placed on the opposite sides of the cut CBD and at the level of the corresponding points in the limb of the anastomosis.

Once the posterior row of the anastomosis is performed, the corresponding opening in the jejunal loop should be significantly smaller than the bile duct opening, because the bowel breach tends to enlarge. In the case of small CBD, a silicone protection stent can be placed but not fixed through the anastomosis. In order to protect the anastomosis by diverting the bile outside, a Voelcker drain can also be chosen. At the end of the procedure, the jejunal loop can be fixed to the hilar plate to avoid any tension at the sutures.

In the setting of a dual-loop reconstructive method, the jejunojejunostomy should be performed at about 40–60 cm from the biliary bypass [2]. When employing the Roux-en-Y reconstruction, we usually perform a side-to-side intracorporeal mechanical isoperistaltic anastomosis with endostapler, closing the enterotomy by using 3-0 polydioxanone double-layer running suture.

10.2.4.3 Hepaticojejunostomy

Before performing hepaticojejunostomy, intraoperative cholangiography and/or laparoscopic ultrasound can be very useful in identifying biliary anatomic variation, and should therefore be considered in these types of biliary bypasses.

If the hepatic duct to anastomose is quite far from the hilum, the procedure does not differ from the previously described technique for choledochojejunostomy (Fig. 10.3a). On the contrary, the management of biliary bypasses close to the

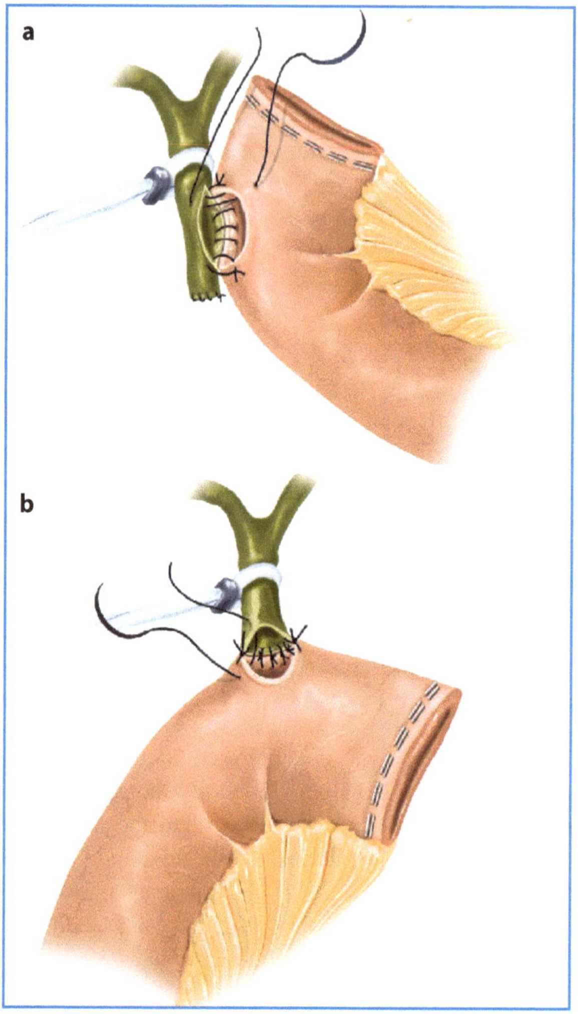

Fig. 10.2 **a** Side-to-side choledocojejunostomy. **b** End-to-side choledocojejunostomy. If the common bile duct is dilated, the posterior row of the anastomosis can be constructed by a single-layer 3-0 poly-dioxanone half-running suture

hilum or involving the hilar bifurcation requires the use of specific procedures. As described in the Hepp-Couinaud approach, if right and left hepatic ducts are still in communication, in order to construct a wide anastomosis, the hilar plate can be lowered to improve access to the left hepatic duct, which can be longitudinally incised on its anterior surface in order to perform a side-to-side anastomosis [10] (Fig. 10.3b). Moreover, the heel of the hepatic confluence can be conveniently cut to obtain an adequate caliber to perform a suitable anastomosis.

10.2.4.4 Cholecystojejunostomy

Cholecystojejunostomy is a procedure mainly applied for palliation of malignant disease in patients with a short life expectancy. Preoperative radiological assessment of cystic duct (CD) patency is unavoidable, as is the evaluation of

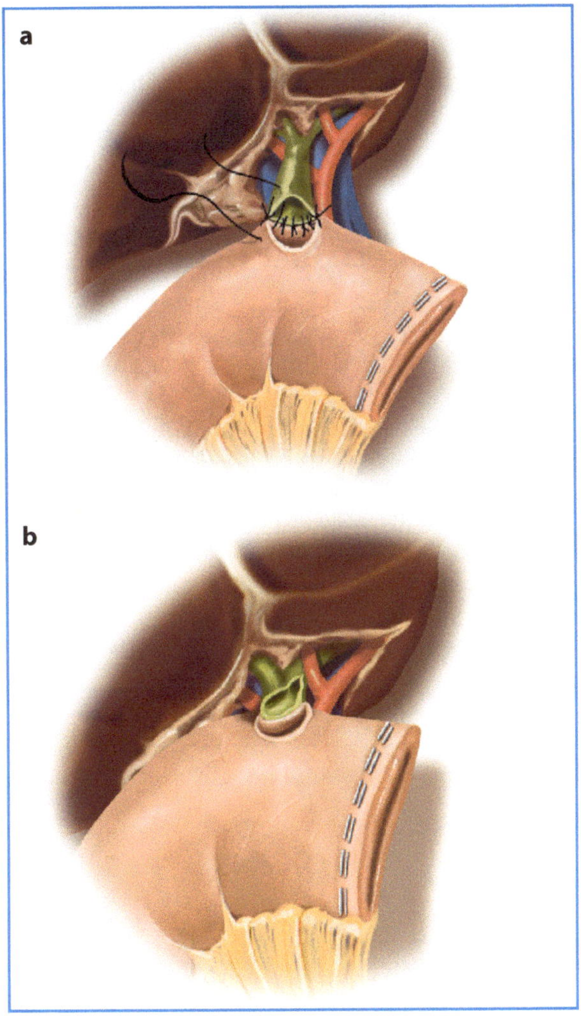

Fig. 10.3 **a** End-to-side hepaticojejunostomy can be accomplished with single-layer 3-0 polydioxanone doublerunning sutures. **b** Side-to-side hepaticojejunostomy: the left hepatic duct can be longitudinally incised according to the Hepp-Couinaud approach

CD insertion in the CBD, which should be at least 1 cm above the obstruction [2]. The biliary-enteric bypass is usually performed between the gallbladder fundus and a jejunal loop, isolated and transposed above the mesocolon, as described above. Usually the limb is fixed to the gallbladder with two opposite stay sutures and opened longitudinally. Both stapled and single-layer sutured, side-to-side 2–3-cm large anastomoses can be performed [2].

10.2.5 Complications

Stricture of the biliary bypass may occur if the anastomosed bile duct is small, in the case of narrow-constructed anastomosis or in cancer relapse. Late closure or bile leakage may occur in cases of inadequate blood supply to the bile duct or to the limb, but also due to excessive tension at the anastomosis. Recurrent jaundice is usually associated with tumor extension or relapse. Cholangitis is usually related to enteric reflux through the anastomosis.

Alternative endoscopic or interventional radiologic decompressive procedures should be considered if the above-mentioned complications occur.

10.3 Minimally Invasive Interventional Biliary Bypass

10.3.1 General Considerations

The primary non-surgical biliary drainage methods are endoscopic retrograde cholangiopancreatography (ERCP) and percutaneous transhepatic biliary drainage (PTBD). Usually ERCP is performed in the case of distal obstruction of the CBD, whereas PTBD is preferably used in the case of proximal biliary obstructions and when ERCP cannot be performed due to anatomical and/or technical reasons. The successful outcome is comparable in both methods and there are no significant differences in terms of mortality [11, 12].

Generally, both procedures are performed under conscious sedation and therefore the use of analgesics to relieve the pain must be evaluated case by case. An adequate antibiotic coverage is still fundamental to prevent the onset of cholangitis and severe sepsis due to the invasive process in cases of excluded bile ducts with stagnant bile.

10.3.2 Procedures

10.3.2.1 Endoscopic Retrograde Cholangiopancreatography

Obstructive jaundice occurs in 70% of patients with pancreatic cancer and in these cases the obstruction of the bile duct is mostly at the level of the distal duct, thus the majority of these patients can be treated with ERCP stenting. The primary benefit of this procedure is substantially related to the absence of any percutaneous access or external drainage system.

Absolute contraindications for the procedure are bleeding diathesis or bleeding disorders and gastrointestinal obstruction (i.e., pharyngeal, esophageal); relative contraindications are active acute pancreatitis, severe cardiopulmonary comorbidity and impossibility to approach the papillary/ampullary regions (i.e., stenosis/duodenal infiltration with anatomic distortion, past surgical procedure on the upper gastrointestinal tract with Roux-en-Y anastomosis).

ERCP can identify both the level and the nature of the obstruction, due to the possibility of collecting samples for biopsy and/or histologic examinations. It is performed using a flexible duodenoscope to reach a stable position of the papillary region, with wire-guided selective papillary and bile duct cannulation, endoscopic sphincterotomy and fluoroscopic retrograde cholangiography. As soon as the biliary stenosis is found and placement of one or more stents is possible, the obstruction can be resolved in the majority of cases. Plastic stents (i.e., polyethylene endoprosthesis) have been used for decades; however, despite the lower cost, usually the onset of a new obstruction occurs in 3–6 months. For this reason, the use of self-expandable metallic stents (SEMS) has become more and more frequent [5]. Reasonably, for all patients who underwent ERCP before complete and exhaustive neoplasm staging, and therefore before a definite treatment decision, the best clinical and most economical strategy can be represented by the use of short-length SEMS, which do not prevent either surgical intervention of pancreatoduodenectomy or a possible new ERCP procedure with placement of a longer or different type of stent [13].

Complications The main potential complications related to ERCP are hemorrhage, cholangitis, pancreatitis and gastrointestinal perforation.

10.3.2.2 Percutaneous Transhepatic Biliary Drainage

PTBD is mostly used in proximal biliary stenosis and/or where the endoscopic drainage cannot be performed due to technical or anatomical reasons and as a non-invasive drainage system.

An absolute contraindication for the procedure is an untreatable bleeding diathesis; relative contraindications are INR >1.5, platelet count lower than 50,000/mm^3, ascites and multiple hepatic cysts and/or other hepatic lesions which do not allow an adequate acoustic ultrasonic window.

In PTBD an ultrasound-guided injection with 18-gauge needle is performed on the liver periphery until reaching the dilated biliary branch, in order to reduce the risk of accidental damage to vascular structures. A hydrophilic guide wire (usually measuring 0.035 inches) is subsequently inserted into the biliary tree as far as the established site, and the biliary drainage is inserted on it. Cholangiography images with administration of water-soluble contrast agent and fluoroscopic examination are obtained during the entire procedure, to obtain a clear anatomic representation of the biliary tree, evaluating the degree and level of the stenosis, as well as the presence of possible anatomic abnormalities.

The placement of one or more SEMS is possible even with percutaneous access, while plastic stents have limited indications, and are mostly employed in cases of benign stenosis of lymphoma.

In the case of a single external biliary drainage, the choice of the access side usually depends on the operator's personal judgement, since either right-side access (subcostal or intercostal) or left-side access (subxiphoid) present advantages and disadvantages. In fact, accessing the biliary tree from the left is generally technically easier and well tolerated by patient and it is preferably used in long-term cases or in cases of ascites due to lesser rate of catheter leakage. The right-sided access, instead, is technically more difficult and presents a higher risk of complications, but it is more effective, allowing the drainage of a higher number of hepatic segments.

With the purpose of anatomically reconstructing the biliary tree, a T-configuration stenting can be favorably chosen, offering the advantage of ensuring drainage of both liver lobes with one single percutaneous access. With the same objectives, also a Y-configuration stenting can be performed, even though this proceeding requires a less convenient double right and left access.

Complications Minor complications related to PTBD are pain, catheter leakage; major complications include acute cholangitis leading to sepsis (potentially fatal), choleperitonitis/bile peritonitis, hemorrhage and pancreatitis. In the case of right intercostal access, pleural effusion and/or pneumothorax can also occur. Catheter displacement is usually more frequent with right-side access [11, 12].

References

1. Gentileschi P, Kini S, Gagner M (2002) Palliative laparoscopic hepatico- and gastrojejunostomy for advanced pancreatic cancer. JSLS 6(4):331–338
2. Toumi Z, Aljarabah M, Ammori BJ (2011) Role of the laparoscopic approach to biliary bypass for benign and malignant biliary diseases: a systematic review. Surg Endosc 25(7):2105–2116
3. Bliss LA, Eskander MF, Kent TS et al (2016) Early surgical bypass versus endoscopic stent placement in pancreatic cancer. HPB (Oxford) 18(8):671–677
4. Berti S, Ferrarese A, Feleppa C et al (2015) Laparoscopic perspectives for distal biliary obstruction. Int J Surg 21(1):S64–S67
5. Hüser N, Michalski CW, Schuster T et al (2009) Systematic review and meta-analysis of prophylactic gastroenterostomy for unresectable advanced pancreatic cancer. Br J Surg 96(7):711–719
6. Winslow ER, Fialkowski EA, Linehan DC et al (2009) "Sideways": results of repair of biliary injuries using a policy of side-to-side hepatico-jejunostomy. Ann Surg 249(3):426–434
7. Taylor BR, Langer B (2005) Procedures for benign and malignant biliary tract disease. In: Souba WW, Fink MP, Jurkovich GJ et al (eds) ACS Surgery: principles and practice. WebMD Professional Publishing, New York
8. Yu H, Wu S, Yu X et al (2015) Single-incision laparoscopic biliary bypass for malignant obstructive jaundice. J Gastrointest Surg 19(6):1132–1138
9. Croce E, Olmi S (2000) Intracorporeal knot-tying and suturing techniques in laparoscopic surgery: technical details. JSLS 4(1):17–22
10. Hepp J, Couinaud C (1956) Approach to and use of the left hepatic duct in reparation of the common bile duct. Presse Med 64(41):947–948 [Article in French]
11. van Delden OM, Laméris JS (2008) Percutaneous drainage and stenting for palliation of malignant bile duct obstruction. Eur Radiol 18(3):448–56
12. Chandrashekhara SH, Gamanagatti S, Singh A, Bhatnagar S (2016) Current status of percutaneous transhepatic biliary drainage in palliation of malignant obstructive jaundice: a review. Indian J Palliat Care 22(4):378–387
13. Chen VK, Arguedas MR, Baron TH (2005) Expandable metal biliary stents before pancreaticoduodenectomy for pancreatic cancer: a Monte-Carlo decision analysis. Clin Gastroenterol Hepatol 3(12):1229–1237

Minimally Invasive Gastric Bypass

11

Andrea Belli and Giulio Belli

11.1 Introduction

Gastric outlet obstruction is unfortunately a common event in patients affected by advanced stage upper gastrointestinal malignancies, and in cases of pancreatic cancer its incidence is estimated to be approximately 15–20% [1]. Symptoms accompanying gastric outlet obstruction such as reflux, nausea, vomiting, abdominal distension (up to occlusion), dehydration and the consequent state of malnutrition can drastically affect patients' quality of life and compromise their life expectancy also by precluding access to medical therapies [2].

In addition, patients affected by pancreatic cancer often present at diagnosis with an impaired performance status, accompanied by a substantial weight loss and a state of malnutrition which can often contribute to morbidity related to the disease or to attempted therapies [3]. In several series, up to 75–85 % of patients with pancreatic cancer present with unresectable disease mainly due to the presence of distant metastases or locally advanced disease with vascular encasement [4]. Even in patients with potentially resectable disease, up to 25–35% of cases can be found to be unresectable at surgery [4] so that life expectancy is still poor for the vast majority of patients with pancreatic cancer. In fact, in non-resected cases median survival is estimated to be approximately 4–6 months [5] from the diagnosis. In this setting, symptom palliation and maintenance of an acceptable quality of life are of crucial importance.

The optimal palliation method should ideally be of minimal impact for the patient, be associated with a low incidence of morbidity and mortality, and should offer long-lasting relief from symptoms thus allowing early tolerance of oral intake [6].

G. Belli (✉)
Department of General and Hepato-Pancreato-Biliary Surgery, S. M. Loreto Nuovo Hospital
Naples, Italy
e-mail: giubelli@unina.it

U. Boggi (Ed), *Minimally Invasive Surgery of the Pancreas*,
Updates in Surgery
DOI: 10.1007/978-88-470-3958-2_11, © Springer-Verlag Italia 2018

11.2 Palliation Strategies

Surgical gastrojejunostomy has been traditionally considered the gold standard for palliation of gastric outlet obstruction in patients affected by periampullary cancer [7] but in the last decade endoscopic stenting with self-expandable metallic stents (SEMSs) has emerged as an effective and less invasive alternative to surgery and progressively gained popularity [8–11].

Several series proved SEMSs to be a safe and effective alternative to surgical palliation. The systematic review by Dormann et al. [12], including more than 600 patients, reported that SEMSs have a technical success rate of 97% and a clinical success (patients able to tolerate oral intake) of 87%. Nevertheless, randomized trials comparing surgical gastrojejunostomy and endoscopic SEMSs have shown conflicting results, with two trials [13, 14] in favor of SEMSs and one favoring surgical gastrojejunostomy [15]. In addition, even if endoscopic SEMSs are effective in relieving short-term symptoms with a shorter hospital stay, they are plagued by a non-negligible incidence of stent occlusion or migration in the long term [15]. Additional endoscopic procedures can be necessary during the patient's residual lifetime and the impact in terms of costs and multiple hospital admissions as well as on global quality of life have still to be investigated, especially in the case of patients with a longer life expectancy.

Only few data on the comparison between open and laparoscopic gastrojejunostomy as well as between laparoscopic gastrojejunostomy and SEMSs are available in the literature. Laparoscopic gastrojejunostomy proved to be safe and effective in several case series [16, 17] and, when compared to the open approach, demonstrated a reduction in intraoperative blood loss, a lower rate of surgical-related complications and a reduced time to tolerate food oral intake as well as a shorter hospital stay [17–20]. The randomized controlled trial by Navarra et al. [21], albeit with the bias of a small sample size (12 patients per arm), confirmed these results but did not report any advantages in terms of hospital stay. A non-negligible conversion rate to laparotomy has also been reported in the literature but the data are mainly related to historical series.

Indeed, the laparoscopic approach carries the general benefits of minimally invasive surgical procedures, which must obviously be pursued in a palliation setting. It may also be speculated that, in resective pancreatic surgery, the laparoscopic approach could potentially reduce the economic impact [22, 23] of surgical gastrojejunostomy when compared to the standard open approach. Table 11.1 summarizes the outcomes of the main studies comparing open and laparoscopic gastrojejunostomy for the treatment of malignant gastric outlet obstruction.

The study by Mehta et al. [13] prospectively compared in a randomized fashion laparoscopic gastrojejunostomy and endoscopic stent placement finding favorable outcomes associated with SEMSs, but the small number of patients included in the trial is a strong limitation of the study. Table 11.2 summarizes the results of the available studies comparing SEMS and minimally invasive gastrojejunostomy.

Table 11.1 Clinical outcomes of main studies comparing open and laparoscopic gastrojejunostomy for malignant gastric outlet obstruction

Author	Year of publication	Type of study	N. of patients		Blood loss	Complications	Time to oral intake	Hospital stay
			open	laparoscopic				
Navarra et al. [21]	2006	RCT	12	12	In favor of laparoscopic GJ	In favor of laparoscopic GJ	In favor of laparoscopic GJ	No differences
Al-Rashedy et al. [18]	2005	RCC	12	15	In favor of laparoscopic GJ	In favor of laparoscopic GJ	Not reported	In favor of laparoscopic GJ
Mittal et al. [20]	2004	RCM	16	14	Not reported	In favor of laparoscopic GJ	In favor of laparoscopic GJ	In favor of laparoscopic GJ
Choi YB [17]	2002	RCM	10	10	Not reported	In favor of laparoscopic GJ	In favor of laparoscopic GJ	In favor of laparoscopic GJ
Bergamaschi et al. [19]	1998	RCC	22	9	In favor of laparoscopic GJ	Not reported	Not reported	In favor of laparoscopic GJ

RCT, randomized controlled trial; *RCC*, retrospective case-control; *RCM*, retrospective case-matched; *GJ*, gastrojejunostomy

Table 11.2 Clinical outcomes of main studies comparing self-expandable metallic stents (SEMSs) and laparoscopic gastrojejunostomy for malignant gastric outlet obstruction (long-term outcomes not investigated)

Author	Year of publication	Type of study	N. of patients		Blood loss	Complications	Time to oral intake	Hospital stay
			open	laparoscopic				
Mehta et al. [13]	2006	RCT	13	14	Not reported	In favor of SEMSs	Not reported	In favor of SEMSs
Mittal et al. [20]	2004	RCM	16	14	Not reported	In favor of SEMSs	In favor of SEMSs	In favor of SEMSs

RCT, randomized controlled trial; *RCM*, retrospective case-matched.

The role of prophylactic gastrojejunostomy in patients with unresectable periampullary cancer is still controversial but a recently published meta-analysis reported that in cases undergoing exploratory laparotomy for planned radical resection and found to be unresectable, prophylactic gastrojejunostomy proved to be effective in reducing the long-term incidence of gastric outlet obstruction without increasing surgical morbidity [24]. Therefore, even though it provides no additional survival benefit, prophylactic gastrojejunostomy seems to be indicated in patients with unresectable periampullary cancer undergoing exploratory laparotomy. In 2016 a review on the diagnostic accuracy of laparoscopy following computed tomography scan for assessing resectability with curative intent of pancreatic and periampullary cancer was published in the Cochrane Database of Systematic Reviews [25]. This review took into account 16 studies comprising a total of 1146 patients and concluded that staging laparoscopy with biopsy and histopathological confirmation of suspicious lesions would avoid an unnecessary laparotomy in 21% of patients scheduled for a radical pancreatic resection.

Consequently, staging laparoscopy is considered a useful option in patients with a diagnosis of resectable or borderline resectable periampullary cancer and scheduled for surgical exploration. In this setting, in cases of unresectable disease at laparoscopy and with the patient already in the operating theater, laparoscopic gastrojejunostomy has nowadays an important role to play.

Further, it should be taken into account that the life expectancy of patients with locally advanced pancreatic cancer is significantly longer than that of patients with metastatic disease and therefore the prolonged survival time can exceed the patency time of SEMSs leading to several hospital readmissions in the long term and minimizing the benefit of shorter hospital stay at the time of the first palliative procedure. Finally, the introduction in clinical practice of new therapeutic regimens such as FOLFIRINOX, which proved in a recent randomized trial to prolong median survival up to 11 months for patients with metastatic pancreatic adenocarcinoma [26], or nab-paclitaxel [27] could shift a proportion of patients towards surgical palliation (preferably laparoscopic). In fact, as reported by the SUSTENT prospective randomized study, gastrojejunostomy can offer better long-term clinical outcomes than endoscopic SEMSs [15].

Therefore, the choice of the optimal palliation strategy has to be tailored on the single patient's condition: SEMS is probably the best option in patients with poor general condition, and a theoretically short life expectancy; surgery, preferably by laparoscopy, represents a valid option for fit patients with a longer life expectancy, especially in the case of unresectable disease diagnosed in the operating theater.

11.3 Personal Experience and Surgical Technique

Between January 2011 and December 2016 at Loreto Nuovo Hospital (Naples, Italy), 14 patients with malignant gastric outlet obstruction and a diagnosis of pancreatic adenocarcinoma were subjected to laparoscopic antecolic and isoperistaltic gastrojejunostomy. Indications for surgery were as follows:

1. patients without evidence of systemic disease, subjected to staging laparoscopy and deemed unresectable (for vascular encasement at laparoscopic US, the presence of subglissonian liver metastases or initial peritoneal carcinomatosis);
2. patients with locally advanced borderline pancreatic cancer with initial symptoms of gastric outlet obstruction and scheduled for neoadjuvant therapies.

The procedure was successfully performed in all cases without intraoperative complications. Blood loss was minimal (mean 90 mL, range 40–180). There were no major complications, but one patient experienced a pneumonia resolved with antibiotic therapy and another a trocar wound infection that was treated conservatively. Two patients experienced symptoms of delayed gastric emptying.

Mean time to free fluid diet was 4 days (range 3–7) and all but the two abovementioned patients had relief of symptoms. Mean hospital stay was 6 days (range 4–15). Our surgical technique is briefly described below.

11.3.1 Operative Technique

The operation is undertaken under general anesthesia, a nasogastric tube is placed and preoperative gastric lavage is indicated in cases of pyloric occlusion with food residue. The patient is placed supine with legs wide apart and in a reverse Trendelenburg position. With the open technique, a blunt Hasson trocar is placed at the umbilicus and pneumoperitoneum is induced at 12 mmHg. The abdomen is inspected and under direct laparoscopic control additional trocars are placed taking into account the individual anatomy of the patient and the requirements of the specific surgical procedure. Generally, 4–5 trocars are placed in the upper abdomen in order to obtain optimal triangulation of the instruments. At least 1 trocar must be 10–12 mm in diameter to allow the introduction of the endoscopic linear stapler that will be used to fashion the gastrojejunostomy.

Exploration of the abdomen is carried out and, after a staging laparoscopy, the mobility of both the stomach and greater omentum is checked in order to be sure that the tissues to be anastomosed are free from neoplastic invasion. The gastrocolic ligament is then opened and the greater omentum retracted cranially. The first jejunal loop is exposed and the appropriate jejunal loop (which can be easily opposed without tension to the stomach) is selected and carefully juxtaposed to the inferior and posterior aspect of the greater curvature of the stomach in an antecolic and isoperistaltic fashion. At least two holding stitches are placed intracorporeally between the jejunum and the stomach in order to hold the loop in place. A safe distance from the tumor should be kept when choosing the anastomotic site. Using electrocautery, two small incisions are made on the antimesenteric wall of the jejunal loop and the gastric wall. A 45- or 60-mm endoscopic linear stapler is introduced into the abdomen and one arm is inserted into the stomach and the other into the lumen of the jejunum. The linear stapler is then closed on the antimesenteric wall of the jejunum and fired. After removal of the stapler, the anastomosis is visually inspected in order to assess luminal patency and to check for any bleeding. Completion of the anastomosis can be carried out either by placing a resorbable running suture or by firing an additional cartridge of endoscopic staples on the residual defect. Once the anastomosis is completed, its patency can be tested by air insufflation or by insertion into the stomach of a dilute methylene blue solution. A nasogastric tube is left in place at the end of the procedure and can be used as a transanastomotic stent to ensure patency of the new gastrojejunal lumen.

References

1. Lopera JE, Brazzini A, Gonzales A et al (2004) Gastroduodenal stent placement: current status. Radiographics 24(6):1561–1573
2. Schmidt C, Gerdes H, Hawkins W et al (2009) A prospective observational study examining quality of life in patients with malignant gastric outlet obstruction. Am J Surg 198(1):92–99
3. Brimhall B, Adler DG (2011) Enteral stents for malignant gastric outlet obstruction. Gastrointest Endosc Clin N Am 21(3):389–403
4. Ghaneh P, Smith R, Tudor-Smith C et al (2008) Neoadjuvant and adjuvant strategies for pancreatic cancer. Eur J Surg Oncol 34(3):297–305
5. Siegel RL, Miller KD, Jemal A (2015) Cancer statistics, 2015. CA Cancer J Clin 65(1):5–29
6. WHO – World Health Organization (1990) Cancer pain relief and palliative care. Report of a WHO Expert Committee. World Health Organ Tech Rep Ser 804:1–75
7. Lillemoe KD, Cameron JL, Hardacre JM et al (1999) Is prophylactic gastrojejunostomy indicated for unresectable periampullary cancer? A prospective randomized trial. Ann Surg 230(3):322–328
8. Maetani I, Akatsuka S, Ikeda M et al (2005) Self-expandable metallic stent placement for palliation in gastric outlet obstructions caused by gastric cancer: a comparison with surgical gastrojejunostomy. J Gastroenterol 40(10):932–937
9. Maetani I, Tada T, Ukita T et al (2004) Comparison of duodenal stent placement with surgical gastrojejunostomy for palliation in patients with duodenal obstructions caused by pancreaticobiliary malignancies. Endoscopy 36(1):73–78
10. Del Piano M, Ballare M, Montino F et al (2005) Endoscopy or surgery for malignant GI outlet obstruction? Gastrointest Endosc 61(3):421–426
11. Espinel J, Sanz O, Vivas S et al (2006) Malignant gastrointestinal obstruction: endoscopic stenting versus surgical palliation. Surg Endosc 20(7):1083–1087
12. Dormann A, Meisner S, Verin N et al (2004) Self-expanding metal stents for gastroduodenal malignancies: systematic review of their clinical effectiveness. Endoscopy 36:543–550
13. Mehta S, Hindmarsh A, Cheong E et al (2006) Prospective randomized trial of laparoscopic gastrojejunostomy versus duodenal stenting for malignant gastric outflow obstruction. Surg Endosc 20(2):239–242
14. Fiori E, Lamazza A, Volpino P et al (2004) Palliative management of malignant antro-pyloric strictures. Gastroenterostomy vs. endoscopic stenting. A randomized prospective trial. Anticancer Res 24(1):269–271
15. Jeurnink SM, Steyerberg EW, van Hooft JE et al; Dutch SUSTENT Study Group (2010) Surgical gastrojejunostomy or endoscopic stent placement for the palliation of malignant gastric outlet obstruction (SUSTENT study): a multicenter randomized trial. Gastrointest Endosc 71(3):490–499

16. Zhang LP, Tabrizian P, Nguyen S et al (2011) Laparoscopic gastrojejunostomy for the treatment of gastric outlet obstruction. JSLS 15(2):169–173
17. Choi YB (2002) Laparoscopic gastrojejunostomy for palliation of gastric outlet obstruction in unresectable gastric cancer. Surg Endosc 16(11):1620–1626
18. Al-Rashedy M, Dadibhai M, Shareif A et al (2005) Laparoscopic gastric bypass for gastric outlet obstruction is associated with smoother, faster recovery and shorter hospital stay compared with open surgery. J Hepatobiliary Pancreat Surg 12(6):474–478
19. Bergamaschi R, Mårvik R, Thoresen JE et al (1998) Open versus laparoscopic gastrojejunostomy for palliation in advanced pancreatic cancer. Surg Laparosc Endosc 8(2):92–96
20. Mittal A, Windsor J, Woodfield J et al (2004) Matched study of three methods for palliation of malignant pyloroduodenal obstruction. Br J Surg 91(2):205–209
21. Navarra G, Musolino C, Venneri A et al (2006) Palliative antecolic isoperistaltic gastrojejunostomy: a randomized controlled trial comparing open and laparoscopic approaches. Surg Endosc 20(12):1831–1834
22. Limongelli P, Belli A, Russo G et al (2012) Laparoscopic and open surgical treatment of left-sided pancreatic lesions: clinical outcomes and cost-effectiveness analysis. Surg Endosc 26(7):1830–1836
23. Limongelli P, Vitiello C, Belli A et al (2014) Costs of laparoscopic and open liver and pancreatic resection: a systematic review. World J Gastroenterol 20(46):17595–17602
24. Huser N, Michalski CW, Schuster T et al (2009) Systematic review and meta-analysis of prophylactic gastroenterostomy for unresectable advanced pancreatic cancer. Br J Surg 96(7):711–719
25. Allen VB, Gurusamy KS, Takwoingi Y et al (2016) Diagnostic accuracy of laparoscopy following computed tomography (CT) scanning for assessing the resectability with curative intent in pancreatic and periampullary cancer. Cochrane Database Syst Rev 7:CD009323
26. Conroy T, Desseigne F, Ychou M et al (2011) PRODIGE Intergroup. FOLFIRINOX versus gemcitabine for metastatic pancreatic cancer. N Engl J Med 364(19):1817–1825
27. Von Hoff DD, Ervin T, Arena FP et al (2013) Increased survival in pancreatic cancer with nab-paclitaxel plus gemcitabine. N Engl J Med 369(18):1691–1703

12 Minimally Invasive Drainage Procedures for Chronic Pancreatitis

Ahmad Hamad, Amer H. Zureikat, and Herbert J. Zeh III

12.1 Introduction

Traditionally, an open operative approach has been preferred in the surgical management of chronic pancreatitis (CP) due to the need for meticulous dissection and reconstruction in an often hostile operative bed. The discovery of laparoscopy has revolutionized the approach to complex surgical conditions ever since it was introduced in the 1980s. In 1994, Gagner and Pomp showed the feasibility of laparoscopic pancreatoduodenectomy (PD) by completing the first laparoscopic pylorus-sparing PD in a patient suffering from chronic pancreatitis, although the patient's postoperative course was complicated by delayed gastric emptying thus prolonging her stay to 30 days [1]. In a series of five laparoscopic distal pancreatectomies and splenectomies for patients with CP, Cuschieri et al. showed the superiority of laparoscopy through improved postoperative patient status and shorter hospital stay, without major complications [2]. After initial resistance, laparoscopy has grown in stature, and is now being routinely used for pancreatic resections and reconstructions, among other surgeries, at high-volume centers, with equivalent rates of mortality and morbidity compared to open procedures [3]. Laparoscopy offers an array of advantages over open surgery including: smaller incisions therefore decreasing blood loss and postoperative pain, expedited functional recovery, and shorter hospital stays.

Recently, the addition of robotic assistance to laparoscopy has redefined minimally invasive surgery by adding the benefit of three-dimensional binocular vision, scaling, stabilization of tremor, reduced operative fatigue, and improved ergonomics from the console-surgeon interface. There is limited data on the outcomes of minimally invasive surgical management for solely benign pancreas conditions such as CP due to continued preference of most surgeons to tackle

H.J. Zeh III (✉)
Department of Surgical Oncology, University of Pittsburgh Medical Center
Pittsburgh, Pennsylvania, USA
e-mail: zehxhx@upmc.edu

U. Boggi (Ed), *Minimally Invasive Surgery of the Pancreas*,
Updates in Surgery
DOI: 10.1007/978-88-470-3958-2_12, © Springer-Verlag Italia 2018

such a condition through an open approach. However, there are large data cohorts that compare open to laparoscopic pancreas surgery in both benign and malignant conditions. Therefore, such studies may be used to provide an insight into the applicability of minimally invasive approaches to CP.

CP has been defined in the past as "a continuing inflammatory disease of the pancreas, characterized by irreversible morphological change, and typically causing pain and/or permanent loss of function" [4]. This chapter will focus on conventional and robotic-assisted laparoscopic procedures for CP and compare them to the open approach. These surgical procedures will include resection-type procedures, drainage procedures, and combination-type procedures involving drainage and resection.

12.2 Minimally Invasive Total Pancreatectomy with Auto Islet Transplantation

The primary indication for minimally invasive total pancreatectomy (TP) with auto islet transplantation (AIT) is to treat refractory or intractable pain in patients with impaired quality of life due to CP in whom medical, endoscopic, or prior surgical therapy have failed [5]. Due to the aggressiveness of this operation and its association with short- and long-term morbidity, this type of procedure is rarely performed, with few reports of a minimally invasive approach. It is indicated for patients with small duct disease without diabetes [6]. The addition of robotic-assisted technology has allowed for a more precise and safe vascular dissection and reconstruction. We have published the largest case series of 10 patients who underwent TP, one of which included an AIT. Three of those patients were suffering from chronic pancreatitis. This study demonstrated the feasibility and safety of TP with or without AIT [6]. Furthermore, Galvani et al. described a case series of six patients with CP who underwent robotic-assisted TP with AIT. No intraoperative complications, conversions to open procedures, postoperative deaths, or major postoperative complications were reported [7].

Briefly our approach to this procedure is as follows [6]. Seven laparoscopic ports are placed, including one 12-mm camera port, three 8-mm robotic ports, one 5-mm port for a self-retaining liver retractor, and two (12-mm and 5-mm) assistant ports. The procedure begins with mobilization of the right colon and duodenum via a medial visceral and Kocher maneuver, respectively. The jejunum is then transected 10 cm from the ligament of Treitz and sutured to the stomach in an antecolic fashion 50 cm downstream to mark the location of the future gastrojejunostomy. Then, in order to enter the lesser sac, the gastrocolic omentum is divided, and the posterior stomach is freed from the anterior surface of the pancreas. Afterwards, the common hepatic artery (CHA), superior border of the pancreas, gastroduodenal artery (GDA), and common bile duct (CBD) are exposed using a robotic hook during dissection of the porta hepatis. The GDA transection is delayed until just prior to specimen extraction in order to reduce warm ischemia time while performing the AIT. The usual TP transection of GDA is performed with a vascular cartridge linear stapler, with enforcement of the stump using a 10-mm clip. Subsequently, the CBD is transected using a linear stapler.

In a TP alone, the neck of the pancreas is divided with an Endo GIA stapler (Covidien, Boulder, CO, USA). As for a TP with AIT, the neck division is delayed in order to preserve islet cell yield. Similar to the GDA, the splenic vein (SV) and artery (SA) are preserved until specimen extraction when they would be transected with vascular staplers. Afterwards, the retroperitoneum is incised laterally to expose the retropancreatic space that includes the splenic vein, splenic artery, and pancreatic body and tail. The entire pancreaticosplenic complex is then completely mobilized by releasing the splenic flexure, and splenorenal and splenocolic ligaments. The pancreas is then released from the superior mesenteric vein (SMV) and portal vein (PV) to expose the superior mesenteric artery (SMA) posteriorly by dividing the inferior and superior pancreaticoduodenal vessels. In order to perform the AIT, the pancreas is then lifted from the retroperitoneum. Heparin is administered intravenously at 50 IU/kg. The SA, GDA, SV are then transected using a vascular stapler in that order, in order to minimize warm ischemia time and maximize the largest number of islet cells. An SV stump is left to allow the infusion of the islets through a 14-gauge catheter. An endoscopic bag is then used to retrieve the specimen. Afterwards, an end-to-side hepaticojejunostomy is created in a "neo-duodenal" fashion using a running suture. A Hoffmeister type, antecolic, end-to-side gastrojejunostomy is then hand sewn in two layers. Finally, the islet cells are infused by gravity into the SV stump, followed by a re-stapled closure of the SV stump.

12.3 Minimally Invasive Lateral Pancreatojejunostomy (Modified Puestow)

In 1954, DuVal published a paper discussing caudal pancreatojejunostomy for chronic relapsing pancreatitis arguing that increased ductal pancreatic pressure contributed to the intractable pain found in patients with chronic pancreatitis [8]. This procedure is therefore commonly indicated for patients with an obstructed or dilated pancreatic duct since it allows its drainage.

Kurian and Gagner were the first to report a series of five cases in which a successful laparoscopic lateral pancreatojejunostomy (LPJ) was performed [9]. However, Tantia et al. and Palanivelu et al. published the two largest series of laparoscopic LPJ in India reporting 17 and 12 patients, respectively. Tantia et al. reported a complication rate of 11.8% which included a wound infection in one patient and an internal hernia in another requiring an operation [10]. Whereas, Palanivelu et al. reported no major postoperative morbidity or mortality, and

83.3% of patients had complete pain relief on median follow-up of 4.4 years [11]. Recently, Khaled et al. described a limited series of five patients with CP undergoing a laparoscopic LPJ with no reported mortality and 80% of patients were pain-free at follow-up of 14 months [12, 13]. In comparison, the conventional open LPJ can be associated with high morbidity rates up to 25% and a mortality rate of less than 5%. There is a single case report of a robotic LPJ performed on a 14-year-old child with idiopathic chronic pancreatitis. There was no mortality or morbidity reported, and the patient remained asymptomatic at 2 years postoperatively [14].

Briefly, our robotic approach to the Puestow procedure is as follows: four robotic ports including a 12-mm supraumbilical camera port, two left sided 8-mm robotic ports (midclavicular and anterior axillary line), and one right-sided midclavicular 8-mm robotic port are place along a transverse line just above the level of the umbilicus. A right upper quadrant (anterior axillary line) 5-mm laparoscopic port is placed for a self-retaining retractor for the stomach. In the right and left lower abdominal quadrants a 5-mm and a 12-mm laparoscopic port are placed for the laparoscopic assistant who stands between the legs. The lesser sac is opened widely with the LigaSure device (Covidien, Boulder, CO, USA) and the stomach is retracted antero-superiorly. A laparoscopic or robotic ultrasound is used to locate the dilated pancreatic duct. The duct is opened longitudinally in its most dilated portion with a robotic scissors and extended proximally and distally with the robotic hook as needed. To create the Roux limb, a defect is created in the mesocolon bare area, and the small bowel is divided approximately 20 to 30 cm (after ensuring the Roux limb can reach the pancreas) beyond the ligament of Treitz using a linear laparoscopic stapler. A side-to-side jejunojejunostomy is created 40 cm distal to transected edge of the Roux limb using a linear 60-mm stapler, and the common enterotomy is closed robotically using two 4-0 v-loc sutures in running fashion. The Roux limb is brought up through the mesocolon and aligned so that the cut edge is facing the spleen. A longitudinally hand-sewn robotic anastomosis is then created between the Roux and the opened pancreatic duct edge using either 4-0 or 3-0 v-loc sutures. The Roux limb is then secured to the mesocolon using interrupted 3-0 silk sutures, and the small bowel hernia defect is approximated using 3-0 silk sutures. A drain is typically left within the lesser sac adjacent to the anastomosis.

12.4 Minimally Invasive Frey Procedure

In essence, the Frey procedure is a hybrid procedure combining both resection and drainage. Therefore, it is indicated for patients with severe pancreatic head inflammation and/or mass, as well as an obstructed or dilated pancreatic duct with a recommended minimum duct width of more than 8 mm for a successful laparoscopic intervention [15]. Tan et al. shared their single-center experience performing the laparoscopic Frey procedure on nine patients as well as comparing it to the open approach performed on 37 patients. They reported seven successful laparoscopic procedures. Two laparoscopic cases were converted to open due to the inability to locate the pancreatic duct. One postoperative complication of postpancreatectomy hemorrhage was reported. All patients who underwent a successful laparoscopic Frey procedure reported improved pain scores at 3-month follow-up [15].

In addition, Killburn et al. described their single-center experience in a series of four consecutive patients undergoing a laparoscopic Frey procedure. Only one postoperative complication was reported with a Clavien-Dindo grade of 4a. The patient was reoperated on due to a leak of the pancreaticojejunal anastomosis with hemorrhage. Within 6 months, all four patients had reported a significant reduction in pain frequency and analgesic requirement [16].

Similar to the robotic LPJ procedure, the robotic Frey procedure utilizes the same port configuration. In addition to the LPJ, the opening of the pancreatic duct extended across the neck towards the genu of the pancreas. At this level, care must be taken to transfix the gastroduodenal artery with 2-0 silk sutures superiorly and inferiorly before dividing the vessel and extending the LPJ towards the neck and genu. Approximately 1.5 grams of the pancreatic head parenchyma is then excavated in depth towards the posterior wall of the duct of Wirsung using the robotic scissors with sparing use of energy, while leaving a 0.5-cm margin from the duodenum to prevent any damage to the biliary duct. Small perforating bleeders can be dealt with using 4-0 or 5-0 proline sutures. The LPJ is then created as done in the Puestow procedure.

12.5 Minimally Invasive Beger Procedure

The Beger procedure is a hybrid procedure similar to the Frey procedure but differs in that is indicated for patients with pancreatic head inflammation and/or mass without pancreatic duct dilation or pancreatic head enlargement.

Available data on the laparoscopic Beger procedure is limited to one case report of a laparoscopic Beger procedure with "Berne modification" in a patient with an inflammatory head mass causing an intrapancreatic common bile duct stricture. There was no reported postoperative morbidity or mortality and the patient was discharged after 5 days. At 16-month follow-up, the patient reported mild pain that was controlled with one-third of the preoperative oral opioid dose [12].

Khaled et al. describe the laparoscopic Beger procedure with "Berne modification" [12]. The head of the pancreas is first encircled by multiple 3-0 vicryl sutures in order to achieve better hemostasis while coring it out. An ultrasonically activated scalpel is then used to core the pancreatic head mass until the pancreatic duct is encountered and opened into the cavity. The bile duct is then opened and the choledochotomy is extended to within the margins of the cored cavity. Using an endostapler, the jejunum is then divided at 75 cm distal to the ligament of Treitz and a side-to-side jejunojejunostomy is then created 60 cm downstream. The Roux limb is then brought up in a retrocolic fashion through the transverse mesocolon in order to create an end-to-side LPJ using a single-layer full-thickness continuous 4-0 PDS suture.

12.6 Conclusions

In the past decade, there has been a trend toward minimally invasive surgery in various pancreatic surgeries due to the relatively higher morbidity and mortality associated with the open approach. Laparoscopic surgery is limited with its current technology using two-dimensional imaging, limited range of instrument motion, and poor surgeon ergonomics [17]. The robotic interface offers various technical advantages that overcome these limitations while permitting a meticulous dissection and reconstruction. However, robotic surgery imposes significant cost and learning curve for surgeons training to adopt this new technology.

In conclusion, conventional and robotic-assisted laparoscopic approaches to chronic pancreatitis are safe and feasible in highly specialized centers, though inferred from limited and small retrospective studies and case reports (Table 12.1). However, further comparative studies on the efficacy of minimally invasive approaches with larger population samples are necessary.

Table 12.1 University of Pittsburgh robotic experience tackling chronic pancreatitis

	Type of robotic procedure		
	Total pancreatectomy [6]	**Frey**	**Puestow**
Number of patients	11	4	8
Mean age (years)	42	46	42
Gender (% of males)	45%	100%	50%
Mean BMI	25.67	25	20.7
Mean LOS (days)	10	6.5	8.4
Pancreatic leaks: number (%) [ISGPF grade]	0	1 (25%) [grade B]	1 (12.5%) [grade A]

BMI, body mass index; *LOS*, length of stay; *ISGPF*, International Study Group on Pancreatic Fistula.

References

1. Gagner M, Pomp A (1994) Laparoscopic pylorus-preserving pancreatoduodenectomy. Surg Endosc 8(5):408–410
2. Cuschieri A, Jakimowicz JJ, van Spreeuwel J (1996) Laparoscopic distal 70% pancreatectomy and splenectomy for chronic pancreatitis. Ann Surg 223(3):280–285
3. Sharpe SM, Talamonti MS, Wang CE et al (2015) Early national experience with laparoscopic pancreaticoduodenectomy for ductal adenocarcinoma: a comparison of laparoscopic pancreaticoduodenectomy and open pancreaticoduodenectomy from the national cancer data base. J Am Coll Surg 221(1):175–184
4. Whitcomb DC, Frulloni L, Garg P et al (2016) Chronic pancreatitis: an international draft consensus proposal for a new mechanistic definition. Pancreatology 16(2):218–224
5. Kesseli SJ, Smith KA, Gardner TB (2015) Total pancreatectomy with islet autologous transplantation: the cure for chronic pancreatitis? Clin Transl Gastroenterol 6:e73
6. Zureikat AH, Nguyen T, Boone BA et al (2015) Robotic total pancreatectomy with or without autologous islet cell transplantation: replication of an open technique through a minimal access approach. Surg Endosc 29(1):176–183
7. Galvani CA, Rodriguez Rilo H, Samame J et al (2014) Fully robotic-assisted technique for total pancreatectomy with an autologous islet transplant in chronic pancreatitis patients: results of a first series. J Am Coll Surg 218(3):e73–e78
8. Duval MK Jr (1954) Caudal pancreatico-jejunostomy for chronic relapsing pancreatitis. Ann Surg 140(6):775–785
9. Kurian MS, Gagner M (1999) Laparoscopic side-to-side pancreaticojejunostomy (Partington-Rochelle) for chronic pancreatitis. J Hepatobiliary Pancreat Surg 6(4):382–386
10. Tantia O, Jindal MK, Khanna S, Sen B (2004) Laparoscopic lateral pancreaticojejunostomy: our experience of 17 cases. Surg Endosc 18(7):1054–1057
11. Palanivelu C, Shetty R, Jani K et al (2006) Laparoscopic lateral pancreaticojejunostomy: a new remedy for an old ailment. Surg Endosc 20(3):458–461
12. Khaled YS, Ammori BJ (2014) Laparoscopic lateral pancreaticojejunostomy and laparoscopic Berne modification of Beger procedure for the treatment of chronic pancreatitis: the first UK experience. Surg Laparosc Endosc Percutan Tech 24(5):e178–e182
13. Khaled YS, Ammori MB, Ammori BJ (2011) Laparoscopic lateral pancreaticojejunostomy for chronic pancreatitis: a case report and review of the literature. Surg Laparosc Endosc Percutan Tech 21(1):e36–e40
14. Meehan JJ, Sawin R (2011) Robotic lateral pancreaticojejunostomy (Puestow). J Pediatr Surg 46(6):e5–e8
15. Tan CL, Zhang H, Li KZ (2015) Single center experience in selecting the laparoscopic Frey procedure for chronic pancreatitis. World J Gastroenterol 21(44):12644–12652
16. Kilburn DJ, Chiow AK, Leung U et al (2017) Early experience with laparoscopic Frey procedure for chronic pancreatitis: a case series and review of literature. J Gastrointest Surg 21(5):904–909
17. Zeh HJ 3rd, Bartlett DL, Moser AJ (2011) Robotic-assisted major pancreatic resection. Adv Surg 45:323–340

Percutaneous Necrosectomy and Sinus Tract Endoscopy for Infected Pancreatic Necrosis

13

Fara Uccelli and Alessandro Zerbi

13.1 Introduction

Acute pancreatitis affects 13–45 cases per 100,000 persons every year and often requires acute hospitalization [1]. The most severe evolution of acute pancreatitis is pancreatic necrosis, which may evolve into infected necrosis in 40–70% of patients, with a mortality rate up to 39% [2–4].

Radiological, endoscopic or surgical treatment may be indicated to remove necrotic tissue in the case of an infected necrotizing pancreatitis. An invasive treatment is indicated when there is a documented infection associated with clinical deterioration. Moreover, invasive treatment may also be indicated without documented infected necrosis if organ failure is present in the case of complications such as abdominal compartment syndrome, acute bleeding, bowel ischemia or obstruction due to mass effect from the necrosis. Invasive procedures should be delayed, if possible, to a minimum of four weeks after initial presentation to allow the collection to become "walled-off" [5].

The first surgical procedure for necrotic pancreatitis was performed by Senn in 1886 [6]; since then, surgery became the standard treatment for necrotizing pancreatitis. Until the 70s the approach was very invasive as pancreatic resection was the procedure of choice. This approach was justified by the belief that by removing the necrotic areas it was possible to prevent those substances derived by pancreatic necrosis from entering the circulation, and to avoid bacterial over-infection. However, such an aggressive approach was related to high mortality rates and did not improve the patient's outcome. Moreover, pancreatic resection

F. Uccelli (✉)
Pancreatic Surgery Unit, Humanitas University, Humanitas Research Hospital,
Rozzano, Italy
e-mail: fara.uccelli@gmail.com

U. Boggi (Ed), *Minimally Invasive Surgery of the Pancreas*,
Updates in Surgery
DOI: 10.1007/978-88-470-3958-2_13, © Springer-Verlag Italia 2018

led to overestimate the necrosis percentage during surgery, with consequently removal of vital pancreatic tissue [7, 8].

More conservative approaches were subsequently developed such as necrosectomy [9]. This technique consisted of the removal of necrotic tissue with sparing of the remaining pancreas. The main limit of necrosectomy is represented by the incomplete removal of partially colliquated necrotic areas. To circumvent such a problem, continuous retro- and endoperitoneal lavage was introduced, mainly in Europe: in the postoperative period, continuous lavage allows continuation of the necrosectomy performed during surgery, thanks to its mechanical and chemical action; in this way pieces of colliquated necrotic tissue can be removed [7, 8, 10]. As an alternative to postoperative continuous lavage to complete necrosectomy, a strategy of scheduled multiple laparotomies (with intermitted closure of the abdominal wall using the zipper technique) or open packing of the lesser sac and scheduled changes of gauzes at 24–48 h intervals (open packing) were introduced, mainly in North American centers [11, 12].

13.2 From Open to Minimally Invasive Necrosectomy

Irrespective of the different postoperative management, the surgical technique of open necrosectomy has not changed much over the years and the most used is the one described by Traverso [13]. This involves a supramesocolic access along the avascular plane between the omentum and the colon, to avoid the contamination of the inferior abdomen [13].

Despite the accuracy of the surgical technique, the mortality of open necrosectomy has always been very high, at the beginning in some cases above 50%. Over the years the mortality decreased gradually to 11% or lower, although it still reaches 39% in some centers. Nowadays, the perioperative mortality for an open necrosectomy in referral centers is largely reported to be in the range of 14–20% [7, 12–17].

With the beginning of laparoscopy some surgeons started to look for less invasive methods for performing necrosectomy.

The first to describe a minimally invasive necrosectomy was Gagner in 1996 [18], who reported on eight patients suffering from infected pancreatic necrosis. Gagner's aim was to perform debridement, necrosectomy and drainage with the same results as open surgery but with a less invasive and traumatic approach and better outcomes. He described three different approaches depending on the type and the location of necrosis. The first approach consisted of a retrogastric/retrocolic debridement and was recommended for early infected fluid or severe sterile pancreatic necrosis. The second approach consisted of a retroperitoneoscopic debridement and was recommended for late infected pancreatic necrosis. The third consisted of a transgastric laparoscopic drainage and debridement. This approach was recommended for infected pseudocysts or late infected pancreatic

Table 13.1 Complications and mortality of minimally invasive necrosectomy in different surgical series

Study	Technique	Number of cases	Success	Complications	Overall mortality
Gagner et al. [18]	Laparoscopic necrosectomy	8	6 (75%)	8 (100%)	0 (0%)
van Sanvoort et al. [24]	Percutaneous drainage	43	15 (35%)	17 (40%)	8 (19%)
Raraty et al. [23]	Retroperitoneal necrosectomy	137	120 (86%)	75 (55%)	26 (19%)
Chang et al. [8]	Retroperitoneal necrosectomy	19	17 (89%)	4 (21%)	3 (16%)
Carter et al. [19]	Retroperitoneal approach	10	8 (80%)	8 (80%)	2 (20%)
Horvath et al. [21]	Combined approach	40	24 (60%)	29 (72%)	2 (5%)

necrosis. All patients had complications, though mortality was 0% and the success rate after the first drainage was around 75% [18].

After Gagner's experience, the minimally invasive technique for necrosectomy gradually began to be used and the minimally invasive retroperitoneal access became a viable alternative when percutaneous drainage was not enough and a surgical approach was needed (Table 13.1).

13.3 Minimally Invasive Percutaneous Necrosectomy

Minimally invasive percutaneous necrosectomy, also called sinus tract endoscopy, is a non-standardized technique. Different approaches with many different tools have been described (Fig. 13.1). Regardless of the technique used, sinus tract endoscopy should be preceded by an accurate computed tomography (CT) study, to identify the location of necrosis and relationships with other abdominal organs.

The radiological drain inserted in the necrosis is often used as a guide in the operating room for the placement of the minimally invasive access. The most common technique is the one described by Carter et al. [19] which uses the laparoscope as a tool to carry out the sinus tract endoscopy. It begins by making a skin incision of 4–5 cm in correspondence to the radiological drain or in its immediate surroundings. One or more ports are then positioned in the incision using the laparoscope (Fig. 13.2). After gas insufflation, necrosectomy is performed through the introduction of long grasp forceps or laparoscopic spoon forceps. Necrotic material is in part removed and copious washing is performed (Fig. 13.3). Finally, percutaneous drains are inserted to drain residual

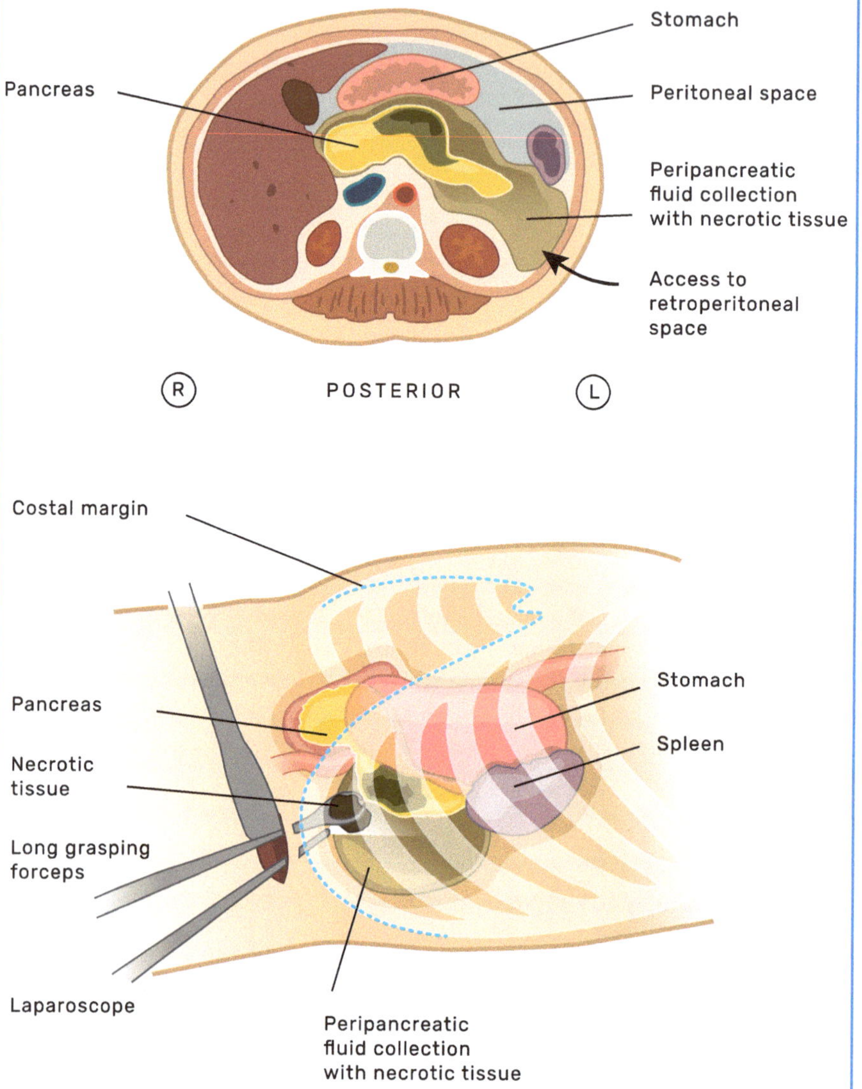

Fig. 13.1 Video-assisted retroperitoneal debridement (Illustration by Marcello Pirovano)

necrotic material: as in open necrosectomy, the purpose of the procedure is not to remove all the necrotic tissue immediately but to facilitate the drainage of necrotic material through percutaneous drains.

This technique appears to be safe and effective, with an overall mortality of 20%. Although the laparoscope is the most used instrument, other techniques with different tools, like the flexible endoscope or the nephroscope, have been described with similar results [20–22].

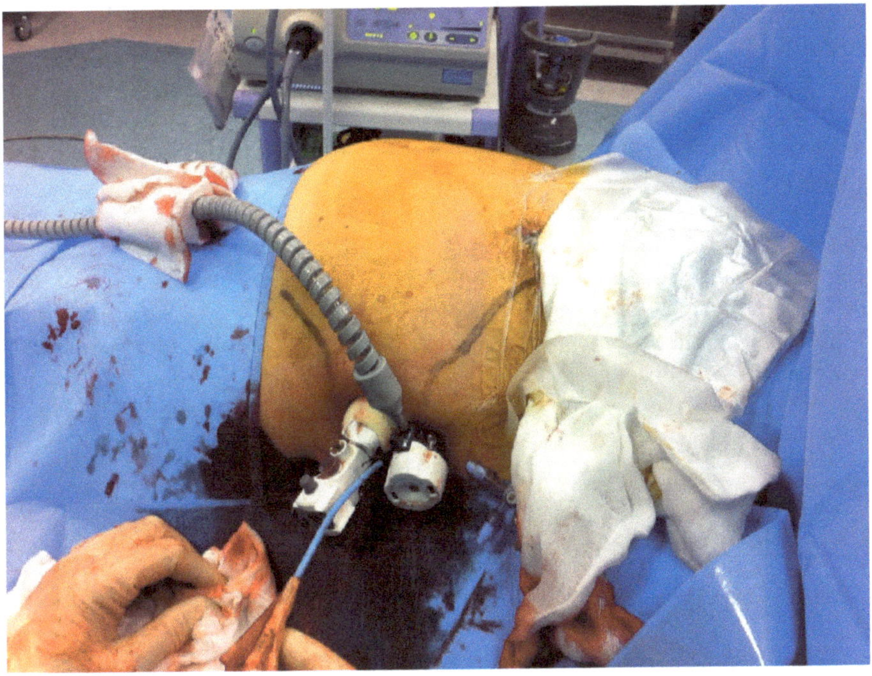

Fig. 13.2 Lateral access for sinus tract endoscopy using radiological drainage as a guide

Sinus tract endoscopy has slowly replaced open necrosectomy, when technically possible. In fact, it has proved to be as effective as the conventional technique but less invasive and burdened with less complications and a lower mortality rate [23].

On the basis of these favorable results, a randomized multicenter study (PANTER) was conducted in the Netherlands in 2010 to compare open surgical

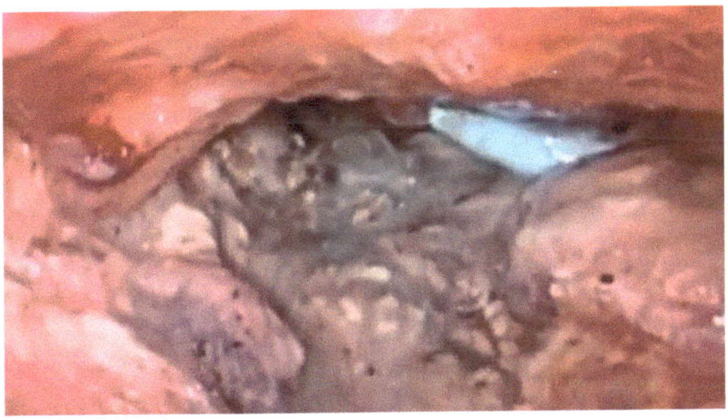

Fig. 13.3 Minimally invasive percutaneous necrosectomy

necrosectomy with the minimally invasive approach (percutaneous drainage and minimally invasive retroperitoneal necrosectomy). The study showed that the best strategy for the treatment of infected necrotic pancreatitis was not laparotomic necrosectomy but the step-up approach, which involved placement of a percutaneous drain followed by minimally invasive retroperitoneal necrosectomy, if necessary [24].

In recent years, progress in endoscopy has slightly reduced the role of sinus tract endoscopy. In fact, the endoscopic transgastric and transduodenal drainage techniques have proved to be safe and effective and they represent a possible alternative to the percutaneous approach [20].

Recent guidelines indicate the minimally invasive step-up approach – i.e., percutaneous or endoscopic drainage followed if necessary by minimally invasive retroperitoneal necrosectomy – as the optimal interventional strategy [25].

13.4 Conclusions

Infected pancreatic necrosis is a severe complication of acute pancreatitis which sometimes still requires surgical treatment. Sinus tract endoscopy has decreased the morbidity and mortality of this surgery compared to the open approach. To date, when technically feasible, a minimally invasive approach should be performed as the gold standard in the surgical treatment of infected pancreatic necrosis.

References

1. Yadav D, Lowenfels AB (2013) The epidemiology of pancreatitis and pancreatic cancer. Gastroenterology 144(6):1252–1261
2. Bello B, Matthews JB (2012) Minimally invasive treatment of pancreatic necrosis. World J Gastroenterol 18(46):6829–6835
3. Trikudanathan G, Attam R, Arain MA et al (2014) Endoscopic interventions for necrotizing pancreatitis. Am J Gastroenterol 109(7):969–981
4. Luigiano C, Pellicano R, Fusaroli P et al (2016) Pancreatic necrosectomy: an evidence-based systematic review of the levels of evidence and a comparison of endoscopic versus non-endoscopic techniques. Minerva Chir 71(4):262–269
5. Working Group IAP/APA Acute Pancreatitis Guidelines (2013) IAP/APA evidence-based guidelines for the management of acute pancreatitis. Pancreatology 13(4 Suppl 2):e1–e15
6. Senn N (1886) The surgery of the pancreas, as based upon experiments and clinical researches. Am J Med Sci 184:423–454
7. Beger HG, Rau BM (2007) New advances in pancreatic surgery. Curr Opin Gastroenterol 23(5):522–534
8. Chang Y-C (2014) Is necrosectomy obsolete for infected necrotizing pancreatitis? Is a paradigm shift needed? World J Gastroenterol 20(45):16925–16934
9. Schröder T, Sainio V, Kivisaari L et al (1991) Pancreatic resection versus peritoneal lavage in acute necrotizing pancreatitis. A prospective randomized trial. Ann Surg 214(6):663–666

10. Becker V, Huber W, Meining A et al (2009) Infected necrosis in severe pancreatitis – Combined nonsurgical multi-drainage with directed transabdominal high-volume lavage in critically ill patients. Pancreatology 9(3):280–286
11. Bradley EL 3rd (1993) A fifteen year experience with open drainage for infected pancreatic necrosis. Surg Gynecol Obstet 177(3):215–222
12. Rodriguez JR, Razo AO, Targarona J et al (2008) Debridement and closed packing for sterile or infected necrotizing pancreatitis. Ann Surg 247(2):294–299
13. Traverso LW, Kozarek RA (2005) Pancreatic necrosectomy: definitions and technique. J Gastrointest Surg 9(3):436–439
14. Götzinger P, Sautner T, Kriwanek S et al (2002) Surgical treatment for severe acute pancreatitis: extent and surgical control of necrosis determine outcome. World J Surg 26(4):474–478
15. Besselink MG, de Bruijn MT, Rutten JP et al (2006) Surgical intervention in patients with necrotizing pancreatitis. Br J Surg 93(5):593–599
16. Mier J, León EL, Castillo A et al (1997) Early versus late necrosectomy in severe necrotizing pancreatitis. Am J Surg 173(2):71–75
17. Babu BI, Sheen AJ, Lee SH et al (2010) Open pancreatic necrosectomy in the multidisciplinary management of postinflammatory necrosis. Ann Surg 251(5):783–786
18. Gagner M (1996) Laparoscopic treatment of acute necrotizing pancreatitis. Semin Laparosc Surg 3(1):21–28
19. Carter CR, McKay CJ, Imrie CW (2000) Percutaneous necrosectomy and sinus tract endoscopy in the management of infected pancreatic necrosis: an initial experience. Ann Surg 232(2):175–180
20. Bakker OJ, van Santvoort HC, van Brunschot S et al (2012) Endoscopic transgastric vs surgical necrosectomy for infected necrotizing pancreatitis: a randomized trial. JAMA 307(10):1053–1061
21. Horvath KD, Kao LS, Wherry KL et al (2001) A technique for laparoscopic-assisted percutaneous drainage of infected pancreatic necrosis and pancreatic abscess. Surg Endosc 15(10):1221–1225
22. Mui LM, Wong SK, Ng EK et al (2005) Combined sinus tract endoscopy and endoscopic retrograde cholangiopancreatography in management of pancreatic necrosis and abscess. Surg Endosc 19(3):393–397
23. Raraty MG, Halloran CM, Dodd S et al (2010) Minimal access retroperitoneal pancreatic necrosectomy: improvement in morbidity and mortality with a less invasive approach. Ann Surg 251(5):787–793
24. van Santvoort HC, Besselink MG, Bakker OJ et al (2010) A step-up approach or open necrosectomy for necrotizing pancreatitis. N Engl J Med 362(16):1491–1502
25. Italian Association for the Study of the Pancreas (AISP), Pezzilli R, Zerbi A et al (2015) Consensus guidelines on severe acute pancreatitis. Dig Liver Dis 47(7):532–543

Minimally Invasive Transduodenal Ampullary Resection

14

Courtney E. Barrows, Ana Sofia Ore, Monica Solis Velasco, and A. James Moser

14.1 Introduction

Local resection of the ampulla was first described by Halsted in 1899 well in advance of A.O. Whipple's first report of successful pancreatoduodenectomy (PD) for ampullary cancer in 1935 [1]. Although PD is the standard treatment for periampullary malignancies, transduodenal ampullary resection (TDAR) is an effective alternative for selected high-risk lesions and benign disease. Recent technical descriptions and short-term outcomes indicate that minimally invasive TDAR offers the oncologic benefits of an open approach with reduced morbidity [2].

TDAR is a technically challenging procedure owing to the complex anatomic relationships between the major/minor papillae and the underlying bile and pancreatic ducts as well as potentially adjacent duodenal diverticula [3]. Given the risk of malignant transformation, complete resection is recommended for most ampullary lesions [4]. An endoscopic approach is the preferred modality for resecting benign ampullary lesions with technically favorable features and low malignant potential and has achieved favorable short-term outcomes in comparison to traditional open TDAR [5].

This chapter reviews indications and comparative outcomes for endoscopic and surgical TDAR with particular attention to the technical aspects of minimally invasive TDAR.

A. J. Moser (✉)
Pancreas and Liver Institute, Beth Israel Deaconess Medical Center, Harvard Medical School
Boston, Massachusetts, USA
e-mail: ajmoser@bidmc.harvard.edu

U. Boggi (Ed), *Minimally Invasive Surgery of the Pancreas*,
Updates in Surgery
DOI: 10.1007/978-88-470-3958-2_14,

14.2 Diagnosis and Staging

Ampulla of Vater neoplasms account for less than 5% of all gastrointestinal tumors [6] and may comprise ampullary adenomas, neuroendocrine tumors, gastrointestinal stromal tumors, lipomas, Brunner's gland hamartomas, paragangliomas, and leiomyomas [3]. Most are discovered incidentally at the time of esophagogastroduodenoscopy (EGD) for unrelated indications [7]. While most ampullary lesions are asymptomatic, common presenting symptoms may include obstructive jaundice, pancreatitis, nonspecific abdominal pain, and gastrointestinal bleeding or anemia [3, 8, 9].

EGD is the first indicated diagnostic intervention to evaluate macroscopic features and permit forceps biopsy to confirm malignancy or dysplasia (Fig. 14.1a). Benign pathology after endoscopic forceps biopsy should be interpreted with caution, as false negative rates range from 19–60% and vary with the size of the as-

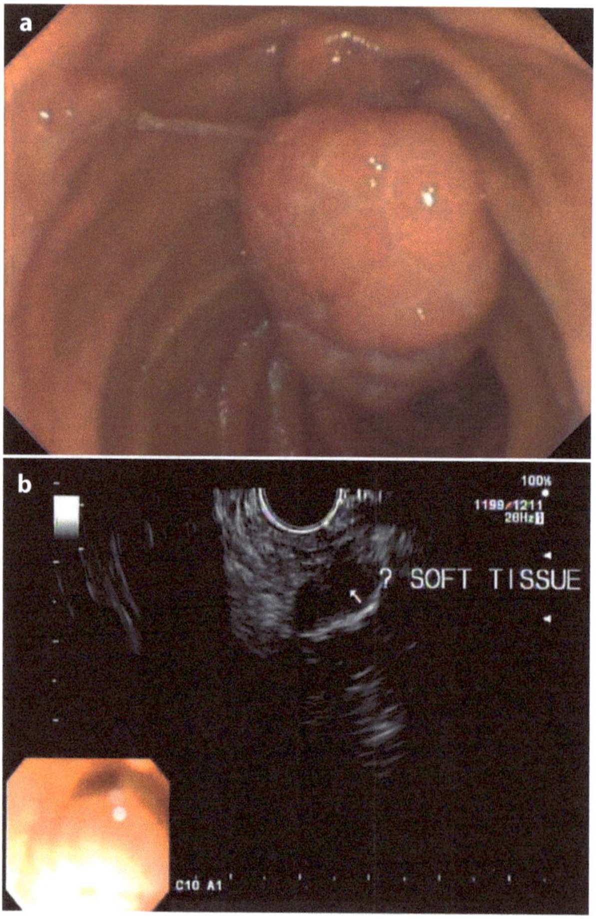

Fig. 14.1 **a** EGD showing a 3-cm partially pedunculated, periampullary adenoma which obstructed views of the biliary orifice. **b** On endoscopic ultrasound (EUS) there appeared to be soft tissue infiltration of the common bile duct, which was dilated to 9 mm. The patient was referred for surgical evaluation and underwent robot-assisted transduodenal ampullary resection (TDAR). Final pathology demonstrated adenoma with high-grade dysplasia, but no evidence of invasive carcinoma

sociated lesion [10]. Endoscopic features may provide sufficient evidence to determine treatment planning. Endoscopic resection is performed in the absence of macroscopic signs of malignancy (see below) for lesions less than 1 cm in diameter without endoscopic ultrasound [10]. Endoscopic ultrasound (EUS) improves local staging of ampullary lesions and detects intraductal extension of the tumor with a high sensitivity/accuracy for T staging in cases of invasive cancer [11].

14.3 Selection Factors for TDAR

Potential surgical approaches vary in complexity and potential morbidity from endoscopic techniques to minimally invasive and open TDAR followed by pancreatoduodenectomy. Published data comparing the outcomes of endoscopic and surgical TDAR have so far included only the open technique. Recent studies evaluating minimally invasive TDAR are confined to short-term outcomes of modest retrospective case series [3, 12–16].

Pancreatoduodenectomy remains the standard of care for ampullary adenocarcinoma due to superior overall survival, lymph node harvest and margin clearance compared to TDAR [17–20]. There is ongoing debate regarding TDAR for T1 ampullary adenocarcinoma in patients with significant comorbid conditions [2, 7, 21].

Current selection criteria favoring TDAR over endoscopic resection include any of the following features:

- Ampullary adenoma with high-grade dysplasia or carcinoma in situ [22, 23].
- Lesions encompassing greater than 1/3 of the duodenal circumference [5, 24]
- Size greater than 2cm given the increased risk of malignancy and morbidity [2, 25]
- Obstructive jaundice [23, 26]
- Macroscopic features suggesting a high likelihood of recurrence or failure of endoscopic resection, such as:
  - Firmness, ulceration, friability, or bleeding [27]
  - Non- or inadequate lift of the periampullary component after submucosal injection to achieve adequate cleavage plane for endoscopic resection [10, 28]
  - Invasion beyond the muscularis layer [27]
- Extension into the common bile duct or pancreatic duct >5 mm by EUS (Fig. 14.1b). Lesser intraductal extension may permit snare ampullectomy [29].

14.4 Technical Aspects of Minimally Invasive TDAR

The following technical aspects of minimally invasive TDAR apply regardless of the laparoscopic or robotic approach.

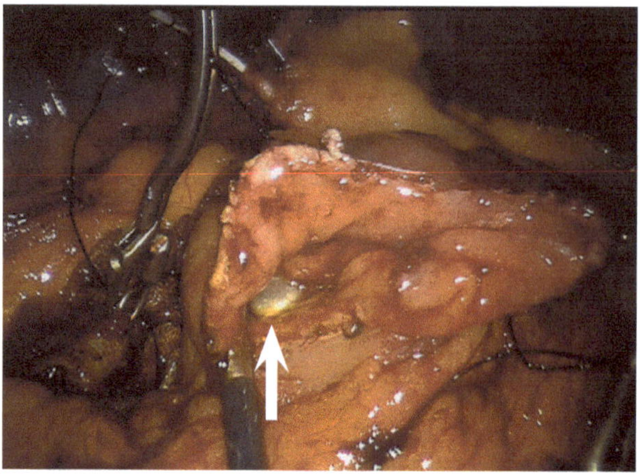

Fig. 14.2 A Fogarty catheter can be used to define the precise location of the ampulla. The image depicts the catheter balloon (*white arrow*) as it exits the ampulla in the lumen of the duodenum (reproduced with permission from [3])

1. *Complete duodenal mobilization* The duodenum is mobilized by dividing its retroperitoneal attachments from the foramen of Winslow to the medial border of the aorta inferiorly in order to assure *en face* exposure of the ampulla and eventual tension-free duodenal closure. The hepatic flexure is mobilized and swung inferiorly and using an energy device in combination with blunt dissection. Gauze sponge pads are placed behind the pancreatic head to rotate the duodenum anteriorly.
2. *Identification of the ampulla* Tailoring the location and length of the duodenotomy is critical to successful exposure of the ampulla without subsequent tension during a planned transverse repair. Whereas the open approach relies on direct palpation of the ampulla through the duodenal wall, intraoperative ultrasound is usually sufficient to identify the ampullary complex by following the intrapancreatic segment of the bile duct to its junction with the pancreatic duct. As required, the cystic duct can be accessed during cholecystectomy to cannulate the distal bile duct, which is then easily identified by ultrasound as it crosses the medial duodenal wall (Fig. 14.2). Intraoperative endoscopy may be used to identify the ampulla but is much less efficient due to the introduction of air into the GI tract, which must be controlled by clamping the proximal jejunum [13].
3. *Exposing the ampulla* (Fig. 14.3) Stay sutures are placed on the medial and lateral surfaces of the duodenum adjacent to the ampulla. Laparoscopic bulldog clamps are used as weights to retract the duodenal wall as a 3–4-cm longitudinal incision is made along the antimesenteric border with cautery scissors. A transfixing suture is placed at the superior aspect of the ampulla and/or stent to expose its inferior border.
4. *Resecting the ampulla* (Fig. 14.4) The mucosa is incised with cautery scissors down to the submucosa 5–10 mm circumferentially around the lesion. Dissection is continued in the submucosal plane, while electrocautery is

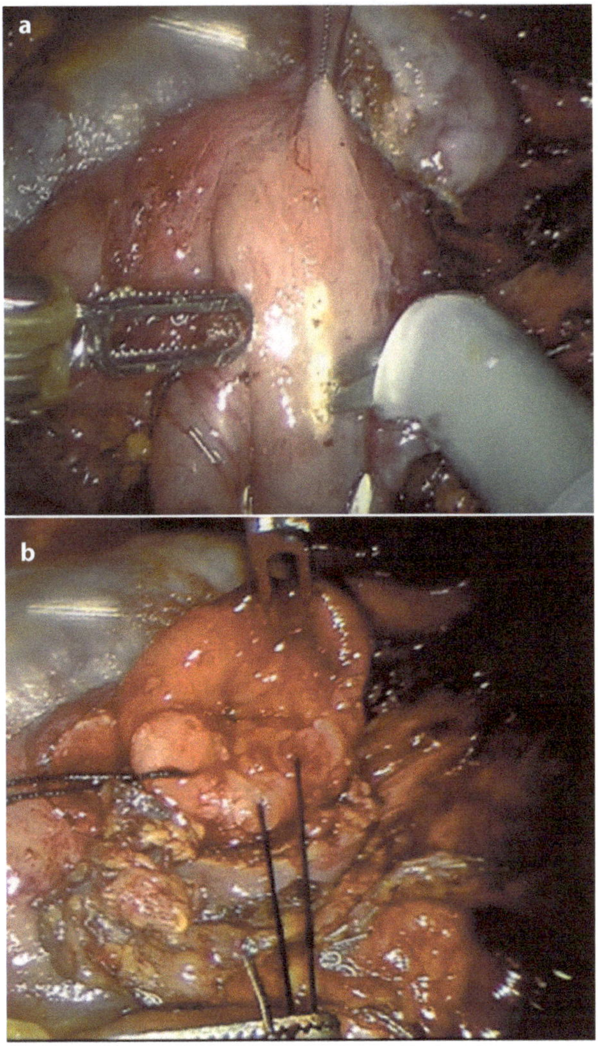

Fig. 14.3 **a** The duodenum is retracted and a 3–4-cm longitudinal incision is made in the duodenum. **b** Once identified, a stay suture is placed through the superior aspect of the ampulla and retracted to facilitate exposure

used to coagulate bridging vessels to maximize visualization and prevent an otherwise obscured field. As the bile duct wall is incised, a fine absorbable polyfilament suture (such as 5-0 vicryl) is placed along its edge to prevent retraction. Identifying the bile duct is simplified when a transcystic catheter is in place. Similarly, a careful search for the adjacent pancreatic duct is made, and the duct is cannulated with a 5-Fr stent in advance of reconstruction. The specimen is retrieved within a specimen bag.

5. *Bile and pancreatic duct reconstruction/sphincteroplasty* The walls of the bile and pancreatic ducts are circumferentially reapproximated to adjacent

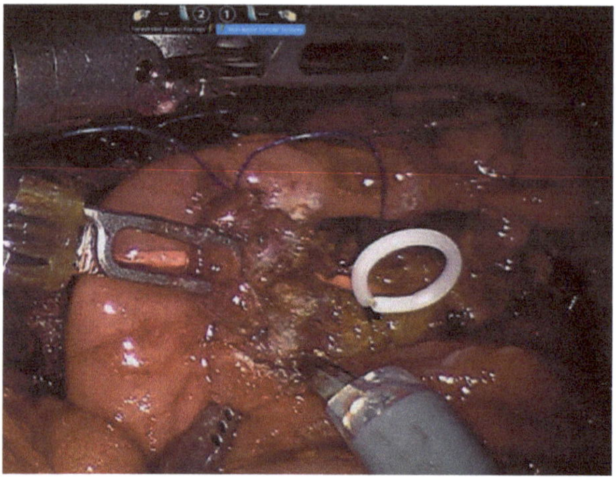

Fig. 14.4 With the robotic grasper retracting the ampullary mass (*left*), the dissection is carried out circumferentially down to the submucosa with the cautery scissors (reproduced with permission from [3])

duodenal mucosa with 5-0 Vicryl sutures. Both anastomoses are preferentially cannulated with biliary and pancreatic duct stents to prevent postprocedure pancreatitis or jaundice. The orifice of the bile duct can be enlarged by dividing the duct along its roof in order to inspect the mucosa for intraductal extension and a proximal bile duct margin can be retrieved for frozen section examination. If the pancreatic duct is difficult to visualize or cannulate, secretin can be administered intraoperatively.

6. *Duodenotomy closure* We close the duodenum preferentially in a transverse manner in two layers. In order to prevent a dog-ear at the corners, we favor a Connell technique using 4-0 v-loc suture followed by seromuscular closure in Lembert fashion. Drain placement is at the surgeon's discretion.
7. *Lymphadenectomy* Lymph node dissection can be performed as indicated for enlarged nodes [13, 21] but is likely an indication of malignancy, for which pancreatoduodenectomy is preferred.
8. *Frozen section analysis* Gross and microscopic clearance is the goal of TDAR. Microscopic examination of circumferential margins obtained through normal-appearing mucosa is of questionable intraoperative benefit except in cases of known high-grade dysplasia or in site carcinoma [13].

14.5 Outcomes of Minimally Invasive TDAR

14.5.1 Postoperative Surveillance

Patients with adenomas and other lesions at risk for recurrence require endoscopic surveillance. Following endoscopic resection, repeat EGD should be performed at three months and one year postpapillectomy. In the absence of no recurrence after two years, further follow-up is based on symptoms [29]. Factors associated with increased risk of recurrence include two or more endoscopic resections needed to achieve complete tumor removal (13-fold greater recurrence risk) and those with FAP or other genetic syndromes [30]. In these cases, longer-term surveillance may be required.

14.5.2 Complications

Endoscopic ampullectomy is the preferred approach for ampullary adenomas without an indication for surgical excision as described above [5]. In the largest series to-date composed of 115 patients, Tsuji et al. [31] described a success rate of 80.9%. The most common postprocedure complications were bleeding (18.2%) and pancreatitis (10.4%). Patients were followed up to one year for long-term complications, yielding 5 cases with papillary stenosis. Predictors of successful endoscopic ampullectomy were lesion size <25 mm and the absence of a genetic predisposition to adenoma formation. In a retrospective review of 109 patients undergoing either endoscopic (n = 68) or surgical ampullectomy (n = 41), Ceppa et al. found that endoscopic was superior to surgical ampullectomy in terms of morbidity, length of stay and readmission rates [6]. Scattered reports advocating for extending the indication of endoscopic ampullectomy to early-stage carcinoma are limited to retrospective, single-institution studies with multiple confounders and suggest higher recurrence rates compared to open TDAR in exchange for more favorable short-term outcomes [29, 32].

Minimally invasive ampullectomy may provide oncologic benefits equivalent to open with improved short-term outcomes. Laparoscopic TDAR for carcinoma in situ or T1 tumors is limited to case reports [14, 33]. The technical challenge of biliary and pancreatic reconstruction during laparoscopic TDAR is significantly alleviated using the robotic technique due to wristed articulation, magnified 3D visualization, and computer-aided reduction of operator tremor for stabilization. Downs-Canner et al. retrospectively reviewed 26 patients with benign and premalignant lesions who underwent robot-assisted duodenal resection, nine of which were ampullectomies. They reported a 15% incidence of grade III and IV Clavien-Dindo complications with zero conversions to open resection [3].

14.6 Conclusions

Minimally invasive TDAR may duplicate the advantages of open ampullectomy in terms of pathological indications and reconstructive options while maintaining the short-term advantages of endoscopic therapy. The robotic technique is particularly well suited to the fine suturing necessary to reconstruct the biliary and pancreatic duct orifices and most closely approximates the open technique.

Future multicenter studies are necessary to gather sufficient prospective evidence of durable benefit given the low incidence of this procedure at any one institution.

Acknowledgements
We are grateful to our non-profit funding partners, without whom this work would not have been possible: the Alliance of Families Fighting Pancreatic Cancer, the Greg and Cathy Griffith Family Foundation, and the John F. Fortney Charitable Pancreatic Cancer Research Foundation.

References

1. Halsted WS (1899) Contributions to the surgery of the bile passages, especially of the common bile-duct. Boston Med Surg J 141(26):645–654
2. Gao Y, Zhu Y, Huang X et al (2016) Transduodenal ampullectomy provides a less invasive technique to cure early ampullary cancer. BMC Surg 16(1):36
3. Downs-Canner S, Van der Vliet WJ, Thoolen SJ et al (2015) Robotic surgery for benign duodenal tumors. J Gastrointest Surg 19(2):306–312
4. Martin JA, Haber GB (2003) Ampullary adenoma: clinical manifestations, diagnosis, and treatment. Gastrointest Endosc Clin N Am 13(4):649–669
5. Patel R, Varadarajulu S, Wilcox CM (2012) Endoscopic ampullectomy: techniques and outcomes. J Clin Gastroenterol 46(1):8–15
6. Ceppa EP, Burbridge RA, Rialon KL et al (2013) Endoscopic versus surgical ampullectomy: an algorithm to treat disease of the ampulla of Vater. Ann Surg 257(2):315–322
7. Askew J, Connor S (2013) Review of the investigation and surgical management of resectable ampullary adenocarcinoma. HPB (Oxford) 15(11):829–838
8. Espinel J, Pinedo E, Ojeda V, Guerra Del Río M (2016) Endoscopic ampullectomy: a technical review. Rev Esp Enferm Dig 108(5):271–278
9. Mansukhani VM, Desai GS, Mouli S et al (2017) Transduodenal ampullectomy for ampullary tumors. Indian J Gastroenterol 36(1):62–65
10. Standards of Practice Committee, Adler DG, Qureshi W, Davila R et al (2006) The role of endoscopy in ampullary and duodenal adenomas. Gastrointest Endosc 64(6):849–854
11. Ridtitid W, Schmidt SE, Al-Haddad MA et al (2015) Performance characteristics of EUS for locoregional evaluation of ampullary lesions. Gastrointest Endosc 81(2):380–388
12. Ahn KS, Han HS, Yoon YS et al (2010) Laparoscopic transduodenal ampullectomy for benign ampullary tumors. J Laparoendosc Adv Surg Tech A 20(1):59–63
13. Marzano E, Ntourakis D, Addeo P et al (2011) Robotic resection of duodenal adenoma. Int J Med Robot 7(1):66–70
14. Rosen M, Zuccaro G, Brody F (2003) Laparoscopic resection of a periampullary villous adenoma. Surg Endosc 17(8):1322–1323
15. Zhang RC, Xu XW, Wu D et al (2013) Laparoscopic transduodenal local resection of periampullary neuroendocrine tumor: a case report. World J Gastroenterol 19(39):6693–6698
16. Borie F, Zarzavadjian Le Bian A (2013) Laparoscopic ampullectomy for an ampullarian adenoma. Surg Endosc 27(11):4385
17. Berberat PO, Kunzli BM, Gulbinas A et al (2009) An audit of outcomes of a series of periampullary carcinomas. Eur J Surg Oncol 35(2):187–191
18. de Castro SM, van Heek NT, Kuhlmann KF et al (2004) Surgical management of neoplasms of the ampulla of Vater: local resection or pancreatoduodenectomy and prognostic factors for survival. Surgery 136(5):994–1002

19. Roggin KK, Yeh JJ, Ferrone CR et al (2005) Limitations of ampullectomy in the treatment of nonfamilial ampullary neoplasms. Ann Surg Oncol 12(12):971–980
20. Maithel SK, Fong Y (2008) Technical aspects of performing transduodenal ampullectomy. J Gastrointest Surg 12(9):1582–1585
21. Amini A, Miura JT, Jayakrishnan TT et al (2015) Is local resection adequate for T1 stage ampullary cancer? HPB (Oxford) 17(1):66–71
22. El Hajj II, Coté GA (2013) Endoscopic diagnosis and management of ampullary lesions. Gastrointest Endosc Clin N Am 23(1):95–109
23. Heidecke CD, Rosenberg R, Bauer M et al (2002) Impact of grade of dysplasia in villous adenomas of Vater's papilla. World J Surg 26(6):709–714
24. Schneider L, Contin P, Fritz S et al (2016) Surgical ampullectomy: an underestimated operation in the era of endoscopy. HPB (Oxford) 18(1):65–71
25. Fanning SB, Bourke MJ, Williams SJ et al (2012) Giant laterally spreading tumors of the duodenum: endoscopic resection outcomes, limitations, and caveats. Gastrointest Endosc 75(4):805–812
26. Ridtitid W, Tan D, Schmidt SE et al (2014) Endoscopic papillectomy: risk factors for incomplete resection and recurrence during long-term follow-up. Gastrointest Endosc 79(2): 289–296
27. Dubois M, Labgaa I, Dorta G, Halkic N (2016) Endoscopic and surgical ampullectomy for non-invasive ampullary tumors: short-term outcomes. BioSci Trends 10(6):507–511
28. Kahaleh M, Shami VM, Brock A et al (2004) Factors predictive of malignancy and endoscopic resectability in ampullary neoplasia. Am J Gastroenterol 99(12):2335–2339
29. Onkendi EO, Naik ND, Rosedahl JK et al (2014) Adenomas of the ampulla of Vater: a comparison of outcomes of operative and endoscopic resections. J Gastrointest Surg 18(9): 1588–1596
30. Posner S, Colletti L, Knol J et al (2000) Safety and long-term efficacy of transduodenal excision for tumors of the ampulla of Vater. Surgery 128(4):694–701
31. Tsuji S, Itoi T, Sofuni A et al (2015) Tips and tricks in endoscopic papillectomy of ampullary tumors: single-center experience with large case series (with videos). J Hepatobiliary Pancreat Sci 22(6):E22–E27
32. Woo SM, Ryu JK, Lee SH et al (2009) Feasibility of endoscopic papillectomy in early stage ampulla of Vater cancer. J Gastroenterol Hepatol 24(1):120–124
33. Honda G, Kurata M, Matsumura H et al (2010) Laparoscopy-assisted transduodenal papillectomy. Dig Surg 27(2):123–126

Role of Minimally Invasive Surgery in the Treatment of Pancreatic Neuroendocrine Tumors

15

Riccardo Ariotti, Francesca Muffatti, Valentina Andreasi, Stefano Partelli, and Massimo Falconi

15.1 Introduction

The laparoscopic approach in pancreatic surgery has been in general considered with caution, because of the inherent technical challenges of pancreatic surgery itself and the risk for postoperative complications [1–13].

Most of the studies, however, report the results achieved in distal pancreatectomy only and they were not specific on the underlying pathology. Whereas in several series adenocarcinomas dominate in the open pancreatic surgery group, benign lesions or tumors with low malignant potential constitute the majority of disease types in the laparoscopic experience.

Pancreatic neuroendocrine tumors (P-NETs) represent *per se* the ideal entities for laparoscopic surgery mainly for two reasons. First, most P-NETs are discovered incidentally when they are small in size and easily resectable [14]. Second, patients with P-NET are usually younger compared with those affected by ductal adenocarcinoma and they have usually a longer life expectancy.

15.2 Pancreatic Neuroendocrine Tumors

P-NETs are classified as either functioning or non-functioning tumors depending on whether or not they present with clinical syndromes associated with excess hormone secretion. Non-functioning tumors are the most frequent type of P-NET.

M. Falconi (✉)
Pancreas Translational and Clinical Research Center, Università Vita e Salute,
San Raffaele Scientific Institute
Milan, Italy
e-mail: falconi.massimo@hsr.it

U. Boggi (Ed), *Minimally Invasive Surgery of the Pancreas*,
Updates in Surgery
DOI: 10.1007/978-88-470-3958-2_15,

They are currently classified into three categories according to the Ki-67 proliferation index: G1 and G2 P-NETs and G3 pancreatic neuroendocrine carcinomas (P-NECs) [15]. G1 and G2 P-NETs usually exhibit a less aggressive behavior than G3 P-NECs [16]. The surgical strategy for P-NETs ranges from enucleation up to total pancreatectomy. Preoperative evaluation should take into account tumor grading, size, localization, relationship between the tumor and the main pancreatic duct, involvement of locoregional anatomical structures, and presence of metastases. The risk of lymph node metastases is usually associated with both tumor grading and size [17, 18]. The larger the tumor (usually P-NETs >2 cm), the higher is the likelihood of associated nodal involvement.

For the detection of primary tumor, computed tomography (CT) or magnetic resonance imaging (MRI) should be used in conjunction with functional imaging, such as ^{68}Gallium positron emission tomography (PET/CT). Endoscopic ultrasound (US) and MRI can accurately determine the relationship of the lesion with the main pancreatic duct, with a sensitivity varying from 80% to 100%, especially when the two techniques are combined [19].

15.3 Surgical Options

Available studies focused on laparoscopic approach for P-NETs are summarized in Table 15.1. Nearly all of them are observational, retrospective studies or comparative analyses of laparoscopic and open cases [20–30].

Different surgical minimally invasive options such as pancreatoduodenectomy (PD) [31], distal pancreatectomy (DP) either spleen-preserving or combined with splenectomy, and enucleation have been described. However, most of the patients underwent DP or enucleation.

Enucleation is a surgical option that has been widely used in patients affected by P-NETs. A recent meta-analysis [32] has compared the outcomes of 1,101 patients who underwent either standard resection or enucleation. Enucleation appeared to be significantly shorter in operative time with a lower risk of blood loss compared to standard resection. Both enucleation and resection had similar mortality and complication rates, but the rate of pancreatic fistula was higher in the enucleation group. On the other hand, enucleation is associated with a significantly reduced incidence of exocrine and endocrine insufficiency.

Enucleation has proven its efficacy in P-NETs especially for small lesions with low malignant potential. An important issue in enucleation is related to lymph node dissection. In most cases, enucleation is performed with either no or limited lymphadenectomy. However, since P-NETs >2 cm are associated with a risk of lymph node metastases up to 56% [17, 18], enucleation should be avoided for lesions >2 cm. Therefore, the role of enucleation is currently limited as the majority of P-NETs <2 cm can be conservatively managed.

Table 15.1 Available studies focused on the laparoscopic approach for P-NETs

Authors	Year	Study type	Period of recruitment	Number of patients	LPS/OPEN
España-Gómez et al. [20]	2009	Retrospective	1995–2007	34	21/13
Gumbs et al. [21]	2008	Retrospective	1992–2006	31	18/13
Hu et al. [22]	2011	Retrospective	2000–2009	89	43/46
Karaliotas, Sgourakis [23]	2009	Retrospective	1999–2008	12	5/7
Kazanjian et al. [24]	2006	Retrospective	1990–2005	70	4/66
Liu et al. [25]	2007	Retrospective	2000–2006	48	7/41
Lo et al. [26]	2004	Retrospective	1999–2002	10	4/6
Roland et al. [27]	2008	Retrospective	1998–2007	37	22/15
Sa Cunha et al. [28]	2006	Retrospective	1999–2005	21	12/9
Zerbi et al. [29]	2011	Prospective	2004–2007	262	21/241
Zhao et al. [30]	2011	Retrospective	1990–2010	292	46/246

P-NETs, pancreatic neuroendocrine tumors; *LPS*, laparoscopic approach; *OPEN*, open approach.

15.4 Technical Aspects

Minimally invasive approaches for P-NETs include both laparoscopic and robot-assisted techniques.

In the last decade, also the robotic approach has been applied to pancreatic resection. In the specific field of P-NETs, a small number of series have been published, and at the present time only case reports or small series included in larger non-specific papers have been published [13, 33, 34]. The role of robotic-assisted pancreatic resection for P-NETs needs further evaluation to determine the possible advantages of this technique and to assess the duration of an adequate learning curve.

From the technical point of view, laparoscopic or robot-assisted pancreatic resection for P-NETs is performed with the same surgical technique used for any other indication to pancreatic surgery. Intraoperative ultrasound (US) is a useful tool during minimally invasive surgery for P-NETs as the nodule often cannot be easily identified. This is particularly true for insulinomas that are usually small in size and not always exophytic. Another specific feature of P-NETs is that they are typically hypervascularized tumors (Fig. 15.1). Therefore, these tumors are

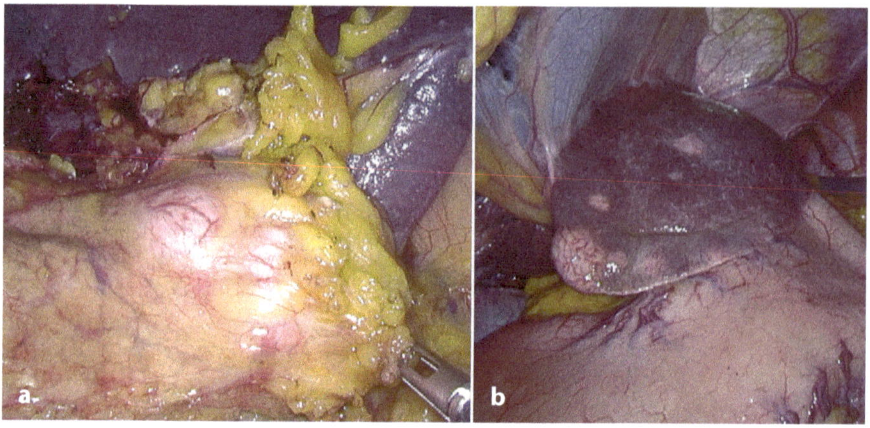

Fig. 15.1 Intraoperative findings of a patient affected by a P-NET of the pancreatic tail (**a**) with multiple liver metastases (**b**)

more prone to bleed. Careful manipulation of the tumor is mandatory in order to avoid bleeding from the tumor surface.

15.5 Surgical Outcomes

A recent meta-analysis comparing open (OPS) and laparoscopic (LPS) pancreatic surgery for P-NETs [14] has shown no differences in operative time between the two groups. On the contrary, laparoscopy has proven to allow a reduction in intraoperative blood loss. Moreover, the meta-analysis showed a significantly lower incidence of overall morbidity and a shorter length of hospital stay in the LPS group.

Despite these better outcomes, the incidence of pancreatic fistula is similar between patients treated with a minimally invasive approach and those who underwent open P-NET resection.

Another meta-analysis confirmed these results, but it pointed out a significant lack of data regarding long-term outcomes [35].

The robot-assisted approach for DP has shown improved lymph node yield for both benign and malignant lesions compared to laparoscopy [36]. Similar results have also been observed after robot-assisted DP for P-NETs, although the role of lymphadenectomy in this setting is still controversial [37].

Haugvik et al. [38] reported a disease-specific 5-year survival of patients who underwent laparoscopic P-NET removal of 90%. Unfortunately, this study did not provide a comparison between patients treated with a minimally invasive approach versus those treated with an open pancreatic resection.

The minimally invasive approach has shown satisfactory outcomes also in the setting of patients affected by type 1 multiple endocrine neoplasia (MEN1) syndrome [39].

MEN1-affected patients with P-NETs represent the ideal candidates for a minimally invasive approach for several reasons. First, the majority of MEN1 patients are young and they have a long life expectancy. Secondly, the majority of them will need further pancreatic resection for recurrent P-NETs during their life. A minimally invasive approach, including preservation of parenchyma and the spleen appears to be a good option to avoid a completion pancreatectomy. This may also have a beneficial effect on the quality of life of these young patients and may reduce long-term problems such as diabetes mellitus, adhesions, and incisional hernias [39].

15.6 Conclusions

Minimally invasive pancreatic surgery is safe and feasible also in patients affected by P-NETs.

Although laparoscopic pancreatic resection for P-NETs has similar short-term outcomes compared to open surgery, there is a substantial lack of data on the oncological safety of this approach. Prospective comparative studies are urgently needed in order to compare long-term outcomes between laparoscopic and open procedures also in patients affected by P-NETs.

References

1. Gagner M, Pomp A (1994) Laparoscopic pylorus-preserving pancreatoduodenectomy. Surg Endosc 8(5):408–410
2. Cuschieri A (1994) Laparoscopic surgery of the pancreas. J R Coll Surg Edinb 39(3):178–184
3. Sussman LA, Christie R, Whittle DE (1996) Laparoscopic excision of distal pancreas including insulinoma. Aust N Z J Surg 66(6):414–416
4. Fernández-Cruz L, Cosa R, Blanco L et al (2007) Curative laparoscopic resection for pancreatic neoplasms: a critical analysis from a single institution. J Gastrointest Surg 11(12):1607–1621; discussion 1621–1622
5. Mabrut JY, Fernández-Cruz L, Azagra JS et al (2005) Laparoscopic pancreatic resection: results of a multicenter European study of 127 patients. Surgery 137(6):597–605
6. Weber SM, Cho CS, Merchant N et al (2009) Laparoscopic left pancreatectomy: complication risk score correlates with morbidity and risk for pancreatic fistula. Ann Surg Oncol 16(10):2825–2833
7. Baker MS, Bentrem DJ, Ujiki MB et al (2009) A prospective single institution comparison of peri-operative outcomes for laparoscopic and open distal pancreatectomy. Surgery 146(4):635–643; discussion 643–645
8. Cho CS, Kooby DA, Schmidt CM et al (2011) Laparoscopic versus open left pancreatectomy: can preoperative factors indicate the safer technique? Ann Surg 253(5):975–980
9. Kooby DA, Gillespie T, Bentrem D et al (2008) Left-sided pancreatectomy: a multicenter comparison of laparoscopic and open approaches. Ann Surg 248(3):438–446
10. Vijan SS, Ahmed KA, Harmsen WS et al (2010) Laparoscopic vs open distal pancreatectomy: a single-institution comparative study. Arch Surg 145(7):616–621

11. Kleeff J, Diener MK, Z'graggen K et al (2007) Distal pancreatectomy: risk factors for surgical failure in 302 consecutive cases. Ann Surg 245(4):573–582
12. Winter JM, Cameron JL, Campbell KA et al (2006) 1423 pancreaticoduodenectomies for pancreatic cancer: a single-institution experience. J Gastrointest Surg 10(9):1199–1210; discussion 1210–1211
13. Strijker M, van Santvoort HC, Besselink MG et al (2013) Robot-assisted pancreatic surgery: a systematic review of the literature. HPB (Oxford) 15(1):1–10
14. Drymousis P, Raptis DA, Spalding D et al (2013) Laparoscopic versus open pancreas resection for pancreatic neuroendocrine tumours: a systematic review and meta-analysis. HPB (Oxford) 16(5):397–406
15. Bosman FT, Carneiro F, Hruban RH et al (eds) (2010) WHO classification of tumors of the digestive system. IARC Press, Lyon
16. Rindi G, Falconi M, Klersy C et al (2012) TNM staging of neoplasms of the endocrine pancreas: results from a large international cohort study. J Natl Cancer Inst 104(10):764–777
17. Partelli S, Gaujoux S, Boninsegna L et al (2013) Pattern and clinical predictors of lymph node involvement in nonfunctioning pancreatic neuroendocrine tumors (NF-PanNETs). JAMA Surg 148(10):932–939
18. Hashim YM, Trinkaus KM, Linehan DC et al (2014) Regional lymphadenectomy is indicated in the surgical treatment of pancreatic neuroendocrine tumors (PNETs). Ann Surg 259(2):197–203
19. Oberg K, Krenning E, Sundin A et al (2016) A Delphic consensus assessment: imaging and biomarkers in gastroenteropancreatic neuroendocrine tumor disease management. Endocr Connect 5(5):174–187
20. España-Gómez MN, Velázquez-Fernández D, Bezaury P et al (2009) Pancreatic insulinoma: a surgical experience. World J Surg 33(9):1966–1970
21. Gumbs AA, Grès P, Madureira F, Gayet B (2008) Laparoscopic vs open resection of pancreatic endocrine neoplasms: single institution's experience over 14 years. Langenbecks Arch Surg 393(3):391–395
22. Hu M, Zhao G, Luo Y, Liu R (2011) Laparoscopic versus open treatment for benign pancreatic insulinomas: an analysis of 89 cases. Surg Endosc 25(12):3831–3837
23. Karaliotas C, Sgourakis G (2009) Laparoscopic versus open enucleation for solitary insulinoma in the body and tail of the pancreas. J Gastrointest Surg 13(10):1869
24. Kazanjian KK, Reber HA, Hines OJ (2006) Resection of pancreatic neuroendocrine tumours: results of 70 cases. Arch Surg 141(8):765–769; discussion 769–770
25. Liu H, Peng C, Zhang S et al (2007) Strategy for the surgical management of insulinomas: analysis of 52 cases. Dig Surg 24(6):463–470
26. Lo CY, Chan WF, Lo CM et al (2004) Surgical treatment of pancreatic insulinomas in the era of laparoscopy. Surg Endosc 18(2):297–302
27. Roland CL, Lo CY, Miller BS et al (2008) Surgical approach and perioperative complications determine short-term outcomes in patients with insulinoma: results of a bi-institutional study. Ann Surg Oncol 15(12):3532–3537
28. Sa Cunha A, Beau C, Rault A et al (2007) Laparoscopic versus open approach for solitary insulinoma. Surg Endosc 21(1):103–108
29. Zerbi A, Capitanio V, Boninsegna L et al (2011) Surgical treatment of pancreatic endocrine tumours in Italy: results of a prospective multicentre study of 262 cases. Langenbecks Arch Surg 396(3):313–321
30. Zhao YP, Zhan HX, Zhang TP et al (2011) Surgical management of patients with insulinomas: result of 292 cases in a single institution. J Surg Oncol 103(2):169–174
31. Boggi U, Amorese G, Vistoli F et al (2015) Laparoscopic pancreaticoduodenectomy: a systematic literature review. Surg Endosc 29(1):9–23
32. Chua TC, Yang TX, Gill AJ, Samra JS (2016) Systematic review and meta-analysis of enucleation versus standardized resection for small pancreatic lesions. Ann Surg Oncol 23(2):592–599

33. Melvin WS, Needleman BJ, Krause KR, Ellison EC (2003) Robotic resection of pancreatic neuroendocrine tumor. J Laparoendosc Adv Surg Tech A 13(1):33–36
34. Fernandez Ranvier GG, Shouhed D, Inabnet WB 3rd (2016) Minimally invasive techniques for resection of pancreatic neuroendocrine tumors. Surg Oncol Clin N Am 25(1):195–215
35. Tamburrino D, Partelli S, Renzi C et al (2017) Systematic review and meta-analysis on laparoscopic pancreatic resections for neuroendocrine neoplasms (PNENs). Expert Rev Gastroenterol Hepatol 1(1):65–73
36. Daouadi M, Zureikat AH, Zenati MS et al (2013) Robot-assisted minimally invasive distal pancreatectomy is superior to the laparoscopic technique. Ann Surg 257(1):128–132
37. Muffatti F, Adamenko O, Partelli S et al (2016) Comparison of robot-assisted and laparoscopic minimally invasive approaches for pancreatic neuroendocrine neoplasms. HPB (Oxford) 18(Suppl 2):e774–e775
38. Haugvik SP, Kaemmerer D, Gaujoux S et al (2016) Pathology and surgical treatment of high-grade pancreatic neuroendocrine carcinoma: an evolving landscape. Curr Oncol Rep 18(5):28
39. Lopez CL, Albers MB, Bollmann C et al (2016) Minimally invasive versus open pancreatic surgery in patients with multiple endocrine neoplasia type 1. World J Surg 40(7):1729–1736

Minimally Invasive Enucleation of Pancreatic Tumors

16

Santiago Sánchez Cabús and Laureano Fernández-Cruz

16.1 Introduction

Among the techniques for parenchyma-preserving pancreatic resection, we have two options: pancreatic enucleation and middle pancreatectomy, with the advantages of better endocrine and exocrine function compared to distal pancreatectomy. Over the years, the feasibility and safety of minimally invasive pancreatic enucleation (MIPE) have been shown. This chapter presents the indications for MIPE and the outcomes of patients undergoing the procedure.

16.2 MIPE: Indications and Contraindications

16.2.1 Indications for Performing MIPE

There is general consensus on the criteria for safe performance of MIPE:

- *Benign or borderline malignant lesions* [1] in the preoperative evaluation, such as pancreatic neuroendocrine tumors (P-NETs), intraductal papillary mucinous neoplasms (IPMN), mucinous cystic neoplasms (MCNs), and selected cases of metastases of renal cell carcinoma.
- *Small lesions*. Generally, the size of the tumor should be ≤3 cm [2–4].
- *Lesions not in contact with the main pancreatic duct*. There must be a minimum distance between the tumor and the main pancreatic duct (MPD) that ranges from 2 to 3 mm, in order to avoid injury to the MPD [5, 6]. The ideal

S. Sánchez Cabús (✉)
Department of Hepato-Pancreato-Biliary Surgery and Transplantation, ICMDiM.
Hospital Clínic de Barcelona
Barcelona, Spain
e-mail: ssanche1@clinic.ub.es

U. Boggi (Ed), *Minimally Invasive Surgery of the Pancreas*,
Updates in Surgery
DOI: 10.1007/978-88-470-3958-2_16, © Springer-Verlag Italia 2018

imaging modalities for determining this distance are computed tomography (CT) scan and magnetic resonance cholangiopancreatography (MRCP) in the preoperative setting, and confirmed by intraoperative ultrasound (IOUS) [7].

16.2.2 Contraindications to MIPE

- Large tumors that take up the majority of the pancreatic tissue.
- Multifocal lesions.
- Infiltrating lesions without a well-defined pseudocapsule.
- Lesions for which enucleation results in injury to the MPD.

16.3 Common Pancreatic Lesions Treated by MIPE

16.3.1 Pancreatic Neuroendocrine Tumors

Minimally invasive surgery and in particular MIPE seems to be an adequate treatment modality for patients with P-NETs, as stated by Fernández-Cruz et al. [8], in view of shorter hospital stay and acceptable pancreas-related complications; however, the postoperative pancreatic fistula (POPF) rate is higher than after pancreatic resection (PR). This group has reported the feasibility and safety of MIPE in non-functioning P-NETs [1], with good oncological results in terms of local recurrence. Recently, Jilesen et al. [9] compared pancreatic enucleation (PE) and PR in patients with P-NETs, and found no significant differences in terms of morbidity and mortality but better endocrine and exocrine function after MIPE. It is noteworthy in this report that patients with a P-NET ≤2 cm in the pancreatic head undergoing pancreatoduodenectomy (PD) had a lymph node involvement rate of 55%. These high figures of lymph node metastases in small tumors are not in agreement with other reports with large number of patients. In this regard, Edil et al. [10] showed a correlation between tumor size and lymph node involvement rate (<1 cm, 14%; 1–1.9 cm, 9%; 2–2.9 cm, 37%; 3–3.9 cm, 56%). We believe that, in non-functioning P-NETs selected for MIPE, lymph node sampling and frozen section examination are mandatory to rule out lymph node metastases; in cases of malignancy, a regional lymphadenectomy should be performed or conversion to open surgery to perform an oncological resection [1, 2, 11].

Among the P-NETs, pancreatic insulinoma is the most common indication for MIPE. Many studies reveal that MIPE for insulinoma is a safe and reproducible procedure with a high cure rate but also with a high POPF rate, particularly as regards lesions in the pancreatic head [8, 12–18]. In addition, recent studies show similar surgical outcomes between PE and surgical pancreatic resection (SPR) [19]. A recent meta-analysis comparing the laparoscopic and the open approach for the treatment of insulinoma has shown a reduced length of hospital stay without significant differences in postoperative mortality, morbidity, POPF, and recurrence or hyperglycemia [20]. In contrast, there are no large studies regarding MIPE in other functioning P-NETs.

Patients with MEN1 syndrome constitute a challenge. Fernández-Cruz et al. [21] showed good results after MIPE in insulinomas associated with MEN1, even though a conversion to open surgery might be indicated for multifocal lesions or tumors located in the pancreatic head. Nell et al. recently published equivalent results after minimally invasive surgery in MEN1 patients comparing the outcomes of robotic surgery (n = 7) with those obtained after laparoscopic surgery (n = 14). However, this report did not specify how many patients were treated by MIPE or by pancreatic resection [22].

16.3.2 Mucinous Neoplasms: IPMN and MCN

Pancreatic enucleation of low-risk branch-duct IPMN located at the head of the pancreas and the uncinate process is a good alternative to PD. Turrini et al. compared PE and PD for low-risk side-branch IPMN and noted a shorter operative time and less blood loss in PE patients [23]. Hwang et al. published a comparative study between PD (10 patients) and PE (4 patients) for branch-duct IPMN, showing similar results [24]. Also, Soejima et al. showed in a comparative study between PD and PE lesser operative time and blood loss in the PE group, as well as a notably reduced rate of endocrine insufficiency (0% vs.42.8%), with equal postoperative complications and maintaining a 0% recurrence rate [25]. Recently, a combined experience from Heidelberg and Stuttgart has been reported on PE for side-branch IPMN, comparing it with PR. Of the 74 patients with PE, 64 branch-duct IPMN revealed 85% low-, 11% moderate-, and 4% high-grade dysplasia on histology. Postoperative morbidity including postoperative POPF was similar in both groups. No mortality occurred after enucleation; after formal resection, one patient died due to multiorgan failure. Both hospital stay (10 vs. 14 days) and rates of postoperative endocrine and exocrine dysfunction were less after enucleation. IPMN-specific recurrence rates (3% vs. 6%) were similar in both groups [26].

There is limited information about the enucleation of MCNs. Ohtsuka et al. recently published their results after laparoscopic resection of MCNs. However only one out of 21 patients included underwent a laparoscopic PE [27].

16.3.3 Other Tumors

Namur et al. reported one single laparoscopic PE for pseudopapillary neoplasm of the pancreas with a postoperative stay of 4 days and without recurrence after a follow-up of 38 months [28]. There are also other reports in the literature of MIPE for different tumors, although the numbers are small [29–31]. The only malignant indication for performing a MIPE in some selected cases, as advocated by some authors, is pancreatic metastases from renal cell carcinoma, since nodal dissection is not mandatory [32, 33].

16.4 Perioperative Outcomes

All MIPE series show a very low mortality rate, except for only one series that reported one death due to acute mesenteric ischemia [4], which accounts for a 4% mortality in that particular report. All other published series either do not explicitly mention mortality or show a uniform immediate mortality rate of 0%.

16.4.1 MIPE Compared to SPR

Compared to SPR, MIPE is associated with reduced blood loss, operative time and postoperative hospital stay without a compromise in either endocrine or exocrine function. Fernández-Cruz et al. noted that POPF was significantly more clinically relevant after MIPE than after other SPR [8]. Cauley et al. compared 45 patients undergoing PE (16 of them laparoscopic PE) for a variety of pancreatic lesions to a matched cohort of 90 patients undergoing PD or distal pancreatectomy (DP), confirming the same results [34]. More recently, two systematic reviews and meta-analyses conducted by Zhou et al. and by Hüttner et al. showed that, the operation time, blood loss, length of hospital stay, and the incidence of endocrine and exocrine insufficiency were all significantly reduced after PE compared with SPR [35, 36].

16.4.2 MIPE Compared to Open PE

MIPE seems to offer advantages over open PE as well. The POPF rate after MIPE is reported in the published series between 0% and 77.8%, with an average POPF rate of about 30–35%, which seems to be similar to open procedures [37]. Some series reported rates between 4% and 25% of clinically relevant POPF, i.e. grades B and C in the International Study Group of Pancreatic Fistula (ISGPF)- classification [38]. Apparently, POPF is more closely related to the distance of the tumor to the MPD than to the surgical approach; Heeger et al.

showed that clinically relevant POPF and overall complications were higher in patients with less than 3 mm between the tumor and the MPD [7]. In addition, there seems to be a significantly increased risk of POPF in patients undergoing MIPE in right-sided pancreatic lesions [39, 40]. However, we believe that in the majority of circumstances the origin of the pancreatic fistula are the small ducts left open in the hole created in the pancreas after the enucleation. A few comparative studies have been recently published showing similar outcomes in terms of POPF: Song et al. published their results in a non-randomized comparative study of 65 patients that showed no differences in outcome between patients undergoing PE and MIPE [5], and Zhang et al. [41] showed that, compared to open PE, MIPE had shorter operating time, lower estimated blood loss, and faster recovery, with comparable preservation of pancreatic function. Concerning robotic PE, Zureikat et al. [42] reported on 10 robotic PE, with an operative time of 204 ± 67 minutes, and a 30% rate of clinical significant complications, a hospital stay of 5 (3–12) days, with a 20% rate of grade B POPF. Moreover, Boggi et al. [43] recently published a series of 12 robotic PE. The results are excellent with reported operative time of 167 ± 177 min, a postoperative hospital stay of 7.0 days (5.3–9.8), and only one patient (8.3%) presenting a grade B POPF, which did not require reintervention. Two other recent comparative studies between open and robotic PE for different pancreatic neoplasms showed better results of robotic PE in terms of blood loss and shorter operative time without differences in morbidity [44, 45].

16.5 Long-term Outcomes

PE is the surgical procedure associated with the maximum preservation of pancreatic tissue. Authors who have evaluated the incidence of postoperative pancreatic endocrine and exocrine insufficiency have shown a very low prevalence of pancreatic insufficiency (around 4–5%), that is, 4–5-fold less compared to DP.

Since patients treated with MIPE usually have benign or low-grade malignant pancreatic lesions, oncologic results in terms of local recurrence in the reported series are excellent. However, most of the series do not explicitly report tumor recurrence and, although for many of them recurrence is 0%, we can find some authors that report a tumor recurrence rate as high as 25% [14]. Recently, a reported recurrence rate of 19% has been reported in patients after PE for non-functioning P-NET, but the number of patients operated with MIPE is not stated [40].

Table 16.1 summarizes the characteristics and outcomes of the main series concerning MIPE, published from 1996 to 2016.

Table 16.1 Characteristics and outcomes of the main published series concerning minimally invasive pancreatic enucleation (MIPE)

Authors	Year	Number of cases	Conversion	Overall complications	Pancreatic fistula	Clinically relevant POPF	Mortality	Operative time	Blood loss	Length of stay	Follow-up	Recurrence	Endocrine insufficiency	Exocrine insufficiency
*Gagner et al. [46, 47]	1996	1	0	n/a	n/a	n/a	0%	180	n/a	4	27	0%	n/a	n/a
*Chapuis et al. [48]	1998	4	25%	25%	25%	25%	0%	160	200	5	n/a	n/a	n/a	n/a
*Berends et al. [49]	2000	9	44.4%	66.6%	50%	n/a	0%	180	<100	7	18	0%	n/a	n/a
*Fernández-Cruz et al. [50]	2002	4	0%	50%	50%	n/a	0%	204	200	5	n/a	n/a	n/a	n/a
*Iihara et al. [51]	2003	6	16.7%	66.6%	60%	n/a	0%	170	15	n/a	n/a	n/a	n/a	n/a
*Edwin et al. [52]	2004	7	n/a	n/a	n/a	n/a	0%	120	100	5.5	n/a	n/a	n/a	n/a
*Jaroszewski et al. [53]	2004	6	50%	33.3%	16%	n/a	0%	n/a	n/a	n/a	29	1	n/a	n/a
*Ayav et al. [54]	2005	19	10.5%	42%	n/a	n/a	0%	115	n/a	11	n/a	n/a	n/a	n/a
*Mabrut et al. [55]	2005	24	12.5%	33.3%	8.3%	n/a	0%	120	n/a	n/a	n/a	0%	n/a	n/a
*Giger et al. [56]	2006	4	25%	n/a	n/a	n/a	0%	155	92.5	5	22	0%	0%	0%
*Fernández-Cruz et al. [57]	2006	15	0%	n/a	40%	n/a	0%	n/a	n/a	n/a	n/a	n/a	n/a	n/a
*Schraibman et al. [58]	2007	5	0%	n/a	n/a	n/a	0%	130	"minimal"	3	n/a	n/a	n/a	n/a
*Sweet et al. [59]	2007	9	22%	77.8%	77.8%	n/a	0%	n/a	n/a	4.4	n/a	n/a	n/a	n/a
*Liu et al. [15]	2007	9	33.3%	22.2%	n/a	n/a	n/a	159	77	11.8	n/a	n/a	n/a	n/a
*Pierce et al. [60]	2007	4	25%	0%	0%	n/a	0%	248	92.5	3	n/a	n/a	n/a	n/a
*Fernández-Cruz et al. [61]	2007	20	5%	40%	35%	15%	0%	120	220	5.5	n/a	n/a	n/a	n/a
*Crippa et al. [62]	2007	4	n/a	43%	38%	n/a	0%	162	n/a	14	n/a	n/a	n/a	n/a

*Fernández-Cruz et al. [8]	2008	21	n/a	42.8%	38%	19%	0%	120	<220	5.5	n/a	n/a	n/a	n/a
*Karaliotas et al. [14]	2009	5	25%	n/a	20%	n/a	0%	121	n/a	11	53	25%	n/a	n/a
*Luo et al. [63]	2009	16	12.5%	n/a	50%	0%	0%	85	205	n/a	19	0%	0%	n/a
*Isla et al. [64]	2009	14	7.1%	n/a	n/a	n/a	n/a	n/a	n/a	n/a	n/a	n/a	n/a	n/a
*Røsok et al. [65]	2010	19	5.2%	n/a	26%	n/a	0%	140	55	n/a	n/a	n/a	n/a	n/a
*Dedieu et al. [4]	2011	23	8.6%	17%	13%	4%	4%	124	64	n/a	53	0%	0%	0%
*Zhao et al. [17]	2011	30	40%	n/a	n/a	n/a	n/a	n/a	n/a	n/a	n/a	n/a	n/a	n/a
*Costi et al. [66]	2012	29	21%	41%	36%	n/a	0%	144	112	18	n/a	n/a	n/a	n/a
*Fernández-Cruz et al. [1]	2012	13	0%	n/a	38%	23%	0%	130	220	6	48	7.6%	n/a	n/a
*Machado et al. [67]	2013	18	n/a	n/a	n/a	n/a	n/a	n/a	n/a	n/a	n/a	n/a	n/a	n/a
*Costi et al. [39]	2013	25	12%	56%	56%	n/a	0%	158	106	18	n/a	n/a	n/a	n/a
‡Zureikat et al. [42]	2013	10	n/a	50%	30%	20%	0%	206	n/a	5	n/a	n/a	n/a	n/a
*Choi et al. [68]	2014	11	0%	9.1%	9.1%	n/a	0%	97.4	35.9	5.5	44.3	0%	n/a	n/a
*Zhang et al. [69]	2015	15	0%	40%	40%	20%	0%	118	80	7.9	39	0%	0%	7.1%
°Thomas et al. [70]	2015	12	0%	n/a	33%	n/a	0%	n/a	n/a	6	33.6	0%	n/a	n/a
*Song et al. [5]	2015	30	0%	10.7%	10.7%	n/a	0%	123.8	n/a	7.8	58.7	n/a	n/a	n/a
‡Boggi et al. [43]	2016	12	0%	8.3%	8.3%	8.3%	0%	167	n/a	7	n/a	n/a	n/a	n/a
‡Jin et al. [44]	2016	31	0%	19%	74.2%	38.7%	0%	100	30	13	19.1	0%	0%	n/a

*Laparoscopic
°Hand-assisted
‡Robotic
POPF, postoperative pancreatic fistula; *n/a*, not available.

References

1 Fernández-Cruz L, Molina V, Vallejos R et al (2012) Outcome after laparoscopic enucleation for non-functional neuroendocrine pancreatic tumours. HPB (Oxford) 14(3):171–176
2 Crippa S, Boninsegna L, Partelli S, Falconi M (2010) Parenchyma-sparing resections for pancreatic neoplasms. J Hepatobiliary Pancreat Sci 17(6):782–787
3 Subar D, Gobardhan PD, Gayet B (2014) Laparoscopic pancreatic surgery: an overview of the literature and experiences of a single center. Best Pract Res Clin Gastroenterol 28(1):123–132
4 Dedieu A, Rault A, Collet D et al (2011) Laparoscopic enucleation of pancreatic neoplasm. Surg Endosc 25(2):572–576
5 Song KB, Kim SC, Hwang DW et al (2015) Enucleation for benign or low-grade malignant lesions of the pancreas: single-center experience with 65 consecutive patients. Surgery 158(5):1203–1210
6 Brient C, Regenet N, Sulpice L et al (2012) Risk factors for postoperative pancreatic fistulization subsequent to enucleation. J Gastrointest Surg 16(10):1883–1887
7 Heeger K, Falconi M, Partelli S et al (2014) Increased rate of clinically relevant pancreatic fistula after deep enucleation of small pancreatic tumors. Langenbecks Arch Surg 399(3):315–321
8 Fernández-Cruz L, Blanco L, Cosa R, Rendón H (2008) Is laparoscopic resection adequate in patients with neuroendocrine pancreatic tumors? World J Surg 32(5):904–917
9 Jilesen AP, Van Eijck CH, Busch OR et al (2016) Postoperative outcomes of enucleation and standard resections in patients with a pancreatic neuroendocrine tumor. World J Surg 40(3):715–728
10 Edil B, Ellison J, Cameron R et al (2011) Even small pancreatic endocrine neoplasm have lymph node metastasis (Abstract). Plenary Presentation at the American Pancreas Club, 45th Annual Meeting. Program, p 55
11 Liang S, Hameed U, Jayaraman S (2014) Laparoscopic pancreatectomy: indications and outcomes. World J Gastroenterol 20(39):14246–14254
12 Dakin GF, Inabnet WB (2004) Multimedia article laparoscopic enucleation of a pancreatic insulinoma. Surg Endosc 18(11):1680
13 Dexter SP, Martin IG, Leindler L et al (1999) Laparoscopic enucleation of a solitary pancreatic insulinoma. Surg Endosc 13(4):406–408
14 Karaliotas C, Sgourakis G (2009) Laparoscopic versus open enucleation for solitary insulinoma in the body and tail of the pancreas. J Gastrointest Surg 13(10):1869
15 Liu H, Peng C, Zhang S et al (2007) Strategy for the surgical management of insulinomas: analysis of 52 cases. Dig Surg 24(6):463–470
16 Sa Cunha A, Beau C, Rault A et al (2007) Laparoscopic versus open approach for solitary insulinoma. Surg Endosc 21(1):103–108
17 Zhao YP, Zhan HX, Zhang TP et al (2011) Surgical management of patients with insulinomas: result of 292 cases in a single institution. J Surg Oncol 103(2):169–174
18 Fernández-Cruz L, Cesar-Borges G (2006) Laparoscopic strategies for resection of insulinomas. J Gastrointest Surg 10(5):752–760
19 Zhang T, Mu Y, Qu L et al (2012) Accurate combined preoperative localization of insulinomas aid the choice for enucleation: a single institution experience over 25 years. Hepatogastroenterology 59(116):1282–1285
20 Su AP, Ke NW, Zhang Y et al (2014) Is laparoscopic approach for pancreatic insulinomas safe? Results of a systematic review and meta-analysis. J Surg Res 186(1):126–134
21 Fernández-Cruz L, Martínez I, Cesar-Borges G et al (2005) Laparoscopic surgery in patients with sporadic and multiple insulinomas associated with multiple endocrine neoplasia type 1. J Gastrointest Surg 9(3):381–388
22 Nell S, Brunaud L, Ayav A et al (2016) Robot-assisted spleen preserving pancreatic surgery in MEN1 patients. J Surg Oncol 114(4):456–461

23 Turrini O, Schmidt CM, Pitt HA et al (2011) Side-branch intraductal papillary mucinous neoplasms of the pancreatic head/uncinate: resection or enucleation? HPB (Oxford) 13(2): 126–131
24 Hwang HK, Park JS, Kim JK et al (2012) Comparison of efficacy of enucleation and pancreaticoduodenectomy for small (<3 cm) branch duct type intraductal papillary mucinous neoplasm located at the head of pancreas and the uncinate process. Yonsei Med J 53(1):106–110
25 Soejima Y, Toshima T, Motomura T et al (2017) Technical feasibility and oncological legitimacy of enucleation of intraductal papillary mucinous neoplasm located at the pancreatic head or uncinate process. Anticancer Res 37(1):321–326
26 Kaiser J, Fritz S, Klauss M et al (2017) Enucleation: a treatment alternative for branch duct intraductal papillary mucinous neoplasms. Surgery 161(3):602–610
27 Ohtsuka T, Takahata S, Takanami H et al (2014) Laparoscopic surgery is applicable for larger mucinous cystic neoplasms of the pancreas. J Hepatobiliary Pancreat Sci 21(5):343–348
28 Namur GN, Ribeiro TC, Souto MM et al (2016) Minimally invasive surgery for pseudopapillary neoplasm of the pancreas. Arq Bras Cir Dig 29(2):97–101
29 Stewart CL, Meguid C, Chapman B et al (2016) Evolving trends towards minimally invasive surgery for solid-pseudopapillary neoplasms. Ann Surg Oncol 23(13):4165–4168
30 Cioffi U, De Simone M, Santambrogio R et al (2003) Laparoscopic enucleation of solitary true pancreatic cyst in an adult. J Gastrointest Surg 7(7):921–924
31 Shi Y, Peng C, Shen B et al (2016) Pancreatic enucleation using the da Vinci robotic surgical system: a report of 26 cases. Int J Med Robot 12(4):751–757
32 Damoli I, Butturini G, Ramera M et al (2015) Minimally invasive pancreatic surgery – a review. Wideochir Inne Tech Maloinwazyjne 10(2):141–149
33 Kuroki T, Eguchi S (2014) Laparoscopic parenchyma-sparing pancreatectomy. J Hepatobiliary Pancreat Sci 21(5):323–327
34 Cauley CE, Pitt HA, Ziegler KM et al (2012) Pancreatic enucleation: improved outcomes compared to resection. J Gastrointest Surg 16(7):1347–1353
35 Zhou Y, Zhao M, Wu L et al (2016) Short- and long-term outcomes after enucleation of pancreatic tumors: an evidence-based assessment. Pancreatology 16(6):1092–1098
36 Hüttner FJ, Koessler-Ebs J, Hackert T et al (2015) Meta-analysis of surgical outcome after enucleation versus standard resection for pancreatic neoplasms. Br J Surg 102(9):1026–1036
37 Inchauste SM, Lanier BJ, Libutti SK et al (2012) Rate of clinically significant postoperative pancreatic fistula in pancreatic neuroendocrine tumors. World J Surg 36(7):1517–1526
38 Bassi C, Dervenis C, Butturini G et al (2005) Postoperative pancreatic fistula: an international study group (ISGPF) definition. Surgery 138(1):8–13
39 Costi R, Randone B, Mal F et al (2013) A critical appraisal of laparoscopic pancreatic enucleations: right-sided procedures (Pancreatic Head, Uncus) are not mini-invasive surgery. Surg Laparosc Endosc Percutan Tech 23(6):524–531
40 Jilesen AP, van Eijck CH, In't Hof KH et al (2015) Postoperative complications, in-hospital mortality and 5-year survival after surgical resection for patients with a pancreatic neuroendocrine tumor: a systematic review. World J Surg 40(3):729–748
41 Zhang RC, Zhou YC, Mou YP et al (2015) Laparoscopic versus open enucleation for pancreatic neoplasms: clinical outcomes and pancreatic function analysis. Surg Endosc 30(7):2657–2665
42 Zureikat AH, Moser AJ, Boone BA et al (2013) 250 robotic pancreatic resections: safety and feasibility. Ann Surg 258(4):554–559
43 Boggi U, Napoli N, Costa F et al (2016) Robotic-assisted pancreatic resections. World J Surg 40(10):2497–2506
44 Jin JB, Qin K, Li H et al (2016) Robotic enucleation for benign or borderline tumours of the pancreas: a retrospective analysis and comparison from a high-volume centre in Asia. World J Surg 40(12):3009–3020
45 Zhang J, Wu WM, You L, Zhao YP (2013) Robotic versus open pancreatectomy: a systematic review and meta-analysis. Ann Surg Oncol 20(6):1774–1780

46 Gagner M, Pomp A, Herrera MF (1996) Early experience with laparoscopic resections of islet cell tumors. Surgery 120(6):1051–1054
47 Gagner M, Pomp A (1997) Laparoscopic pancreatic resection: is it worthwhile? J Gastrointest Surg 1(1):20–25
48 Chapuis Y, Bigourdan JM, Massault PP et al (1998) Videolaparoscopic excision of insulinoma. A study of 5 cases. Chirurgie 123(5):461–467 [Article in French]
49 Berends FJ, Cuesta MA, Kazemier G et al (2000) Laparoscopic detection and resection of insulinomas. Surgery 128(3):386–391
50 Fernández-Cruz L, Sáenz A, Astudillo E et al (2002) Outcome of laparoscopic pancreatic surgery: Endocrine and nonendocrine tumors. World J Surg 26(8):1057–1065
51 Iihara M, Obara T (2003) Recent advances in minimally invasive pancreatic surgery. Asian J Surg 26(2):86–91
52 Edwin B, Mala T, Mathisen Ø et al (2004) Laparoscopic resection of the pancreas: a feasibility study of the short-term outcome. Surg Endosc 18(3):407–411
53 Jaroszewski DE, Schlinkert RT, Thompson GB, Schlinkert DK (2004) Laparoscopic localization and resection of insulinomas. Arch Surg 139(3):270–274
54 Ayav A, Bresler L, Brunaud L et al (2005) Laparoscopic approach for solitary insulinoma: a multicentre study. Langenbecks Arch Surg 390(2):134–140
55 Mabrut JY, Fernandez-Cruz L, Azagra JS et al (2005) Laparoscopic pancreatic resection: results of a multicenter European study of 127 patients. Surgery 137(6):597–605
56 Giger U, Michel JM, Wiesli P et al (2006) Laparoscopic surgery for benign lesions of the pancreas. J Laparoendosc Adv Surg Tech A 16(5):452–457
57 Fernández-Cruz L, Pardo F, Cugat E et al (2006) Análisis del Registro Nacional Español de la Cirugía Laparoscópica del Páncreas. Cirugía Española 79(5):293–298 [Article in Spanish]
58 Schraibman V, Goldenberg A, de Matos Farah JF et al (2007) Laparoscopic enucleation of pancreatic insulinomas. J Laparoendosc Adv Surg Tech A 17(4):399–401
59 Sweet MP, Izumisato Y, Way LW et al (2007) Laparoscopic enucleation of insulinomas. Arch Surg 142(12):1202–1204; discussion 1205
60 Pierce RA, Spitler JA, Hawkins WG et al (2007) Outcomes analysis of laparoscopic resection of pancreatic neoplasms. Surg Endosc 21(4):579–586
61 Fernández-Cruz L, Cosa R, Blanco L et al (2007) Curative laparoscopic resection for pancreatic neoplasms: a critical analysis from a single institution. J Gastrointest Surg 11(12):1607–1621
62 Crippa S, Bassi C, Salvia R et al (2007) Enucleation of pancreatic neoplasms. Br J Surg 94(10):1254–1259
63 Luo Y, Liu R, Hu MG et al (2009) Laparoscopic surgery for pancreatic insulinomas: a single-institution experience of 29 cases. J Gastrointest Surg 13(5):945–950
64 Isla A, Arbuckle JD, Kekis PB et al (2009) Laparoscopic management of insulinomas. Br J Surg 96(2):185–190
65 Røsok BI, Marangos IP, Kazaryan AM et al (2010) Single-centre experience of laparoscopic pancreatic surgery. Br J Surg 97(6):902–909
66 Costi R, Randone B, Mal F et al (2013) Laparoscopic minor pancreatic resections (enucleations/atypical resections). A long-term appraisal of a supposed mini-invasive approach. Wideochir Inne Tech Maloinwazyjne 8(2):117–129
67 Machado MA, Surjan RC, Goldman SM et al (2013) Laparoscopic pancreatic resection. From enucleation to pancreatoduodenectomy. 11-year experience. Arq Gastroenterol 50(3):214–218
68 Choi KS, Chung JC, Kim HC (2014) Feasibility and outcomes of laparoscopic enucleation for pancreatic neoplasms. Ann Surg Treat Res 87(6):285–289
69 Zhang RC, Zhou YC, Mou YP et al (2016) Laparoscopic versus open enucleation for pancreatic neoplasms: clinical outcomes and pancreatic function analysis. Surg Endosc 30(7):2657–2665
70 Thomas E, Matsuoka L, Alexopoulos S et al (2015) Laparoscopic hand-assisted parenchymal-sparing resections for presumed side-branch intraductal papillary mucinous neoplasms. J Laparoendosc Adv Surg Tech A 25(8):668–671

Central Pancreatectomy: from Open to Minimally Invasive

17

Calogero Iacono, Fabio Bagante, Andrea Ruzzenente, and Alfredo Guglielmi

17.1 Introduction

Open central pancreatectomy (the Dagradi-Serio-Iacono operation) was performed for the first time in 1982 by Dagradi and Serio to remove a functioning neuroendocrine tumor (insulinoma) located in the neck of the pancreas [1]. Central pancreatectomy is a parenchyma-sparing operation allowing the removal of benign and low-grade malignant lesions from the neck and the proximal body of the pancreas (Fig. 17.1). To promote the widespread acceptance of this novel technique, Iacono et al. completed exocrine and endocrine pancreatic function tests demonstrating that central pancreatectomy, when performed for appropriate indications and with an accurate surgical technique, was associated with almost no postoperative variation of pancreatic functions [2–4]. In particular, compared with pancreatoduodenectomy and distal pancreatectomy, central pancreatectomy resulted in a lower rate of postoperative endocrine (e.g., diabetes) and exocrine insufficiency, while additional advantages were associated with preservation of the spleen (fewer infectious and thromboembolic complications) as well as of the biliary and upper digestive tracts [2, 3]. In a systematic review by Iacono and al., between 1988 and 2010, 94 studies described 963 patients who underwent central open pancreatectomy [3].

While the vast majority of patients underwent open surgery, from 2002, when the first laparoscopic central pancreatectomy was performed by Baca et al. [5], a laparoscopic approach was used in 18 patients, while robotic-assisted central pancreatectomy was performed on 12 patients [3].

C. Iacono (✉)
Department of Surgery, Unit of Hepato-Pancreato-Biliary Surgery, University of Verona, School of Medicine
Verona, Italy
e-mail: calogero.iacono@univr.it

U. Boggi (Ed), *Minimally Invasive Surgery of the Pancreas*, Updates in Surgery
DOI: 10.1007/978-88-470-3958-2_17, © Springer-Verlag Italia 2018

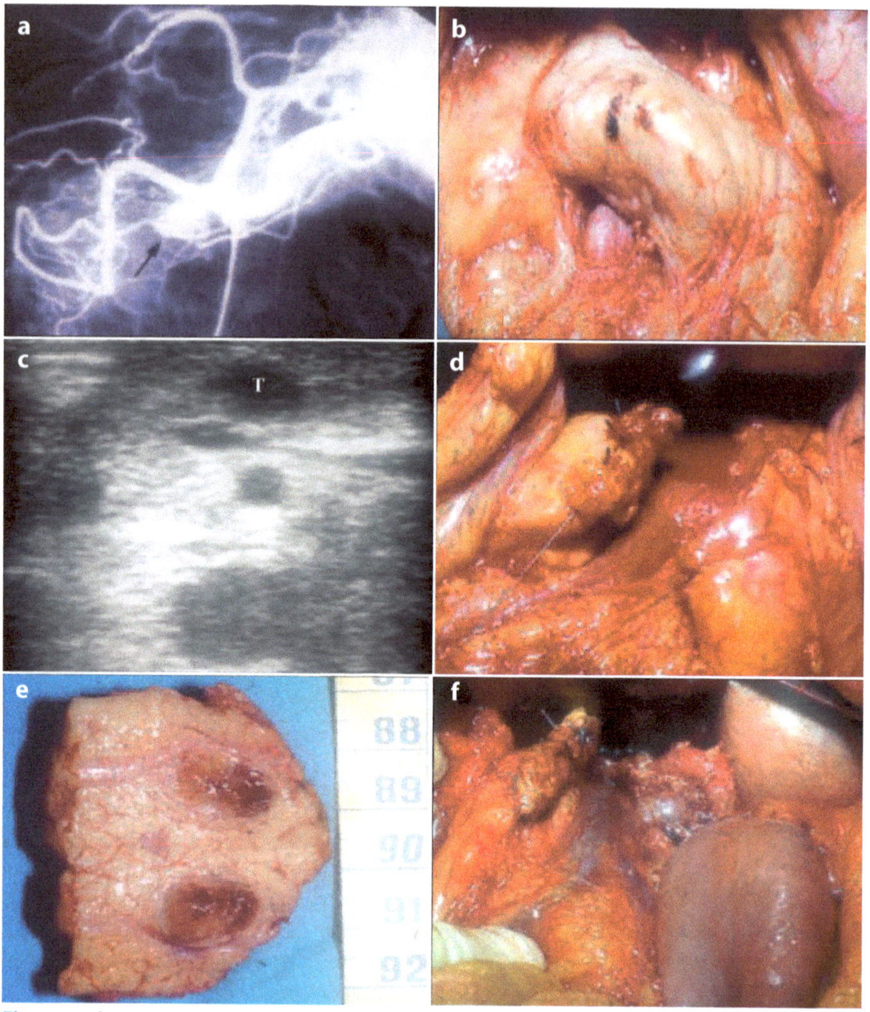

Fig. 17.1 Open central pancreatectomy in a patient with insulinoma syndrome. **a** Angiography showing a small hypervascular lesion in the neck of the pancreas (*black arrow*). **b** Intraoperative appearance with no evidence of the lesion. **c** Intraoperative ultrasonography shows the tumor (*T*) inside the pancreatic parenchyma. **d** Proximal and distal pancreatic stumps after resection of the neck. **e** Specimen of the central pancreatectomy showing the insulinoma close to the Wirsung duct. **f** Final appearance of central pancreatectomy, the cephalic stump is sutured and the distal stump is anastomized with a Roux-en-Y jejunal loop

In a recent report on USA trends in postoperative outcomes of minimally invasive versus open pancreatic surgery, the rate of minimally invasive pancreatic resection increased from 3% in 2002 to 14% in 2012 [6]. Moreover, minimally invasive pancreatectomies were associated with lower rates of postoperative morbidity and shorter length of stay compared to open resections.

17.2 Minimally Invasive Central Pancreatectomy: Laparoscopic and Robotic-Assisted Approaches

Regarding minimally invasive central pancreatectomy, in 2013 Machado et al. reported that since 2005 a total 51 central pancreatectomies were performed laparoscopically, 21 (41%) patients underwent total laparoscopy, 27 (53%) required robotic assistance, 1 (2%) required hand assistance, and 2 (4%) patients required conversion to open central pancreatectomy [7]. In 32 (63%) patients, reconstruction was performed using a pancreatogastrostomy, while in 18 (35%) cases reconstruction involved a Roux-en-Y pancreatojejunostomy. The mean operative time was 356 minutes, mortality was zero, morbidity rate was high mainly because of pancreatic fistula (46%), but no patient presented exocrine or endocrine insufficiency [7]. Recently, Senthilnathan et al. reported the long-term outcomes of 14 patients who underwent laparoscopic central pancreatectomy from October 2004 to September 2013 in a single institution for tumors located in the body and neck of pancreas less than 3 cm in size and with a radiologically benign-looking tumor [8]. The mean operative time was 239.7 min and overall mean length of stay was about 8 days. Surgical margins were negative in all cases and there were no deaths or major postoperative complications. On long-term follow-up, two patients developed diabetes while no patients developed any detectable exocrine deficiency. Of note, no patients relapsed during a median follow-up of 44 months [8].

During central pancreatectomy, pancreatoenterostomy is the most technically difficult step to perform laparoscopically and the postoperative pancreatic fistula (POPF) rate is as high as in open central pancreatectomy. For these reasons, several authors have proposed novel pancreatic anastomosis techniques in addition to the standard pancreatojejunostomy and pancreatogastrostomy. Specifically, Jiao et al. reported the short-term outcomes of four patients undergoing laparoscopic long-sleeve pancreatogastrostomy (LPG), a novel technique resembling the pancreatogastrostomy with gastric partition proposed by Fernandez-Cruz as a pancreatic anastomosis technique after open pylorus-preserving pancreatoduodenectomy [9, 10]. As reported by the authors, the pancreatic stump at the body-tail was mobilized laparoscopically to free it at least 1 cm away from the splenic vein, and a vertical band gastroplasty was then created with a 60-mm Endo GIA stapler (TriStaple, tan cartridge; Covidien, Hampshire, UK) more than 3 cm away from the lesser gastric border to ensure gastric outlet patency. A long sleeve gastric tube measuring at least 6 cm in length in the greater curvature of stomach was then prepared and made ready for an end-to-end pancreatogastrostomy. A pancreatic stent was inserted into the pancreatic duct across the anastomosis whenever the pancreatic duct was visible, and a continuous running suture with 2/0 PDS was applied laparoscopically to the posterior wall and interrupted sutures to the anterior wall for an end-to-end LPG. With a median follow-up of 27.5 months, there was no mortality and one patient had a grade A postoperative pancreatic fistula (POPF) that was managed conservatively [9]. A different approach, already used in the open technique [3], has been proposed by Francone et al. reporting double pancreatojejunostomy in a pure laparoscopic central pancreatectomy for a non-functioning pancreatic neuroendocrine neoplasm located in the pancreatic neck. By realizing a double pancreatojejunostomy, the authors obtained to cover both cut pancreatic surfaces draining pancreatic juice from both the proximal and distal main ducts. Of note, during a follow-up of 18 months the patients did not have disease recurrence or exocrine and endocrine pancreas insufficiencies [11]. Recently, Hong et al. reported the short-term outcomes of 10 consecutive patients undergoing laparoscopic central pancreatectomy with binding pancreatogastrostomy for cystic serous adenoma, intraductal papillary mucinous neoplasm, of neuroendocrine tumor, and solid pseudopapillary tumor of pancreas [12]. Binding pancreatogastrostomy was previously described by the same group as a novel pancreatic reconstruction technique in which the stump of the pancreas was inserted into the stomach and held in place with two purse-string sutures which do not penetrate the pancreas [13]. As reported by the authors, the distal pancreas stump was further freed by dissecting it from the splenic artery and splenic vein for about 3 cm as preparation for anastomosis, followed by closing the cutting surface with stitch sutures. An approximately 3-cm opening was made on the posterior wall of the stomach and an additional 3–5-cm opening was made on the anterior gastric wall, a full-layer purse suture was made at the opening of posterior wall of the stomach, and the pancreatic stump was dragged into the stomach for about 2 cm under direct observation. By tying the purse suture, the gastric wall was "binded" to the pancreatic stump, followed by closing the anterior gastric wall [13]. Postoperatively, one patient had a POPF and one had delayed gastric emptying, which were managed with conservative treatment, while upper gastrointestinal bleeding occurred in one patient who required a second surgical operation. During a follow-up ranging from 7 to 40 months, no patients had recurrence, and no patients developed any detectable exocrine or endocrine deficiency [13].

Regarding the surgical outcomes of laparoscopic central pancreatectomy, Song et al. compared 26 patients who underwent laparoscopic central pancreatectomy, 14 open central pancreatectomy, and 96 patients undergoing extended laparoscopic distal pancreatectomy [14].

The authors reported that even if the tumor sizes in the laparoscopic central pancreatectomy (2.2 cm) and open central pancreatectomy (2.9 cm) groups were smaller than in the extended laparoscopic distal pancreatectomy (4.0 cm) group, the mean operation time in the laparoscopic central pancreatectomy group (350 min) was longer than both open central pancreatectomy (270 min) and extended laparoscopic distal pancreatectomy groups (211 min). Regarding the short-term outcomes, there were more surgical complications in the laparoscopic central pancreatectomy (39%) and open central pancreatectomy groups (50%) than in the extended laparoscopic distal pancreatectomy group (15%); however, the mean length of stay was 14 days for the laparoscopic central pancreatectomy group, which was significantly shorter than the 22.4 days for the open central pancreatectomy group. Interestingly, endocrine pancreatic insufficiency was less frequent after laparoscopic central pancreatectomy than after extended laparoscopic distal pancreatectomy (11.5% vs. 30.8%) [14]. Of note, these results were analogous to those from the systematic review and meta-analysis comparing open central pancreatectomy with open distal pancreatectomy [3].

In 2004, Giulianotti et al. described the first robotic-assisted central pancreatectomy [15]. Among the three patients who underwent robotic-assisted central pancreatectomy, one patient developed a POPF, which was managed conservatively, and length of stay was 9 days for two patients and 27 days for one patient. Of note, during a mean follow-up of 44 months no endocrine or exocrine pancreatic insufficiencies were observed [15].

Robotic-assisted surgery is recognized as the most advanced minimally invasive surgical approach given its magnified three-dimensional visualization and Endowrist instruments permitting greater range of motion and enhanced dexterity. The robotic-assisted pancreatectomies have demonstrated to offer several advantages over open and laparoscopic pancreatic surgery including reduced postoperative pain, lower estimated blood loss, and shorter hospital stay [16, 17].

Regarding central pancreatectomy, recently a Chinese group compared the short-terms outcomes of 50 patients who underwent robotic-assisted central pancreatectomy with 50 patients who underwent open central pancreatectomy in a randomized clinical trial [18]. Operative time (160 min for robotic-assisted vs. 193 min for open, $p = 0.002$), blood loss (50 mL for robotic-assisted vs. 200 mL for open, $p \leq 0.001$), and clinical POPF rate (18% for robotic-assisted vs. 36.0% for open, $p = 0.043$) were lower in robotic-assisted central pancreatectomy. Of note, robotic-assisted central pancreatectomy was associated with a significantly shorter length of stay compared to open central pancreatectomy, 15.6 and 21.7 days ($p = 0.002$), respectively [18].

17.3 Indications

Reviewing the current literature on minimally invasive central pancreatectomy, the indications for laparoscopic and robotic-assisted central pancreatectomy greatly reflect those for open central pancreatectomy. In particular, symptomatic serous cystadenoma, mucinous cystadenoma, solid cystic pseudopapillary tumors, and selected cases of intraductal papillary mucinous neoplasm (IPMN) were the lesions most frequently resected using a minimally invasive approach. Of note, the conditions for which central pancreatectomy is more appropriate have a greater incidence rate in young and heathy patients who could benefit from the advantages of a minimally invasive approach, such as smaller incisional scar resulting in superior cosmetic results.

Conversely, the authors reported smaller lesion size (<2–3 cm) in the minimally invasive central pancreatectomy group compared with lesions between 2 and 5 cm in size in the open group.

17.4 Laparoscopy Technique

As in the open procedure, minimally invasive central pancreatectomy requires two steps, first resecting the central pancreatic segment and then the reconstructive part to oversew the cephalic stump and perform the digestive anastomosis with the distal stump.

In the laparoscopic procedure, the patient is placed in the supine position or a reverse Trendelenburg position. Four trocars are placed under direct scope vision: two 5-mm trocars (one on the right flank for the operator's left hand and one on the left flank for surgical assistance) and two 12-mm trocars (one on the umbilicus for the operator's right hand and one on the right lower quadrant of the abdomen for the laparoscope) are used. The gastrocolic omentum is divided for entrance to the lesser sac. The superior mesenteric vein (SMV) and portal vein (PV) are identified at the inferior border of the pancreatic neck and dissected over the retropancreatic PV making a tunnel in front of the SMV. On completion of the tunnel, a tape is passed through to provide traction on the pancreas. By pulling the tape upwards, the pancreatic neck is dissected proximally and distally for approximately 2 cm. For transection of the proximal pancreas with a safe resection margin, endoscopic linear staplers are usually used while distal pancreatic transection is performed with a harmonic scalpel or linear stapler. The pancreatic duct is isolated and transected. To release the distal stump of the pancreas, small branches of splenic vein and artery to and from the pancreas, respectively, are clipped or ligated and then transected. This dissection is extended up to 2 cm away from the distal section line. After completing the resection, the specimen is placed in an entrapment bag and removed through the 12-mm umbilical port. For the reconstructive step, the most common anastomosis is end-to-side invaginated pancreatojejunostomy with a double-layer suture. A 2-layer end-to-side pancreatojejunostomy with polypropylene 5-0 interrupted suture is used for the external seromuscular layer of the jejunum while a polypropylene 4-0 continuous suture is used for the full-layer jejunal anastomosis with the pancreas. As previously reported, different pancreatoenteric anastomoses have been proposed and the pancreatogastrostomy is reported as the most frequent technique after pancreatojejunostomy [7].

17.5 Robotic-Assisted Technique

After the first robotic-assisted central pancreatectomy was described, further modifications of the robotic technique were reported by Addeo et al. and Kang et al. [15, 19–21]. Compared with open and laparoscopic central pancreatectomy, the robotic approach might benefit from high range of instrument motion (almost 540°), elimination of tremor, improved dexterity and surgeon comfort, as well as 3D binocular visualization and high magnification (20×–30×) [22].

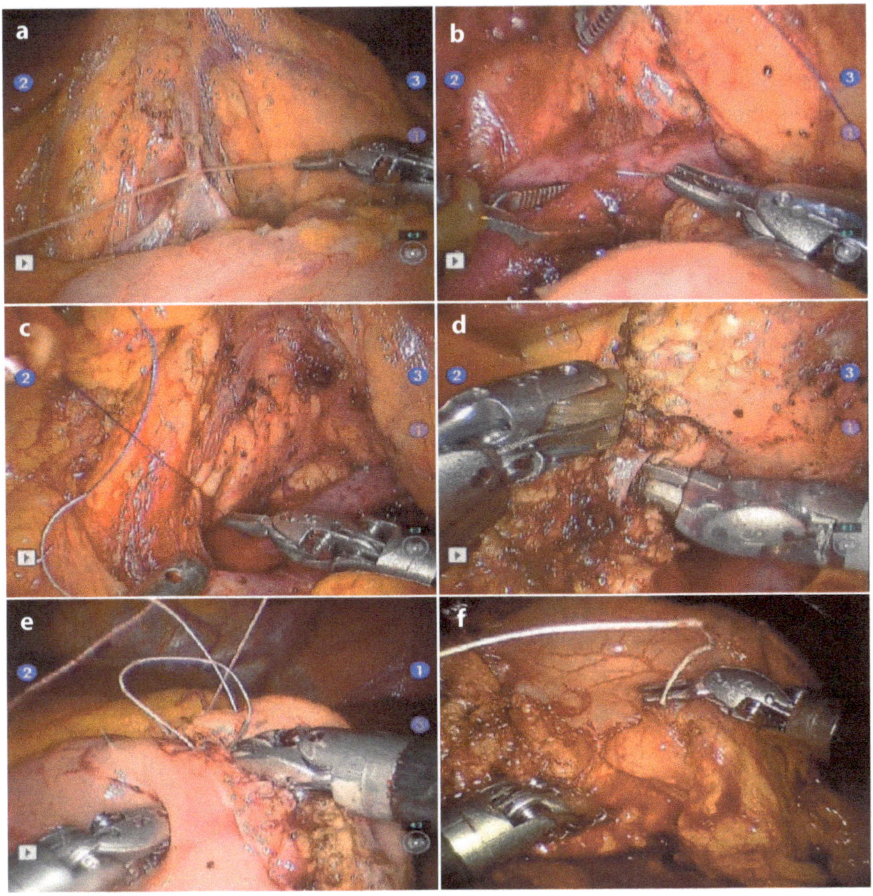

Fig. 17.2 **a** After entering the lesser sac the pancreas is elevated. Small posterior vessels are selectively ligated. **b** A tunnel is developed behind the neck of the pancreas. Small pancreatic veins are secured by fine polypropylene sutures. **c** Before dividing the pancreas, transverse pancreatic arteries are fixed by polypropylene sutures. **d** During pancreatic transection the main pancreatic duct is identified and cut sharply. **e** Pancreatojejunostomy. **f** Pancreatogastrostomy. (Courtesy of Prof. Ugo Boggi)

Robotic-assisted central pancreatectomy requires that patients are placed supine with the legs apart while the operative table is positioned at 20° in the reverse Trendelenburg position, slightly tilted to the left side. The da Vinci surgical system is docked over the head of the patient, with two operating arms on the patient's left side. Four trocars are placed for access by the robotic arms, and an additional 12-mm trocar is placed for the assistant's access. The lesser sac is entered by opening the gastrocolic ligament, and the posterior gastric wall is lifted and retracted cranially exposing the pancreas. While the anterior surface of the portal vein dissected at the superior edge of the pancreatic body, the SMV is exposed at the inferior edge of the pancreatic neck. After a retropancreatic tunnel is created under the pancreatic neck by gentle dissection, the pancreatic neck is transected using an endoscopic stapler or an ultrasonic scalpel. As frequently reported, interrupted stitches of polypropylene 4-0 are applied to the proximal stump selectively achieving an adequate hemostasis. The distal pancreas is then dissected between the pancreas and splenic vessels to obtain a free resection margin. Accurately, small branches of splenic vein and artery to and from the pancreas, respectively, are clipped or ligated and then transected. The transection of the pancreatic body is then performed on the left side of the lesion using the robotic ultrasonic scalpel. Reconstruction can be performed by either pancreatojejunostomy or pancreatogastrostomy, based on individual patient factors and surgeon's preference (Fig. 17.2).

17.6 Conclusions

Central pancreatectomy can be selected carefully as an appropriate surgical option for benign and borderline malignant lesions limited to the pancreatic body/neck area. Function-preserving minimally invasive pancreatic surgery would also enhance the feasibility and safety of minimally invasive (laparoscopic) central pancreatectomy. Moreover, a robotic surgical system may allow surgeons to perform complex and difficult laparoscopic procedures more easily, effectively, and precisely. Further studies and follow-up data are needed to address the real benefits of the robot in this advanced laparoscopic era.

References

1. Iacono C, Ruzzenente A, Bortolasi L, Guglielmi A (2014) Central pancreatectomy: the Dagradi Serio Iacono operation. Evolution of a surgical technique from the pioneers to the robotic approach. World J Gastroenterol 20(42):15674–15681
2. Iacono C, Bortolasi L, Serio G (1998) Is there a place for central pancreatectomy in pancreatic surgery? J Gastrointest Surg 2(6):509–516; discussion 516–517
3. Iacono C, Verlato G, Ruzzenente A et al (2013) Systematic review of central pancreatectomy and meta-analysis of central versus distal pancreatectomy. Br J Surg 100(7):873–885
4. Iacono C, Bortolasi L, Facci E et al (2007) The Dagradi-Serio-Iacono operation central pancreatectomy. J Gastrointest Surg 11(3):364–376
5. Baca I, Bokan I (2003) Laparoscopic segmental pancreas resection and pancreatic cystadenoma. Chirurg 74(10):961–965 [Article in German]
6. Okunrintemi V, Gani F, Pawlik TM (2016) National trends in postoperative outcomes and cost comparing minimally invasive versus open liver and pancreatic surgery. J Gastrointest Surg 20(11):1836–1843
7. Machado MA, Surjan RC, Epstein MG, Makdissi FF (2013) Laparoscopic central pancreatectomy: a review of 51 cases. Surg Laparosc Endosc Percutan Tech 23(6):486–490
8. Senthilnathan P, Gul SI, Gurumurthy SS et al (2015) Laparoscopic central pancreatectomy: our technique and long-term results in 14 patients. J Minim Access Surg 11(3):167–171

9. Jiao LR, Gall TM, Sodergren MH, Fan R (2016) Laparoscopic long sleeve pancreaticogastrostomy (LPG): a novel pancreatic anastomosis following central pancreatectomy. Hepatobiliary Surg Nutr 5(3):245–248
10. Fernández-Cruz L, Cosa R, Blanco et al (2008) Pancreatogastrostomy with gastric partition after pylorus-preserving pancreatoduodenectomy versus conventional pancreatojejunostomy: a prospective randomized study. Ann Surg. 248(6):930–938
11. Francone E, Berti S, Celoria GM et al (2016) Double pancreaticojejunostomy in pure laparoscopic central pancreatectomy: an uncommon reconstructive strategy. Minerva Chir 71(2):156–158
12. Hong D, Liu Y, Peng S et al (2016) Binding pancreaticogastrostomy in laparoscopic central pancreatectomy: a novel technique in laparoscopic pancreatic surgery. Surg Endosc 30(2):715–720
13. Peng SY, Wang JW, Hong DF et al (2011) Binding pancreaticoenteric anastomosis: from binding pancreaticojejunostomy to binding pancreaticogastrostomy. Updates Surg 63(2):69–74
14. Song KB, Kim SC, Park KM et al (2015) Laparoscopic central pancreatectomy for benign or low-grade malignant lesions in the pancreatic neck and proximal body. Surg Endosc 29(4):937–946
15. Giulianotti PC, Sbrana F, Bianco FM et al (2010) Robot-assisted laparoscopic middle pancreatectomy. J Laparoendosc Adv Surg Tech A 20(2):135–139
16. Zhou JY, Xin C, Mou YP et al (2016) Robotic versus laparoscopic distal pancreatectomy: a meta-analysis of short-term outcomes. PLoS One 11(3):e0151189
17. Stauffer JA, Asbun HJ (2015) Minimally invasive pancreatic surgery. Semin Oncol 42(1):123–133
18. Chen S, Zhan Q, Jin JB et al (2017) Robot-assisted laparoscopic versus open middle pancreatectomy: short-term results of a randomized controlled trial. Surg Endosc 31(2):962–971
19. Addeo P, Marzano E, Nobili C et al (2011) Robotic central pancreatectomy with stented pancreaticogastrostomy: operative details. Int J Med Robot 7(3):293–297
20. Kang CM, Kim DH, Lee WJ, Chi HS (2011) Initial experiences using robot-assisted central pancreatectomy with pancreaticogastrostomy: a potential way to advanced laparoscopic pancreatectomy. Surg Endosc 25(4):1101–1106
21. Cheng K, Shen B, Peng C et al (2013) Initial experiences in robot-assisted middle pancreatectomy. HPB (Oxford) 15(4):315–321
22. Zeh HJ 3rd, Bartlett DL, Moser AJ (2011) Robotic-assisted major pancreatic resection. Adv Surg 45:323–340

18 Minimally Invasive Distal Pancreatectomy for Pancreatic Cancer

Riccardo Casadei, Claudio Ricci, Giovanni Taffurelli, Carlo Alberto Pacilio, and Francesco Minni

18.1 Introduction

The first description of laparoscopic distal pancreatectomy (LDP) was reported by Cuschieri et al. [1] and Gagner et al. [2] in 1996 for chronic pancreatitis and islet cell tumors, respectively. The first robotic distal pancreatectomy (RDP) was reported by Melvin et al. in 2003 for a neuroendocrine tumor in the tail of the pancreas [3]. Since these reports, LDP and RDP have been increasingly utilized for benign and borderline lesions in the body and tail of the pancreas However, while there is sufficient evidence to support the use of the minimally invasive approach for resection of benign and borderline lesions in the body and tail of the pancreas [4–7], its use for patients with adenocarcinoma of the distal pancreas has been rarely reported and its validity is still unclear. Recent data from a national database showed an incidence of LDP for PDAC of 12.6% [8]. This datum increased to 31% when robotic distal pancreatectomy was considered [9]. The aims of performing a minimally invasive distal pancreatectomy (MIDP) are: 1) to allow the same clinical and oncological results as open distal pancreatectomy with 2) a smaller incision, earlier postoperative recovery, less postoperative pain and earlier return to normal life.

18.2 Surgical Techniques

The two goals of pancreatic resection for adenocarcinoma are complete resection of the tumor with a margin of normal tissue (R0), and resection of regional

R. Casadei (✉)
Department of Medical and Surgical Sciences (DIMEC), University of Bologna, S.Orsola-Malpighi Hospital
Bologna, Italy
e-mail: riccardo.casadei@unibo.it

U. Boggi (Ed), *Minimally Invasive Surgery of the Pancreas*, Updates in Surgery
DOI: 10.1007/978-88-470-3958-2_18,

nodes adopting an early vascular control and a "no–touch" technique in order to obtain a radical oncological resection with minimal risk of tumor dissemination and seeding.

These general principles have been translated from open to minimally invasive distal pancreatectomy by Strasberg et al. [10] who proposed a radical anterograde modular pancreatosplenectomy (RAMPS) to resolve these problems. A RAMPS is conducted properly as an anterior RAMPS or posterior RAMPS, depending on the extent of penetration of the tumor [11, 12]. However, these principles were adopted rarely as reported in the two meta-analyses about LDP in pancreatic cancer [13, 14].

18.2.1 Laparoscopic Approach

The technique of laparoscopic distal pancreatectomy can vary widely between different surgeons and centers. The medial approach was the first described and has become the standard technique. Several other techniques have been reported including the lateral approach, retroperitoneal and hand-assisted versions [15].

In the medial approach, after general anesthesia, the patient is positioned supine with a 20° head-up and foot-down tilt (reverse Trendelenburg position) and 30° degree right lateral decubitus with the patient's hip at the break in the table. The surgeon stands between the patient's lower limbs, with the first assistant holding the laparoscope on the right side, the second assistant on the left side, and the scrub nurse on the right side by the feet of the patient (Fig. 18.1). Trocar placement should be adapted to both the size of the patient and the location of the tumor (body or tail). Usually, four to five trocars are placed in a semicircular fashion centered around an umbilical camera, as shown in Fig. 18.1. After an open sub/supraumbilical cut-down, a 12-mm trocar is inserted and pneumoperitoneum established. A 30° laparoscope is inserted. Three additional trocars are inserted under vision; the primary access port (10–12 mm) is located on the left midclavicular line between the umbilical and left flank port; the secondary access port (5 mm or 10–12 mm) at the left anterior axillary line, 3–5 cm under the costal margin and another 5-mm one in the epigastrium, in the subxiphoid area, used to retract the stomach and the liver. An additional 5 mm or 10–12 mm working port is placed between the right anterior axillary line and midclavicular line just cephalad to the umbilicus as it will facilitate lymphadenectomy at the hepatic artery and celiac trunk.

The lateral approach is less frequently used for pancreatic cancer. It is performed mainly for benign or borderline lesions of the tail of the pancreas. Briefly, the patient is kept supine and positioned in a 30° right lateral decubitus with the hip at the break in the table; the surgeon, the first assistant and the scrub nurse stand to the right of the patient. Usually, four or five trocars are placed [16].

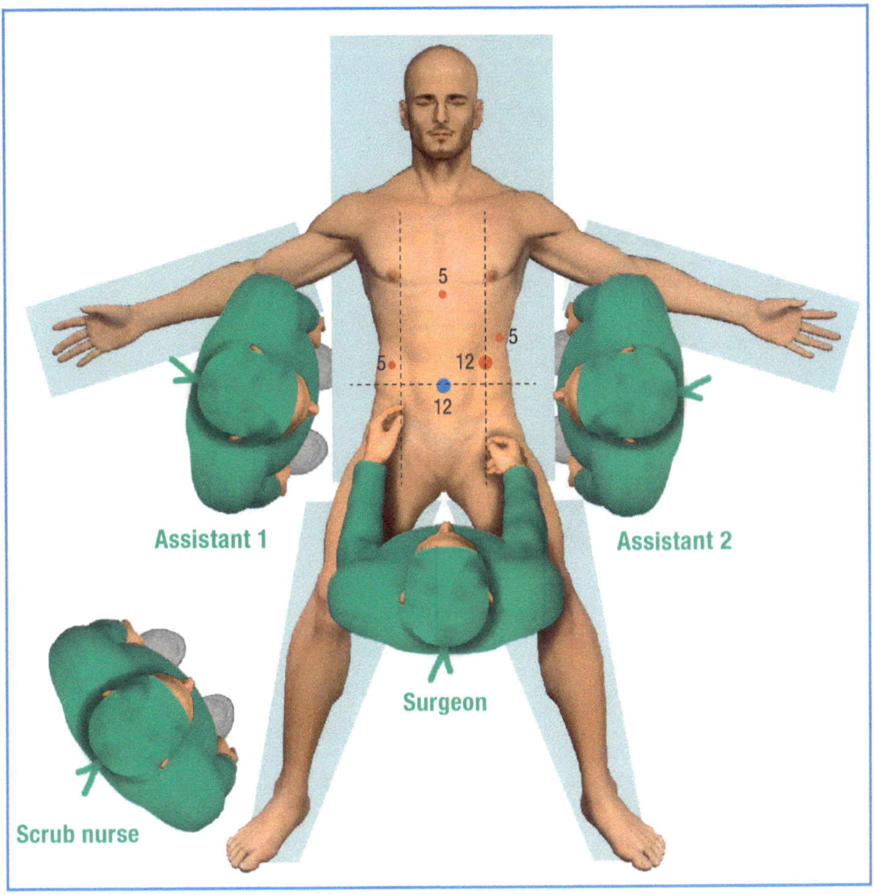

Fig. 18.1 Position of the patient, surgeons, and scrub nurse, with trocar placement for laparoscopic distal pancreatectomy for pancreatic cancer

18.2.2 Robotic Approach

Robotic distal pancreatectomy (RDP) cases were performed with the da Vinci system (Si or Xi models). The patient is placed supine and the operative table is oriented 20° in the reverse Trendelenburg position and tilted to the right side by about 20°. Typically, 5 ports are used (3, 8-mm; 2, 12-mm) as well as 3 robotic arms and 1 laparoscopic port (an accessory port for the assistant). The optic port is placed in the periumbilical area. The assistant port (10–12 mm) is inserted in the right pararectal region. The other ports are placed in a semicircular fashion centered around the umbilical camera as shown in Fig. 18.2. After port placement and induction of pneumoperitoneum, the robot is docked into position. At the end of the operation, once the gland is divided and hemostasis secured, the robot is undocked and the specimen extracted in a plastic bag laparoscopically.

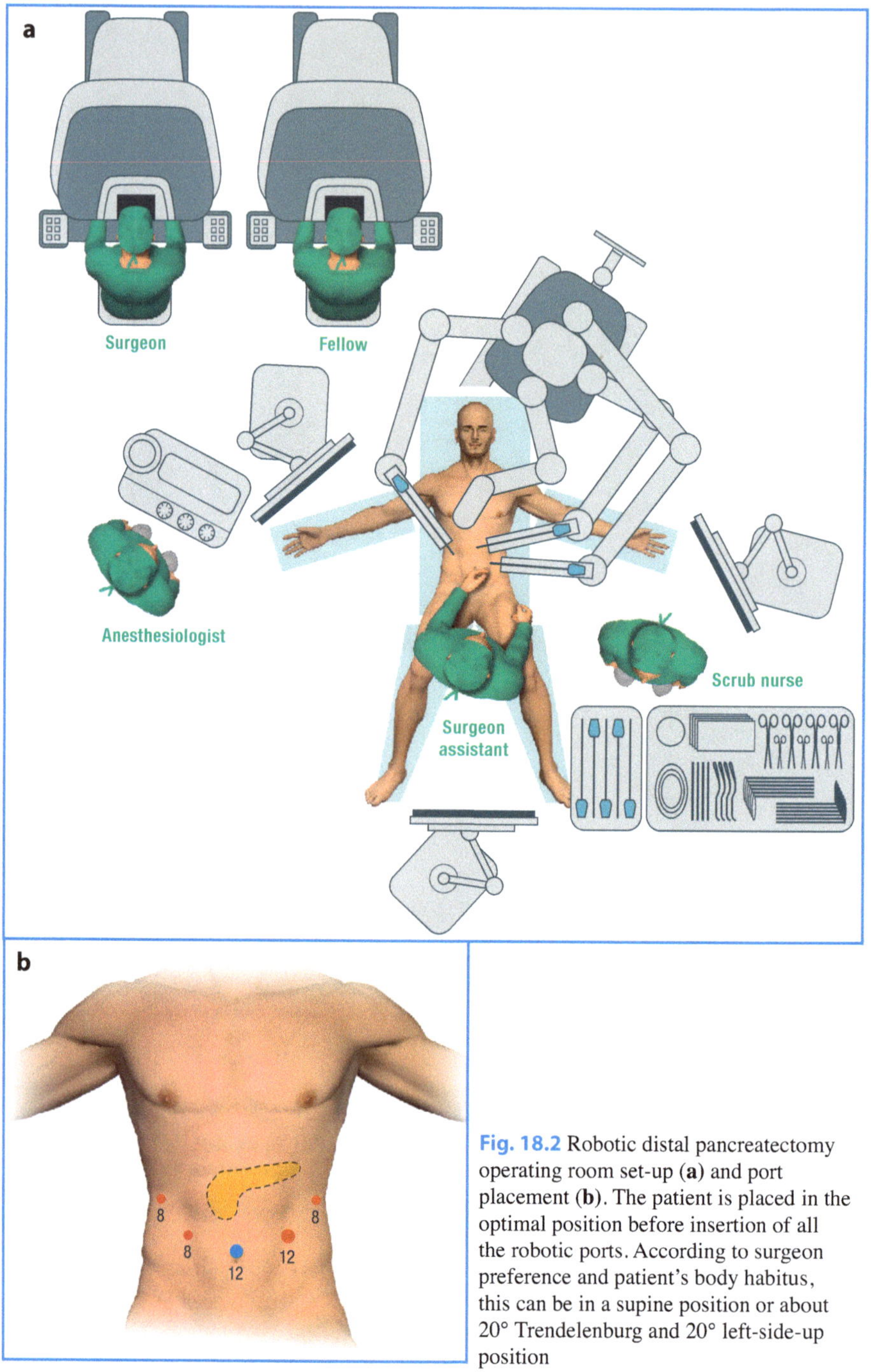

Fig. 18.2 Robotic distal pancreatectomy operating room set-up (**a**) and port placement (**b**). The patient is placed in the optimal position before insertion of all the robotic ports. According to surgeon preference and patient's body habitus, this can be in a supine position or about 20° Trendelenburg and 20° left-side-up position

18.2.3 Operative Technique

Regarding the operative technique, three points should be emphasized.

1. The surgical steps of distal pancreatectomy are the same in the laparoscopic and robotic approach.
2. The following steps are recommended in all patients by several authors [11, 12, 15] and by the DIPLOMA (distal pancreatectomy, minimally invasive or open, for malignancy) trial as the standard for a minimally invasive distal pancreatectomy in pancreatic cancer: (a) radical anterograde modular pancreatosplenectomy (RAMPS) with Gerota's fascia resection or, whenever the posterior margin of the tumor seems to involve the adrenal gland, posterior RAMPS, including resection of involved organs (e.g., adrenal gland or kidney); (b) splenectomy; (c) lymphadenectomy according to the ISGPS (International Study Group on Pancreatic Surgery) guidelines [17].
3. Dissection is performed using a diathermy hook, ultrasonic device, 5–10 mm clip applicators or hem-o-lok. Transection of the pancreas is preferably performed with a stapler even though cut-sewing techniques are accepted.

A 30° telescope, inserted in the first trocar, allows visualization of all of the abdominal cavity to exclude liver or peritoneal metastases. The gastrocolic ligament and short gastric vessels are divided with the ultrasonic device allowing access to the anterior surface of the pancreas. The splenocolic ligament is divided and the splenic flexure mobilized to permit a complete exposure of the pancreatic tail. Intraoperative ultrasonography is used at this stage to delineate the tumor, identify its relationship to the splenic vessels and define the level of resection needed. The stomach can be lifted with a suture to allow a good exposure of the pancreas or it can be retracted with a retractor inserted in the 5-mm port in the epigastrium. Mobilization of the distal pancreas begins from the inferior border, in an area distant from the neoplasm, usually with caudocranial direction, and continues down until Gerota's fascia that represents the posterior plane. Gerota's fascia is incised and lifted and the dissection is joined from below towards the superior pancreatic margin. The superior margin is dissected and Gerota's fascia is incised at the same level. A tape is pulled through this plane to lift the pancreas. The dissection of the inferior margin and the development of the posterior plane are continued towards the splenic/superior mesenteric vein junction. Then, a second tape is passed under the pancreas to the right of the neoplasm with the aim of creating a clear dissection plane from the retroperitoneum. The pancreas is transected at the neck keeping a clear margin from the lesion, using a linear stapler device. The splenic artery is divided at its origin with two endoscopic clips; the splenic vein at its junction with the superior mesenteric vein. Depending on the relation to the tumor, the inferior mesenteric vein is transected or left intact. Lymphadenectomy including stations 10, 11 and 18 has to be performed.

Stations 8 and 9 are harvested only if the cancer is confined to the body of the pancreas. Finally, the spleen is divided from its remaining retroperitoneal attachment and the specimen is removed from a small incision, usually a Pfannenstiel incision, in an impermeable extraction bag.

18.3 Results

18.3.1 Laparoscopic Distal Pancreatectomy

The results of recent systematic reviews and meta-analyses demonstrate the safety and feasibility of a LDP, showing that LDP is not inferior to open distal pancreatectomy (ODP), at least for benign and low-grade malignant disease [4–7, 18]. However, when adopting the minimally invasive approach for resection of pancreatic ductal adenocarcinoma (PDAC), there are many doubts that the oncological standards of the open approach can be achieved. Thus, the oncological efficiency of the minimally invasive approach for malignant lesions in the pancreas is still open to debate. To our knowledge, there are two systematic reviews and meta-analyses that compared LDP with ODP for pancreatic ductal adenocarcinoma (PDAC) [13, 14].

The first [13], published in 2015, included five comparative case-control studies involving 261 patients who underwent a distal pancreatectomy, of whom 80 (30.7%) undergoing LDP, and 181 (69.3%) undergoing ODP. The outcomes of clinical interest confirmed the safety of LDP. In fact, overall mortality, morbidity, postoperative pancreatic fistula, reoperation, and number of patients eligible for adjuvant therapy were similar between LDP and ODP. In addition, the laparoscopic group had longer operative times ($P = 0.04$), lesser blood loss ($P = 0.01$), a shorter hospital stay ($P < 0.001$) and smaller tumor size ($P = 0.04$). Finally, the outcomes of oncological interest showed the safety and feasibility of the LDP in PDAC. In fact, the R0 resection rate was similar between the two groups ($P = 0.53$), as were the mean harvested lymph nodes ($P = 0.33$), and the laparoscopic approach did not affect the overall survival rate ($P = 0.32$).

In the second systematic review and meta-analysis [14], published in 2016, 11 non-randomized studies were included (1506 participants, of whom 353 undergoing LDP and 1153 undergoing ODP). All of these studies were retrospective cohort-like studies or case-control studies. The outcomes of clinical interest did not show any differences between LDP and ODP: postoperative mortality was 0.5% versus 1%; postoperative morbidity 8.8% versus 5.1%; clinically relevant pancreatic fistula 7.7% versus 6.6%, etc. Mean length of hospital stay was shorter by 2.43 days in the laparoscopic group than in the open group. The calculated oncological measures were only the R status, recurrences rate and long-term mortality, and they proved to be non statistically significant between the two groups.

Conversion rate varies widely between different surgeons and centers (mean conversion rate 22%; range 0–66%) [11]. In the multicenter study of Kooby et al. [19], the conversion rate was 17% (4 out of 23 LDPs) and the reasons for conversion were hemorrhage in one patient, failure to progress in two patients, and concern for margin adequacy in the fourth. In the single-center study reported by Magge et al. [20], five patients out of 23 (18%) underwent conversion to ODP and all conversions occurred during the first 12 attempted minimally invasive resections for PDAC. More recently, probably due to an increasing expertise in performing LDP, other authors reported a conversion rate of 0% [11, 13].

18.3.2 Robotic Distal Pancreatectomy

Several authors [21, 22] reported the safety and feasibility of robotic distal pancreatectomy and three recent meta-analyses compared LDP with RDP showing similar clinical results. In addition, RDP showed less blood loss and a better rate of splenic preservation compared with LDP [23–25]. However, these studies included all types of pancreatic tumors, not only PDAC. There are no studies that considered RDP only for PDAC. Nevertheless, in the published studies RDP was performed in a higher percentage of cases (11–30%) of PDAC than LDP. Oncologic adequacy parameters reported in the meta-analysis of Gavriilidis et al. [24] reported a similar R0 margin status and number of harvested lymph nodes in the two groups considered. Waters et al. [26] first compared RDP with ODP, showing similar postoperative outcomes and the same oncological safety. More recently, Lee et al. [27] reported a study that compared RDP with ODP, taking into account only patients affected by PDAC. The oncological results (R status and positive nodes) were similar between RDP and ODP but the authors considered only four RDP versus 249 ODP. Conversion rates are reported to range from 0% to 38% [23] and are related mainly to inadequate exposure and tumor proximity to major vessels. Other reasons include tumor invading adjacent organs (excluding the spleen), margin assessment, adhesions, and bleeding. Reported risk factors for conversions to an open procedure are gender (male patients) and patients with more visceral fat mass [26]. In interpreting these results, it should be taken into account that these studies have several limitations. First, the data utilized included only retrospective case-control studies, leading to the potential introduction of additional selection and information bias. No randomized controlled trials have compared MIDP versus ODP. Thus, observed differences may be a result of confounding due to minimally invasive operation on less extensive cancer and open surgery on more extensive cancer. Second, the number of cases reported is small and is not sufficient to allow correct conclusions. Third, the information regarding hospital volume in pancreatic surgery is rarely reported. In fact, pancreatic laparoscopic/robotic surgery not only requires specific technical training, but also specific and scientific knowledge of pancreatic diseases. Four, the laparoscopic technique was different in the studies evaluated. Finally, the overall quality of evidence was very low. Other limitations are the learning curve and the costs of the procedures. Regarding the learning curve in LDP, Ricci et al. [28] showed that the main indicator for establishing completion of the learning curve was the operative time. The authors noted that it decreased with the increase in the number of procedures and established that after 17 procedures the learning curve was completed if performed by surgeons experienced with advanced laparoscopic procedures and at a high-volume center for pancreatic surgery. The completed learning curve reduced the operative time by 18%. Regarding the learning curve in RDP, Napoli et al. [29], based on the reduction of operative times (421.1±20.5 vs. 248.9±9.3 min; $p < 0.0001$), reported that completion of the learning curve was achieved after 10 operations. Shakir et al. [30], on the contrary, reported that reductions of the operative time were observed after the first 20 and 40 cases (from 311 to 266 and 210 minutes, respectively). In addition, the authors showed that RDP outcomes were optimized after 40 cases. Regarding the costs of the LDP, Ricci et al. [31] showed that LDP is more expensive than ODP but it allows for a better quality of life and especially an earlier return to normal life. Thus, the higher cost of LDP is acceptable in terms of cost-effectiveness to Italian and European health care services. The costs related to RDP are mainly due to the da Vinci system. Waters et al. [26] showed that the operative costs of RDP were higher than ODP but the costs of the hospital stay were lower. Thus, the authors suggested that a robotic approach to distal pancreatectomy is cost-effective.

In summary, despite its limitations, MIDP seems safe, feasible and oncologically effective as compared with ODP, suggesting that MIDP could be an acceptable approach for resection of pancreatic ductal adenocarcinoma of the left pancreas.

References

1. Cuschieri A, Jakimowicz JJ, van Spreeuwel J (1996) Laparoscopic distal 70% pancreatectomy and splenectomy for chronic pancreatitis. Ann Surg 223(3):280–285
2. Gagner M, Pomp A, Herrera MF (1996) Early experience with laparoscopic resections of islet cell tumors. Surgery 120(6):1051–1054
3. Melvin WS, Needleman BJ, Krause KR, Ellison EC (2003) Robotic resection of pancreatic neuroendocrine tumor. J Laparoendosc Adv Surg Tech A 13(1):33–36
4. Nigri GR, Rosman AS, Petrucciani N et al (2011) Metaanalysis of trials comparing minimally invasive and open distal pancreatectomies. Surg Endosc 25(5):1642–1651
5. Venkat R, Edil BH, Schulick RD et al (2012) Laparoscopic distal pancreatectomy is associated with significantly less overall morbidity compared to the open technique: a systematic review and meta-analysis. Ann Surg 255(6):1048–1059
6. Pericleous S, Middleton N, McKay SC et al (2012) Systematic review and meta-analysis of case-matched studies comparing open and laparoscopic distal pancreatectomy: is it a safe procedure? Pancreas 41(7):993–1000
7. Mehrabi A, Hafezi M, Arvin J et al (2015) A systematic review and meta-analysis of laparoscopic versus open distal pancreatectomy for benign and malignant lesions of the pancreas: it's time to randomize. Surgery 157(1):45–55

8. Sulpice L, Farges O, Goutte N et al; ACHBT French Pancreatectomy Study Group (2015) Laparoscopic distal pancreatectomy for pancreatic ductal adenocarcinoma: time for a randomized controlled trial? Results of an all-inclusive national observational study. Ann Surg 262(5):868–874
9. Adam MA, Choudhury K, Goffredo P et al (2015) Minimally invasive distal pancreatectomy for cancer: short-term oncologic outcomes in 1733 patients. World J Surg 39(10):2564–2572
10. Strasberg SM, Drebin JA, Linehan D (2003) Radical antegrade modular pancreatosplenectomy. Surgery 133(5):521–527
11. Abu Hilal M, Richardson JR, de Rooij T et al (2016) Laparoscopic radical 'no-touch' left pancreatosplenectomy for pancreatic ductal adenocarcinoma: technique and results. Surg Endosc 30(9):3830–3838
12. Kuroki T, Eguchi S (2015) Laparoscopic distal pancreatectomy for pancreatic ductal adenocarcinoma. Surg Today 45(7):808–812
13. Ricci C, Casadei R, Taffurelli G et al (2015) Laparoscopic versus open distal pancreatectomy for ductal adenocarcinoma: a systematic review and meta-analysis. J Gastrointest Surg 19(4):770–781
14. Riviere D, Gurusamy KS, Kooby DA et al (2016) Laparoscopic versus open distal pancreatectomy for pancreatic cancer. Cochrane Database Syst Rev 4:CD011391
15. Strickland M, Hallet J, Abramowitz D et al (2015) Lateral approach in laparoscopic distal pancreatectomy is safe and potentially beneficial compared to the traditional medial approach. Surg Endosc 29(9):2825–2831
16. Casadei R, Ricci C, D'Ambra M et al (2010) Laparoscopic versus open distal pancreatectomy in pancreatic tumours: a case-control study. Updates Surg 62(3–4):171–174
17. Tol JA, Gouma DJ, Bassi C et al; International Study Group on Pancreatic Surgery (2014) Definition of a standard lymphadenectomy in surgery for pancreatic ductal adenocarcinoma: a consensus statement by the International Study Group on Pancreatic Surgery (ISGPS). Surgery 156(3):591–600
18. Ricci C, Casadei R, Taffurelli G et al (2016) Laparoscopic distal pancreatectomy: many meta-analyses, few certainties. Updates Surg 68(3):225–234
19. Kooby DA, Hawkins WG, Schmidt CM et al (2010) A multicenter analysis of distal pancreatectomy for adenocarcinoma: is laparoscopic resection appropriate? J Am Coll Surg 210(5):779–785
20. Magge D, Gooding W, Choudry H et al (2013) Comparative effectiveness of minimally invasive and open distal pancreatectomy for ductal adenocarcinoma. JAMA Surg 148(6):525–531
21. Cirocchi R, Partelli S, Coratti A et al (2013) Current status of robotic distal pancreatectomy: a systematic review. Surg Oncol 22(3):201–207
22. Boggi U, Napoli N, Costa F et al (2016) Robotic-assisted pancreatic resections. World J Surg 40(10):2497–2506
23. Huang B, Feng L, Zhao J (2016) Systematic review and meta-analysis of robotic versus laparoscopic distal pancreatectomy for benign and malignant pancreatic lesions. Surg Endosc 30(9):4078–4085
24. Gavriilidis P, Lim C, Menahem B et al (2016) Robotic versus laparoscopic distal pancreatectomy – The first meta-analysis. HPB (Oxford) 18(7):567–574
25. Zhou JY, Xin C, Mou YP et al (2016) Robotic versus laparoscopic distal pancreatectomy: a meta-analysis of short-term outcomes. PLoS One 11(3):e0151189
26. Waters JA, Canal DF, Wiebke EA ct al (2010) Robotic distal pancreatectomy: cost effective? Surgery 148(4):814–823
27. Lee SY, Allen PJ, Sadot E et al (2015) Distal pancreatectomy: a single institution's experience in open, laparoscopic, and robotic approaches. J Am Coll Surg 220(1):18–27
28. Ricci C, Casadei R, Buscemi S et al (2015) Laparoscopic distal pancreatectomy: what factors are related to the learning curve? Surg Today 45(1):50–56
29. Napoli N, Kauffmann EF, Perrone VG et al (2015) The learning curve in robotic distal pancreatectomy. Updates Surg 67(3):257–264

30. Shakir M, Boone BA, Polanco PM et al (2015) The learning curve for robotic distal pancreatectomy: an analysis of outcomes of the first 100 consecutive cases at a high-volume pancreatic centre. HPB (Oxford) 17(7):580–586
31. Ricci C, Casadei R, Taffurelli G et al (2015) Laparoscopic distal pancreatectomy in benign or premalignant pancreatic lesions: is it really more cost-effective than open approach? J Gastrointest Surg 19(8):1415–1424

19 Spleen-Preserving Distal Pancreatectomy with and without Preservation of the Splenic Vessels

Alessandro Esposito, Luca Landoni, Luca Casetti, Stefano Andrianello, Giovanni Butturini, Roberto Salvia, and Claudio Bassi

19.1 Introduction

Preservation of the spleen during distal pancreatectomy was first proposed [1] to reduce possible infectious and hematologic complications that often occur after splenectomy, such as postsplenectomy sepsis, abdominal abscesses, pulmonary complications and thrombocytosis [2–4]. Without performing splenectomy, a complete clearance of the retroperitoneum and adequate lymph node retrieval cannot be obtained, and for this reason spleen-preserving distal pancreatectomy can only be carried out in the case of benign or borderline disease of the body and tail of the pancreas. The main indications are usually non-functioning neuroendocrine tumors smaller than 20 mm [5], insulinomas, serous cystadenomas and mucinous cysts, such as intraductal papillary mucinous neoplasms and mucinous cystadenomas, without signs of imminent malignant degeneration. Different techniques for spleen preservation have been described. The Warshaw procedure [6] requires ligation of the splenic vessels both at the level of the pancreatic transection margin and at the level of the splenic hilum leaving the blood supply to the spleen through the short gastric and left gastroepiploic vessels. In recent years, this procedure has gained popularity especially among laparoscopic surgeons since it is probably more straightforward, faster and associated with lesser blood loss as the pancreatic tail must not be detached from the splenic vessels.

C. Bassi (✉)
Department of General and Pancreatic Surgery, The Pancreas Institute, University of Verona Hospital Trust
Verona, Italy
e-mail: claudio.bassi@univr.it

U. Boggi (Ed), *Minimally Invasive Surgery of the Pancreas*,
Updates in Surgery
DOI: 10.1007/978-88-470-3958-2_19, © Springer-Verlag Italia 2018

However, there is some concern about a conspicuous incidence of splenic infarction and gastric varices [7–9]. On the other hand, splenic vessel preservation, known as the Kimura procedure [10], is more technically challenging and even though theoretically it should maintain an intact blood supply to the spleen, patency of the splenic vein and artery could be compromised [11, 12].

19.2 Operative Technique

We always use two different monitors placed on the right and left side of the patient, just above the shoulders (Fig. 19.1). The patient is placed in a supine position, 20–30° reverse Trendelenburg, 15–20° right-tilted, with the left arm abducted and the legs spread apart. The operating surgeon is positioned between patient's legs; the first assistant is on the left of the operating surgeon and the

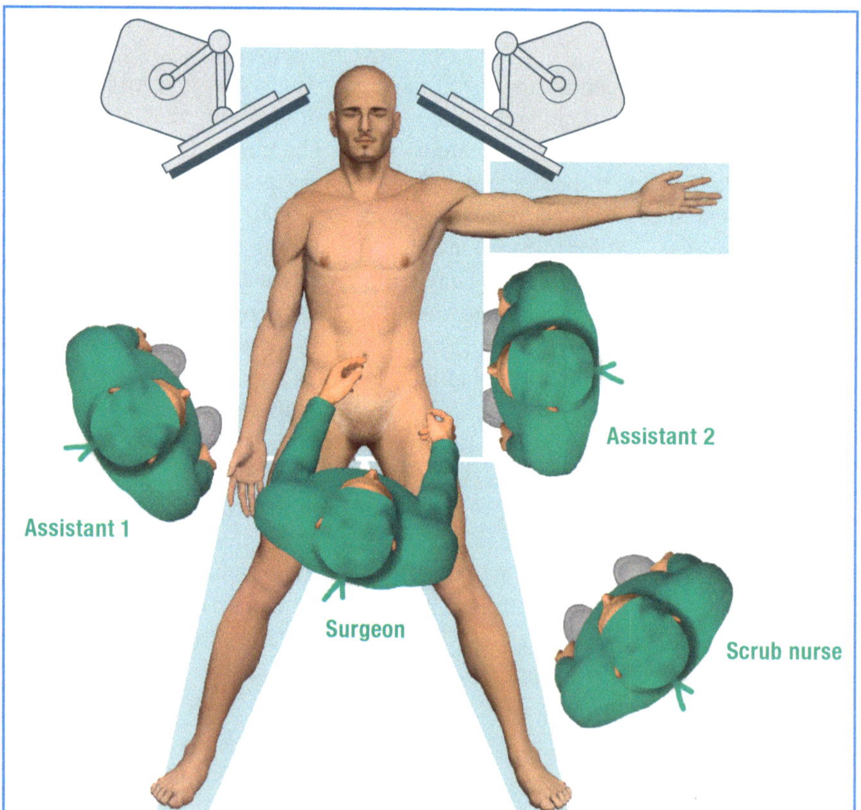

Fig. 19.1 Surgical team during spleen-preserving distal pancreatectomy: operating surgeon between the patient's legs; first assistant on the right of the patient; second assistant on the left; scrub nurse on the left, behind the second assistant

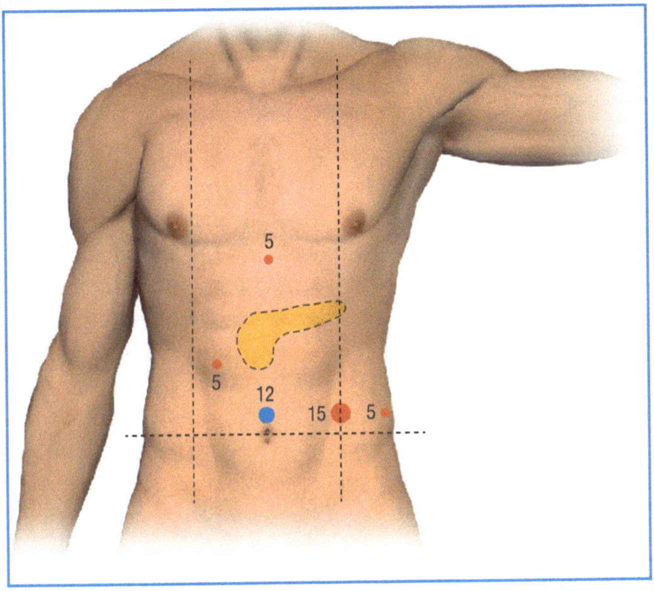

Fig. 19.2 Placement of trocars for spleen-preserving distal pancreatectomy

second assistant is on the left side of the patient. The scrub nurse is on the right side of the operating surgeon. Four ports are used: one 12-mm optical port above the umbilicus, one 5-mm operating trocar in the epigastrium, one 5-mm operating trocar in the right hypochondrium and one 15-mm operating trocar in the left hypochondrium at the level of the lateral aspect of the rectus abdominis muscle or at the level of the midclavicular line. If necessary, another 5-mm trocar may be placed in the left hypochondrium, lower and 10 cm more lateral than the last one described, with the function to retract caudally the splenic flexure in difficult cases (Fig. 19.2). We prefer a 30° scope and the most used instruments are a fenestrated grasper, scissors, monopolar hook, bipolar forceps, blunt dissector, ultrasonic dissector and clip applier. The procedure begins with access to the lesser sac by transecting the gastrocolic ligament from the level of the pancreatic neck to the splenic hilum. At this time, intraoperative ultrasound can be very useful if the lesion is not immediately recognized. Moreover, ultrasound is mandatory to assess the position of the tumor relative to the splenic vessels to confirm the operative strategy for splenic vessel management. We recommend not to routinely lower the splenic flexure by transecting the splenocolic ligament in order to maintain a good blood supply to the spleen. The stomach is retracted cephalad using a grasper introduced through the epigastric port to expose the pancreas. The stomach can also be suspended by using a Penrose drain passed through the lesser sac. Using the monopolar hook and ultrasonic dissector, dissection is continued at the level of the inferior border of the pancreas exposing the superior mesenteric vein. The retropancreatic tunnel is started with blunt dissection at the inferior border of the pancreas detaching the pancreatic neck from the superior mesenteric vein. Then, dissection with the monopolar hook and ultrasonic dissector is continued at the superior border of the pancreas exposing the hepatic artery, splenic artery and portal vein. Lifting the stomach, the left gastric vein can be exposed and used as a landmark to discriminate the common hepatic artery from the splenic artery that can usually be recognized on the lateral aspect of the left gastric vein. The splenic artery is isolated and placed on a vessel loop. The cephalad portion of the retropancreatic tunnel is then completed and pancreatic neck is passed with the blunt dissector and placed on an umbilical tape. By lifting the pancreatic neck, the splenic vein can be recognized, dissected and isolated through a combination of blunt dissection and monopolar hook and eventually placed on a vessel loop as well. Sometimes, on lifting the pancreatic neck, the splenic vein may be excessively retracted cephalad making its dissection difficult. In such cases, the splenic vein can be more easily isolated before completing the retropancreatic tunnel. Intraoperative ultrasound can be used to accurately measure pancreatic thickness. The pancreas is then transected by performing a formal distal pancreatectomy or a parenchyma-sparing procedure sectioning at least 20 mm from the macroscopic borders of the lesion. In the case of pancreatic remnants thinner than 20 mm we usually prefer an endostapler with reinforced suture line (Endo GIA Reinforced Reload with Tri-Staple Technology, violet or black cartridge, Covidien). In the case of thicker pancreatic remnants, or if the retropancreatic tunnel is not suitable for introduction of the device, the endostapler might not be a valid and safe option. In these cases, we prefer to directly transect the pancreas with the ultrasonic dissector. Both techniques can ensure a good level of hemostasis. In the case of splenic vessel preservation, a meticulous dissection is performed by lifting the pancreas and detaching the posterior aspect of the gland from the splenic vessels and from the retroperitoneal surface using a monopolar hook, blunt dissection and ultrasonic dissection. Small branches from the pancreas to the splenic vessels should be carefully identified and coagulated with the ultrasonic dissector or bipolar forceps or ligated using clips. After completing the mobilization from medially to laterally, the pancreatic body/tail specimen is placed into an endobag and extracted from the umbilical port incision or, in the case of large cystic lesions, from a Pfannenstiel incision.

In the Warshaw procedure, the splenic artery and veins are transected at the level of the celiac trunk and at the level of the superior mesenteric vein/portal vein axis, respectively. The left gastric vein should be preserved if possible. Proximal splenic vessel transection must be performed before sectioning the pancreas. Proceeding with the dissection from medial to lateral, the splenic vessels are ligated again at the level of the splenic hilum preserving the left gastroepiploic vessels. Vessel transection is usually performed using clips, vascular staplers, or polymeric locking ligation systems (hem-o-lok, Weck closure system). Color and viability of the spleen is then checked to assess the adequacy of blood supply. If there is a clear risk of massive splenic infarction, splenectomy is carried out. Splenic vessel resection is usually carried out if splenic vessel dissection from the pancreas is not safe or in the case of uncontrolled bleeding that usually occurs while resecting large masses. Other possible settings that increase the efforts needed to achieve complete detachment of the splenic vessels from the pancreatic tail are the presence of tight adhesions between the lesion and the vessels and excessive coiling or kinking of the splenic artery. For these reasons, it is mandatory to obtain complete control of splenic vessels before proceeding with pancreas transection and mobilization.

The surgical procedure ends with the placement of either Penrose or closed suction drains at the level of the pancreatic transection margin.

19.3 Issues in Splenic Vessel Resection or Preservation

Laparoscopic spleen-preserving distal pancreatectomy, both with splenic vessel resection or preservation, is a widely reported surgical technique [2, 3, 6, 7, 9–17]. Currently, the only accepted indication is for benign or at least borderline lesions of the tail of the pancreas even though there is no trial demonstrating the long-term oncologic outcomes of the latter. For this reason, the first critical issue regards appropriate patient selection through a complete preoperative work-up able to correctly diagnose lesions such as low-grade neuroendocrine tumors, benign or borderline cystic lesions or solid pseudopapillary tumors. The Warshaw technique should be a faster and more straightforward technique. It is often carried out when preservation of the splenic vessels fails due to uncontrolled bleeding, and for this reason it should be associated with greater intraoperative blood loss. Moreover, the reduced arterial blood supply to the spleen should increase the risk of splenic infarction and the venous blood flow, shifted from the splenic vein to the short gastric vessels, should produce gastric varices with possible upper gastrointestinal bleeding. Splenic vessel preservation, instead, should maintain viability of the spleen, but it is a more technically-demanding procedure with longer operative times. The splenic artery varies among patients with marked differences in tortuosity of the vessel from the origin to the splenic hilum. The splenic vein, by contrast, is invariably straight but often embedded in the body of the pancreas receiving branches that are very fine and easily injured. These theories, however, are not so consistent with the literature. Quite large series do not report any difference in terms of intraoperative blood loss or operative time when comparing splenic vessel preservation or resection [7, 13]. Nevertheless, evidence about long-term follow-up may be required to prove the safety of splenic vessel resection since results from large surgical series show that the incidence of splenic abscess or infarction could be low (9–14.2%) even in the case of vessel resection [17]. The number of short gastric vessels is somewhat variable. Their sufficiency in perfusing the spleen could be evaluated by clamping the splenic vessels at the level of distal resection, before attempting pancreatic tail dissection from the splenic vein and artery. In the event of uncontrolled bleeding, this test of splenic viability could be precluded since the splenic vessels are immediately ligated. Failed spleen preservation requiring splenectomy significantly prolongs the operative time and increases the rate of massive bleeding, transfusions, conversion to open surgery and surgical morbidity [15]. This suggests that spleen preservation is probably beneficial for patients undergoing distal pancreatectomy. The shift of venous return through the short gastric vessels is responsible for the specific risk of developing gastric varices. Most series show that a fairly large portion of patients will develop gastric varices after splenic vessel resection (30–70%), but the risk of bleeding has been reported to be low (<5%) [7, 13, 18–20].

Although only few reports have been published in the last decade, splenic vessel resection or preservation during spleen-preserving distal pancreatectomy seems to share similar surgical outcomes with regard to operative time, blood loss and length of hospital stay and, in expert hands, even similar results in terms of spleen viability [17]. The robotic approach seems to increase the rate of splenic vessel preservation when compared with conventional laparoscopy since it is more effective in vessel dissection [15]. Splenic vessel preservation, however, should always be attempted since it certainly ensures the most physiological blood supply to the spleen; the procedure must be switched to vessel resection in the event of difficult resections or uncontrolled bleeding.

References

1. Gagner M, Pomp A, Herrera MF (1996) Early experience with laparoscopic resections of islet cell tumors. Surgery 120:1051–1054
2. Shoup M, Brennan MF, McWhite K et al (2002) The value of splenic preservation with distal pancreatectomy. Arch Surg 137(2):164–168
3. Aldridge MC, Williamson RC (1991) Distal pancreatectomy with and without splenectomy. Br J Surg 78(8):976–979
4. Koukoutsis I, Tamijmarane A, Bellagamba R et al (2007) The impact of splenectomy on outcomes after distal and total pancreatectomy. World J Surg Oncol 5:61
5. Falconi M, Eriksson B, Kaltsas G et al (2016) Consensus guidelines update for the management of functional p-NETs (F-p-NETs) and non-functional p-NETs (NF-p-NETs). Neuroendocrinology 103(2):153–171
6. Vezakis A, Davides D, Larvin M, McMahon MJ (1999) Laparoscopic surgery combined with preservation of the spleen for distal pancreatic tumors. Surg Endosc 13(1):26–29
7. Butturini G, Inama M, Malleo G (2012) Perioperative and long-term results of laparoscopic spleen-preserving distal pancreatectomy with or without splenic vessels conservation: a retrospective analysis. J Surg Oncol 105(4):387–392
8. Miura F, Takada T, Asano T et al (2005) Hemodynamic changes of splenogastric circulation after spleen-preserving pancreatectomy with excision of splenic artery and vein. Surgery 138(3):518–522
9. Fernández-Cruz L, Martínez I, Gilabert R et al (2004) Laparoscopic distal pancreatectomy combined with preservation of the spleen for cystic neoplasms of the pancreas. J Gastrointest Surg 8(4):493–501
10. Kimura W, Inoue T, Futakawa N et al (1996) Spleen-preserving distal pancreatectomy with conservation of the splenic artery and vein. Surgery 120(5):885–890

11. Yoon YS, Lee KH, Han HS et al (2009) Patency of splenic vessels after laparoscopic spleen and splenic vessel-preserving distal pancreatectomy. Br J Surg 96(6):633–640
12. Yoon YS, Lee KH, Han H-S et al (2014) Effects of laparoscopic versus open surgery on splenic vessel patency after spleen and splenic vessel-preserving distal pancreatectomy: a retrospective multicenter study. Surg Endosc 29(3):583–588
13. Zhou ZQ, Kim SC, Song KB et al (2014) Laparoscopic spleen-preserving distal pancreatectomy: comparative study of spleen preservation with splenic vessel resection and splenic vessel preservation. World J Surg 38(11):2973–2979
14. Inoko K, Ebihara Y, Sakamoto K et al (2015) Strategic approach to the splenic artery in laparoscopic spleen-preserving distal pancreatectomy. Surg Laparosc Endosc Percutan Tech 25(4):e122–e125
15. Chen S, Zhan Q, Chen JZ et al (2015) Robotic approach improves spleen-preserving rate and shortens postoperative hospital stay of laparoscopic distal pancreatectomy: a matched cohort study. Surg Endosc 29(12):3507–3518
16. Ntourakis D, Marescaux J, Pessaux P (2015) Robotic spleen preserving distal pancreatectomy: how I do it (with video). World J Surg 39(1):292–296
17. Yu X, Li H, Jin C et al (2015) Splenic vessel preservation versus Warshaw's technique during spleen-preserving distal pancreatectomy: a meta-analysis and systematic review. Langenbecks Arch Surg 400(2):183–191
18. Carrère N, Abid S, Julio CH et al (2007) Spleen-preserving distal pancreatectomy with excision of splenic artery and vein: a case-matched comparison with conventional distal pancreatectomy with splenectomy. World J Surg 31(2):375–382
19. Miura F, Sano K, Amano H et al (2011) Is spleen-preserving distal pancreatectomy with excision of the splenic artery and vein feasible? Surgery 150(3):572
20. Tien YW, Liu KL, Hu RH et al (2010) Risk of varices bleeding after spleen-preserving distal pancreatectomy with excision of splenic artery and vein. Ann Surg Oncol 17(8):2193–2198

Minimally Invasive Pancreatectomy plus Islet Autotransplantation for Benign Tumors of the Pancreatic Neck and Body

20

Francesca Aleotti, Rita Nano, Paola Maffi, Lorenzo Piemonti, Massimo Falconi, and Gianpaolo Balzano

20.1 The Emerging Surgical Problem of Benign Pancreatic Lesions

Thanks to the rapid evolution of diagnostic techniques as well as to their more widespread use, there has been a continuous rise in the number of patients diagnosed with pancreatic lesions, particularly benign/borderline lesions, such as intraductal papillary mucinous neoplasms (IPMN), serous/mucinous cystadenomas, and neuroendocrine tumors. These pancreatic incidentalomas, encountered during diagnostic assessment or follow-up for other clinical conditions, must be carefully evaluated to decide about surgical treatment or follow-up. According to recent estimations, more than one million Italian people may have such benign pancreatic lesions; only a strict minority of those lesions will evolve to malignancy. Therefore, the risk of undergoing unnecessary surgery and dying from the complications of this surgery is indeed higher than the risk of dying as a result of malignant transformation. In fact, though the mortality rate of pancreatic resections has dropped under 3–5% in high-volume centers, it remains higher than 10% in low-volume hospitals. A recent paper evaluating the outcome of pancreatic cancer surgery in Italy found that about 90% of hospitals offering surgery to patients with pancreatic cancer were in the very-low-volume and low-volume categories. Beyond surgical complications, the second problem of pancreatic resections is pancreatic insufficiency, both exocrine and endocrine. In particular, the onset of postsurgical diabetes – pancreatogenic diabetes mellitus, or type 3c

G. Balzano (✉)
Pancreas Translational and Clinical Research Center, Università Vita e Salute,
San Raffaele Scientific Institute
Milan, Italy
e-mail: balzano.gianpaolo@hsr.it

U. Boggi (Ed), *Minimally Invasive Surgery of the Pancreas*,
Updates in Surgery
DOI: 10.1007/978-88-470-3958-2_20, © Springer-Verlag Italia 2018

diabetes mellitus (T3cDM) – may impact quality of life, and it is often an underestimated consequence of pancreatic surgery. We have prospectively evaluated 651 patient candidates for pancreatic surgery, finding that the risk of developing diabetes after left pancreatectomy was 21%, which increased to 30–50% during follow-up. This risk was associated with classic risk factors of type 2 DM (age, family history, body mass index) and the amount of pancreas removed (subtotal pancreatectomies and distal resections are at higher risk of developing T3cDM). While the loss of exocrine parenchyma, resulting in lipid malabsorption, can be relatively easily compensated for by the oral administration of pancreatic enzyme capsules, T3cDM most often necessitates subcutaneous insulin injections along with a perpetual strict control of blood sugar levels. Moreover, T3cDM has often been linked to a so-called "brittle" diabetes that is at higher risk of both hypo- and hyperglycemic events. This is of course most frequent in patients who have undergone total pancreatectomy but it should be considered that all parenchyma resections cause not only a loss of insulin-producing β cells, but also of the counter-regulatory components of Langerhans' islets (i.e., glucagon-secreting α cells).

20.2 Minimally Invasive Distal Pancreatectomy

The question of whether laparoscopy is superior to the open approach in distal pancreatectomy is still a subject of debate. Its advantages are linked to a more rapid postoperative recovery with a shorter hospital stay and reduced postoperative pain, as well as better esthetic results. Much of the concern regarding these techniques is that there is to date insufficient literature (in terms of randomized controlled trials) demonstrating similar oncological long-term outcomes in patients undergoing surgery for pancreatic adenocarcinoma. As oncological concerns are not applicable to benign or borderline neoplasms of the left pancreas, these lesions should therefore represent the ideal disease to be treated with minimally invasive surgery. Furthermore, pancreatic adenocarcinoma is rare in young patients, showing a growing incidence with age, whereas benign lesions can affect patients of all ages, especially female patients in the case of cystadenomas. Young patients with benign and borderline pancreatic lesions are therefore the ideal candidates for minimally invasive distal pancreatectomy, and are those more often requesting minimally invasive surgery.

20.3 Islet Autotransplantation to Improve Glycemic Control after Pancreatic Resections

As pancreatic surgery became progressively safer, the decrease in mortality rates corresponded with an increased interest in postoperative morbidity rates and quality of life. Diabetes is certainly the major long-term disabling consequence of pancreatic resections, because of its impact on everyday life, possible acute events (such as hypoglycemic episodes) and long-term complications (such as nephropathy, neuropathy and retinopathy). Differently from patients with malignancy, whose life-expectancy is unfortunately short, diabetes may have heavy effects on patients with benign or borderline lesions.

The first autologous transplant of endocrine pancreatic islets was performed at the University of Minnesota in 1977. It was initially developed for those patients with chronic pancreatitis for whom total pancreatectomy was proposed. Since then, the University of Minnesota, along with a few other centers worldwide, has published data regarding large series of patients, demonstrating that a majority of patients receiving islet autotransplantation (IAT) achieved islet graft function. The most important factor associated with the rate of insulin independence appears to be the number of islet cells transplanted/kg. The initial criteria for patient eligibility set by Minnesota included only patients with chronic pancreatitis; no mention was made of patients with other benign lesions, and pancreatic malignancy was a specific contraindication. Since then a few case reports and case series have been published documenting the use of IAT in patients with benign tumors or even with pancreatic or periampullary malignancy.

The first systematic use of IAT in patients with disease other than chronic pancreatitis took place at our institution, starting in 2008. Since then, 58 patients received IAT at San Raffaele Hospital. We have applied this technique in patients receiving resection for chronic pancreatitis, but also in other patient groups:

a) patients undergoing completion pancreatectomy for pancreatic fistula after pancreatoduodenectomy (PD);
b) patients initially treated by PD, but in whom a pancreatic anastomosis was considered too risky, and who therefore underwent completion pancreatectomy during the same operation;
c) patients undergoing extended distal pancreatectomy for benign/borderline lesions located at the pancreatic neck or proximal body, as discussed in this chapter; the alternative procedure for these patients would have been either extended distal pancreatectomy without IAT or central pancreatectomy, which is, however, burdened by an increased risk of clinically significant pancreatic fistulas.

20.3.1 Methods of Islet Isolation

Ricordi first described the method of islet isolation in 1988 to enhance the disassembling of the pancreatic tissue via a combined enzymatic and mechanical digestion while preserving endocrine cell cluster integrity (Fig. 20.1). Briefly, the pancreatic duct is cannulated with a 14–20G catheter and distended by intraductal infusion of a cold collagenase solution. After digestion at 37°C

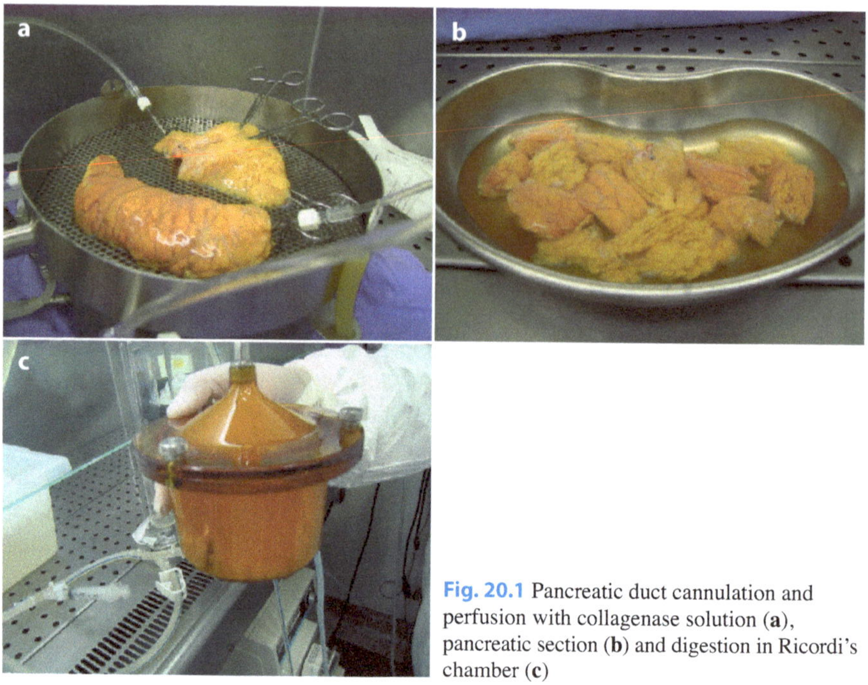

Fig. 20.1 Pancreatic duct cannulation and perfusion with collagenase solution (**a**), pancreatic section (**b**) and digestion in Ricordi's chamber (**c**)

in a modified Ricordi chamber, islets are purified in a cell processor using a continuous gradient. Purified islet fractions are counted and their numbers expressed as number of islets normalized to IEQ (islet equivalent: volume of 150 μm diameter sphere). Evidence of no microbial contamination, as documented by a negative Gram stain of the islet preparation immediately before transplant and by negative microbial cultures reported at the time of infusion should be mandatory. When IAT is applied to the patients discussed in this chapter, i.e., patients treated by distal pancreatectomy because of benign or borderline tumors, islets are infused the day after operation by an angiographic procedure, through percutaneous transhepatic cannulation of the portal vein with an 18-Gauge catheter, under ultrasonographic and fluoroscopic guidance (Fig. 20.2). Patency of the portal vein and portal pressure is recorded before and after the infusion. In those patients in whom infusion into the portal vein is contraindicated, such as patients with hepatic lesions or cirrhosis, islets can be infused in the bone marrow at the level of the superior-posterior iliac crest under local anesthesia. The use of the bone marrow as a safe and efficient alternative site for islet transplantation has been assessed by our group.

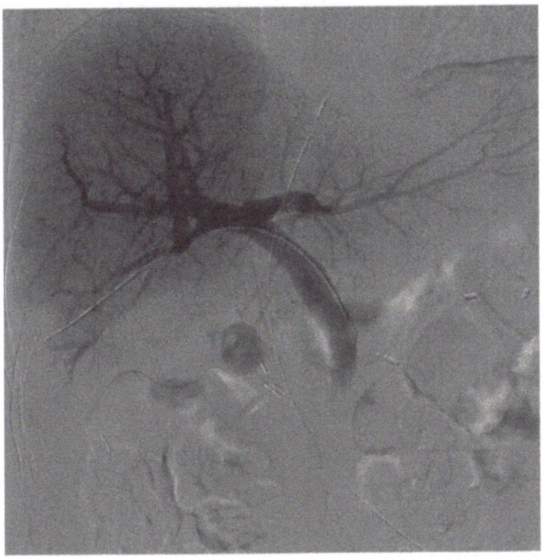

Fig. 20.2 Transhepatic islet infusion under fluoroscopic guidance

20.3.2 Results of Distal Pancreatectomy and Islet Autotransplantation

In our center, 19 patients were candidates for extended distal pancreatectomy and IAT owing to body-neck benign or borderline tumors. Of these, in two cases it was not possible to proceed with the transplant, because of an insufficient islet yield in one case and an intraoperative finding of intraductal papillary mucinous neoplasm with severe dysplasia in the other. Therefore 17 patients completed the procedure. Six of them underwent minimally invasive surgery. Demographics, operative results and pathologic data of the population are reported in Table 20.1. Nine (53%) of 17 patients had minor postpancreatectomy complications, none had major complications (i.e., Clavien-Dindo >2). Complications related

Table 20.1 Patients undergoing distal pancreatectomy plus islet autotransplantation

Number of patients	19
Age	58 ± 13 years
Sex (M/F)	6/13
Pathology	10 cystic lesions 7 NETs 1 chronic pancreatitis 1 other (gastric GIST)
Postoperative complications	9 (52.9%): all minor complications
PostIAT complications	2 (11.7%)

IAT, islet autotransplantation; *NET*, neuroendocrine tumor; *GIST*, gastrointestinal stromal tumor.

to IAT occurred in two (11.7%) patients: one left branch portal vein thrombosis, successfully treated with anticoagulation therapy, and one liver bleed, which resolved spontaneously. The median postoperative hospital stay was 9 days. All patients were disease free at their last scheduled follow-up visit (731–109 days). The median number of infused islets was 1036 (594–1565) IEQ/kg. A total of 94% of patients achieved and maintained insulin independence, while one patient needed small doses of insulin immediately after surgery (median 0.16 U/kg/day). Two patients developed mild hyperglycemia and were successfully treated with oral hypoglycemic agents and lifestyle modification, respectively. At the last follow-up visit, all patients had a stable HbA1c (5.8% [5.3–6.1%]) and showed sustained insulin production (fasting C-peptide: 1.61 ng/mL [1.31–1.87]), with no significant change from presurgical levels. Of note, no patients experienced hypoglycemic episodes.

20.4 Discussion and Conclusions

Benign pancreatic lesion of the pancreatic neck might require extensive surgery, possibly leading to pancreatogenic diabetes. The incidence of new-onset diabetes after distal pancreatectomy is probably underestimated: the analysis of diabetes occurrence in hemipancreatectomized living-donors for pancreas transplantation showed an unexpectedly high rate of glucose metabolism impairment, with 25% of donors having overt diabetes or glucose intolerance [1] and 40% having abnormalities of glucose metabolism 3–10 years after donation [2]. An additional important aspect to consider when assessing the burden of diabetes after partial pancreatectomy is the duration of postsurgical follow-up: while shortly after partial pancreatectomy, 8–23% of patients have pancreatogenic diabetes, this proportion increases to 30–50% during the follow-up [3]. Recently, we reported that 21% of the patients undergoing partial pancreatectomy experienced new-onset diabetes and 30% of those with diabetes prior to surgery had worsening of glucose control [4]: because median follow-up was 2.2 years, we may have underestimated the true incidence of pancreatogenic diabetes. Central pancreatectomy has been proposed as a surgical strategy for the treatment of benign neoplasms of the pancreatic body-neck [5–8], as a technique to prevent pancreatic insufficiency. However, central pancreatectomy has even a higher risk of pancreatic fistula compared to distal pancreatectomy [7, 9] and, in central pancreatectomy the fistula occurring at the anastomotic site will be an active one. Further, in cases of benign lesion, the distal pancreas is usually soft with a non-dilated duct, increasing the probability of a clinically significant pancreatic fistula.

Islet autotransplantation is a promising strategy for reducing the risk of diabetes onset after pancreatic resection. IAT may be an alternative to central pancreatectomy to preserve the endocrine function of the distal pancreas without increasing the fistula risk. The expected complications of transhepatic islet infusion are low, mainly related to minor intra- and perihepatic bleeding and transient portal thrombosis [10, 11]. Ris et al. [12] reported their experience in open distal pancreatectomy and IAT in 25 patients over a 17-year period. At a median follow-up of 90 months, all patients were insulin independent.

In our case series, minimally invasive distal pancreatectomy with IAT proved to be a substantially safe procedure, both regarding postoperative and postprocedural complications and long-term oncological safety. Only one patient developed insulin-dependent diabetes.

A concern regarding this strategy is the possibility of occult malignancy in the normal pancreas segment to be processed for IAT. Careful pre- and intraoperative work-up, including endoscopic ultrasound is essential for accurate patient selection. In our protocol, the presence of any multifocal pancreatic neoplasm at preoperative imaging or intraoperative evaluation, including multifocal benign intraductal-papillary mucinous neoplasm or a diagnosis (suspected or ascertained) of multiple endocrine neoplasm is an exclusion criterion. Further, pancreatic specimens are sent for frozen section analysis of the margin, with a margin of 1 cm from the processed portion of the gland. In our series, this procedure guaranteed that patients were disease-free with a median follow-up of 2 years.

The ultimate goal of our technique is to reduce the morbidity of extended pancreatic resection required for patients with benign pancreatic tumor of the body-neck. The minimally invasive treatment in combination with IAT will provide an improvement in the early and late postoperative quality of life of these patients.

References

1. Kendall DM, Sutherland DE, Najarian JS et al (1990) Effects of hemipancreatectomy on insulin secretion and glucose tolerance in healthy humans. N Engl J Med 322(13):898–903
2. Kumar AF, Gruessner RW, Seaquist ER (2008) Risk of glucose intolerance and diabetes in hemipancreatectomized donors selected for normal preoperative glucose metabolism. Diabetes Care 31(8):1639–1643
3. Maeda H, Hanazaki K (2011) Pancreatogenic diabetes after pancreatic resection. Pancreatology 11(2):268–276
4. Balzano G, Dugnani E, Pasquale V et al (2014) Clinical signature and pathogenetic factors of diabetes associated with pancreas disease (T3cDM): a prospective observational study in surgical patients. Acta Diabetol 51(5):801–811
5. Balzano G, Zerbi A, Veronesi P et al (2003) Surgical treatment of benign and borderline neoplasms of the pancreatic body. Dig Surg 20(6):506–510
6. Orsenigo E, Baccari P, Bissolotti G, Staudacher C (2006) Laparoscopic central pancreatectomy. Am J Surg 191(4):549–552
7. Efron DT, Lillemoe KD, Cameron JL, Yeo CJ (2004) Central pancreatectomy with pancreaticogastrostomy for benign pancreatic pathology. J Gastrointest Surg 8(5):532–538
8. Hirono S, Tani M, Kawai M et al (2009) A central pancreatectomy for benign or low-grade malignant neoplasms. J Gastrointest Surg 13(9):1659–1665

9. Balzano G, Zerbi A, Cristallo M, Di Carlo V (2005) The unsolved problem of fistula after left pancreatectomy: the benefit of cautious drain management. J Gastrointest Surg 9(6):837–842
10. Kawahara T, Kin T, Kashkoush S et al (2011) Portal vein thrombosis is a potentially preventable complication in clinical islet transplantation. Am J Transplant 11(12):2700–2707
11. Villiger P, Ryan EA, Owen R et al (2005) Prevention of bleeding after islet transplantation: lessons learned from a multivariate analysis of 132 cases at a single institution. Am J Transplant 5(12):2992–2998
12. Ris F, Niclauss N, Morel P et al (2011) Islet autotransplantation after extended pancreatectomy for focal benign disease of the pancreas. Transplantation 91(8):895–901

Laparoscopic Distal Pancreatectomy with En Bloc Splenectomy

21

Alessandro Coppola, Damiano Caputo, Felice Giuliante, and Roberto Coppola

21.1 Introduction

In recent years, the widespread application of minimally invasive surgery has gradually expanded to several surgical fields, and has become the gold standard of care for many surgical diseases [1]. The advantages of minimally invasive surgery for diseases of the pancreas are still under evaluation. Nowadays, there is a widespread use of laparoscopic and robotic techniques also in pancreatic surgery, and several reports confirm the feasibility and safety of this approach.

At the beginning of the laparoscopic era only patients with benign or functional diseases were considered candidates for a laparoscopic approach [2]. The oncological appropriateness of this approach compared to the open approach was debated for a long time. Technological and instrumental improvements as well as an increased experience have extended the feasibility of performing more complex surgical procedures such as distal pancreatectomy and pancreatoduodenectomy. In addition, recent advances in surgical techniques and perioperative management have facilitated safe and successful pancreatic resections, which represent the first step for a cure for patients with pancreatic malignancies.

Pancreatoduodenectomy and distal pancreatectomy are the two common surgical procedures performed to treat pancreatic diseases.

Laparoscopic pancreatoduodenectomy (LPD) requires a high level of laparoscopic skill, a clear understanding of the anatomy and a high level of expertise in open pancreatic surgery. For these reasons, the use of the laparoscopic approach for surgery of the head of the pancreas is still debatable.

R. Coppola (✉)
Department of Surgery, Campus Bio-Medico University of Rome
Rome, Italy
e-mail: r.coppola@unicampus.it

U. Boggi (Ed), *Minimally Invasive Surgery of the Pancreas*,
Updates in Surgery
DOI: 10.1007/978-88-470-3958-2_21, © Springer-Verlag Italia 2018

For laparoscopic distal pancreatectomy (LDP), the complexity of the surgery is significantly less and the operation requires a lesser level of laparoscopic skills when compared to pancreatoduodenectomy. LDP does not require any pancreatic, biliary or gastrointestinal reconstruction, which is an important Achilles' heel for LPD.

The first report of LDP was published in 1994 by Cuschieri [3]. From the beginning, LDP has shown equivalent postoperative outcomes to open distal pancreatectomy (ODP), with other advantages in regards to less intraoperative blood loss, less postoperative pain and a shorter hospitalization.

Benign lesions, neuroendocrine tumors and borderline lesions were the first indications for LDP reported in the literature [2, 4]. Nowadays malignant diseases of the body and tail of the pancreas are also approached with the laparoscopic technique. Several reports have investigated the oncological safety of LDP compared with open operation, finding similar outcomes in terms of radical resection rate, lymph node retrieval and overall survival. However, most of these reports analyzed retrospective data with considerable differences in patient selection. A significant bias, especially at the beginning of the laparoscopic era, was that advanced cancers were still treated with an open approach [5].

A recent paper reporting on 20 years' experience with the treatment of distal pancreatic adenocarcinoma at the Mayo Clinic (Jacksonville, FL, USA) confirmed less blood loss and need for blood transfusion, shorter hospital stay and a faster time to initiate chemotherapy in patients treated with LDP compared to ODP [6]. No significant difference was found in survival due to the fact that survival is influenced more by the biology of the pancreatic cancer than by the surgical technique adopted. However, strong evidence on the oncological results of LDP by means of randomized trials with long-term follow-up is still lacking.

A useful guide for selecting patients for LDP was proposed by Lee et al. [7], who presented, in 2014, the so-called Yonsei criteria. The Yonsei criteria were developed to identify patients eligible for a laparoscopic approach. They advocate using the laparoscopic approach only if the cancer is confined into the pancreas with an intact fascia layer between the pancreas and the left adrenal gland and at least 1 cm clearance from the celiac axis. These criteria are used as recommendations but many surgeons do not always follow them strictly. In fact, several papers report multivisceral laparoscopic resections, in relation to the experience of the center.

21.2 Surgical Technique for Laparoscopic Distal Pancreatectomy

Historically, distal pancreatectomy included removal of the spleen due to the close relation between the body-tail of the pancreas and the splenic vessels. Preservation of the spleen is still largely debated in distal pancreatectomy. In the case of benign lesions, spleen preservation should be considered in order to avoid immunological deficit, leukocytosis, thrombocytosis and postsplenectomy sepsis.

Benoist and colleagues et al. [8] reported that spleen preservation was associated with more surgical complications when compared to distal pancreatectomy with splenectomy.

A different conclusion was reported in a retrospective review from the Memorial Sloan-Kettering Cancer Center, comparing distal pancreatectomy with and without splenectomy. The authors concluded that preserving the spleen was associated with a reduction in perioperative infectious complications, severe complications, and length of hospital stay [9].

Spleen preservation during distal pancreatectomy can be performed following two different techniques. Kimura et al. [10] proposed a technique for preservation of the splenic vessels in open distal pancreatectomy; this technique was later modified for the laparoscopic approach. Warshaw [11] proposed another spleen preservation technique with ligation of the splenic vessels. Both techniques are not free from complications such as spleen infarction for the Warshaw technique or postoperative bleeding for the Kimura technique.

A Consensus Conference in Laparoscopic Surgery for Pancreatic Neoplasms was held in Amsterdam in June 2016, during the 24th International Congress of the European Association for Endoscopic Surgery (EAES) [12]. The conclusion was that LDP is a feasible and safe alternative to the open approach in the treatment of both benign and malignant pancreatic lesions, providing advantages in terms of reduced blood loss, enhanced postoperative recovery and shorter hospital stay.

The spleen-preserving approach is strongly recommended for benign tumors, but there is no agreement for this technique in invasive cancer. Kawaguchi et al. described his experience in a small number of cases of pancreatic adenocarcinoma treated with splenic vessel ligation and spleen preservation with extensive lymphadenectomy, reporting no difference in terms of 5-year survival compared to distal pancreatectomy with splenectomy [13].

According to the EAES consensus, in patients with adenocarcinoma of the pancreas, splenectomy is recommended to achieve an adequate oncologic margin and lymph node clearance. However, for patients with benign or low-grade malignant tumors in the body/tail of the pancreas, preservation of the spleen with its immune function reduces the risk of overwhelming postsplenectomy infection and other complications related to the splenectomy procedure itself. Moreover, some authors reported that splenectomy may have a negative influence on long-term survival along with an increased risk of other cancers [14].

According to Strasberg et al., the greatest advantage surgery can offer patients with pancreatic adenocarcinoma is radicality of the resection. To achieve this, it is mandatory to resect the pancreatic tail *en bloc* with the spleen and all the lymph nodes around the splenic vessels and splenic hilum. In 2003, Strasberg described his surgical approach, called radical antegrade modular pancreatosplenectomy (RAMPS), which aimed to improve radicality of resection for left-side pancreatic

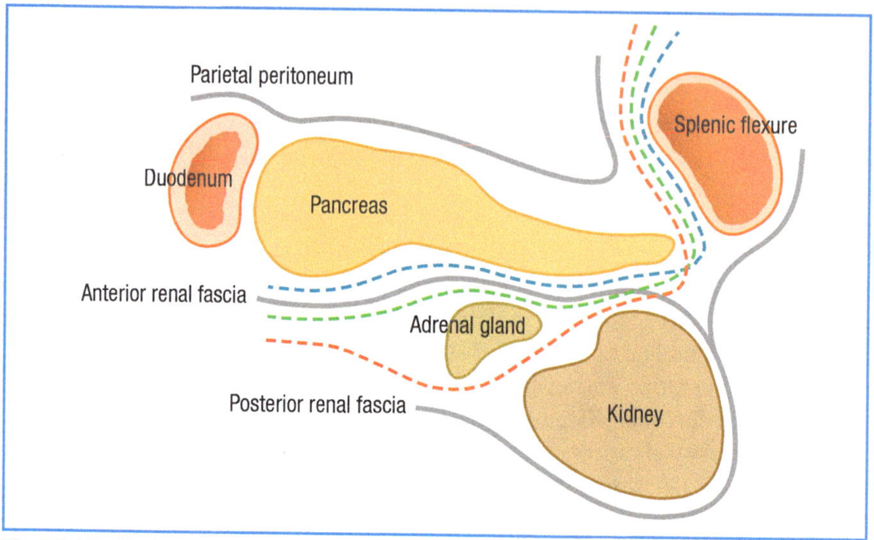

Fig. 21.1 Radical antegrade modular pancreatosplenectomy (RAMPS) planes: *blue line*, standard distal pancreatectomy plane of resection; *green line*, anterior RAMPS plane of resection; *orange line*, posterior RAMPS plane of resection

tumors [15]. With this technique, the horizontal dissection plane from right to left allows a radical resection of regional lymph nodes (Fig. 21.1).

In LDP, right-to-left resection is very commonly performed, and application of the RAMPS approach to LDP seems to achieve good results [7]. In a recent paper, Kim et al. [16] described his laparoscopic RAMPS technique and reported favorable results in terms of negative posterior margin, lymph node retrieval and also better disease-free and overall survival. The magnified view obtained with laparoscopy allows a better visualization of the correct anatomical dissection plane, which improves the radicality of the resection.

Another example of a useful alternative surgical technique is the "clockwise technique" described by Asbun et al. in 2011 [17]. For this technique, the patient is placed in a modified right lateral position. The surgeon stands to the right of the operating table. There are five steps to this technique, which is performed using four trocars (Fig. 21.2):

1. mobilization of the splenic flexure of the colon and exposure of the pancreas;
2. dissection along the inferior edge of the pancreas and choosing the site for pancreatic division;
3. pancreatic parenchymal division and ligation of the splenic vein and artery;
4. dissection along the superior edge of the pancreas;
5. mobilization of the spleen and specimen removal.

Similar to the RAMPS technique also the "clockwise technique" affords wide exposure of the pancreas and the plane of dissection can be chosen to include or exclude the left adrenal gland, the Gerota's fascia, or the superior leaflet of the transverse colon mesentery.

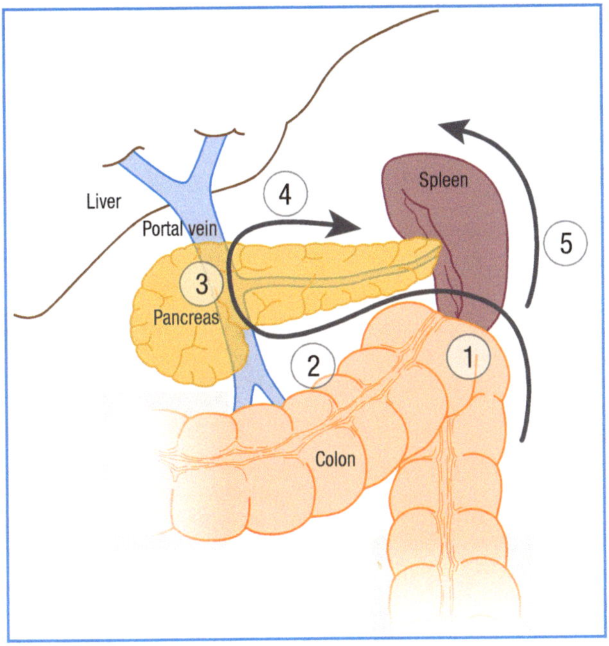

Fig. 21.2 The five steps of the Asbun clockwise technique

21.3 Postoperative Management and Complications

Many studies have reported that following an LDP the incidence of postoperative pancreatic fistula is the same as in open surgery, ranging between 0 to 34% [5]. No differences were reported when comparing the fistula rates in pancreatic resection with or without splenectomy.

The correct management of the pancreatic stump is not supported by validated recommendations or guidelines [18]. Several methods for closure of the pancreatic stump are described in the literature, such as the duct ligation, ultrasonic and stapler closure, fibrin glue occlusion, meshes and pancreatoenteric anastomosis [19, 20]. The suture of the pancreatic stump can be reinforced with tissue sealants but also this technique is still debated [21]. In 2012 Montorsi et al. [22] published a multicenter Italian randomized controlled trial on the efficacy of an absorbable fibrin sealant patch after distal pancreatic resection. In this trial 20% percent of the resections were performed laparoscopically and no differences in terms of postoperative pancreatic fistula were found.

The use of surgical abdominal drains and the timing of their removal are controversial. In the majority of the surgical experiences the use of drains is strongly recommended, although some authors have proposed a selective use of the drains. The rationale for this second position is that an abdominal drain can easily be itself the cause of infection of a postoperative fluid collection close to the pancreatic stump.

In conclusion, laparoscopic distal pancreatectomy with *en bloc* splenectomy is a safe and feasible technique that the surgeon can adopt also in case of malignancies of the body and tail of the pancreas. Splenectomy is not strictly recommended but is still indicated in the treatment of borderline tumors or premalignant diseases such as intraductal papillary mucinous neoplasms.

References

1. Zhang M, Fang R, Mou Y et al (2015) LDP vs ODP for pancreatic adenocarcinoma: a case matched study from a single-institution. BMC Gastroenterol 15:182
2. Venkat R, Edil BH, Schulick RD et al (2012) Laparoscopic distal pancreatectomy is associated with significantly less overall morbidity compared to the open technique: a systematic review and meta-analysis. Ann Surg 255(6):1048–1059
3. Cuschieri A (1994) Laparoscopic surgery of the pancreas. J R Coll Surg Edinb 39(3):178–184
4. Klompmaker S, van Zoggel D, Watkins AA et al (2016) Nationwide evaluation of patient selection for minimally invasive distal pancreatectomy using American College of Surgeons' National Quality Improvement Program. Ann Surg [Epub ahead of print] doi:10.1097/SLA.0000000000001982
5. de Rooij T, Klompmaker S, Abu Hilal M et al (2016) Laparoscopic pancreatic surgery for benign and malignant disease. Nat Rev Gastroenterol Hepatol 13(4):227–238
6. Stauffer JA, Coppola A, Mody K et al (2016) Laparoscopic versus open distal pancreatectomy for pancreatic adenocarcinoma. World J Surg 40(6):1477–1484
7. Lee SH, Kang CM, Hwang HK et al (2014) Minimally invasive RAMPS in well-selected left-sided pancreatic cancer within Yonsei criteria: long-term (>median 3 years) oncologic outcomes. Surg Endosc 28(10):2848–2855
8. Benoist S, Dugué L, Sauvanet A et al (1999) Is there a role of preservation of the spleen in distal pancreatectomy? J Am Coll Surg 188(3):255–260
9. Shoup M, Brennan MF, McWhite K et al (2002) The value of splenic preservation with distal pancreatectomy. Arch Surg 137(2):164–168
10. Kimura W, Inoue T, Futawaka N et al (1996) Spleen-preserving distal pancreatectomy with conservation of the splenic artery and vein. Surgery 120(5):885–890
11. Warshaw AL (1988) Conservation of the spleen with distal pancreatectomy. Arch Surg 123(5):550–553
12. Edwin B, Sahakyan MA, Abu Hilal M et al (2017) Laparoscopic surgery for pancreatic neoplasms: the European Association for Endoscopic Surgery clinical consensus conference. Surg Endosc 31(5):2023–2041
13. Kawaguchi Y, Fuks D, Nomi T et al (2015) Laparoscopic distal pancreatectomy employing radical en bloc procedure for adenocarcinoma: technical details and outcomes. Surgery 157(6):1106–1112
14. Linet MS, Nyrén O, Gridley G et al (1996) Risk of cancer following splenectomy. Int J Cancer 66(5):611–616
15. Strasberg SM, Drebin JA, Linehan D (2003) Radical antegrade modular pancreatosplenectomy. Surgery 133(5):521–527
16. Kim EY, Hong TH (2017) Initial experience with laparoscopic radical antegrade modular pancreatosplenectomy for left-sided pancreatic cancer in a single institution: technical aspects and oncological outcomes. BMC Surg 17(1):2
17. Asbun HJ, Stauffer JA (2011) Laparoscopic approach to distal and subtotal pancreatectomy: a clockwise technique. Surg Endosc 25(8):2643–2649
18. Reeh M, Nentwich MF, Bogoeversuski D et al (2011) High surgical morbidity following distal pancreatectomy: still an unsolved problem. World J Surg 35(5):1110–1117

19. Blansfield JA, Rapp MM, Chokshi RJ et al (2011) Novel method of stump closure for distal pancreatectomy with a 75% reduction in pancreatic fistula rate. J Gastrointest Surg 16(3):524–528
20. Diener MK, Seiler CM, Rossion I et al (2011) Efficacy of stapler versus hand-sewn closure after distal pancreatectomy (DISPACT): a randomized, controlled multicentre trial. Lancet 377(9776):1514–1522
21. Fingerhut A, Veyrie N, Ata T et al (2008) Use of sealants of pancreatic surgery: critical appraisal of the literature. Dig Surg 26(1):7–14
22. Montorsi M, Zerbi A, Bassi C et al (2012) Efficacy of an absorbable fibrin sealant patch (TachoSil) after distal pancreatectomy: a multicenter, randomized, controlled trial. Ann Surg 256(5):853–859; discussion 859–860

Robotic Spleen-Preserving Distal Pancreatectomy with and without Preservation of the Splenic Vessels

22

Sergio Alfieri, Antonio Pio Tortorelli, and Roberta Menghi

22.1 Introduction

In patients with adenocarcinoma of the body and tail of the pancreas, distal pancreatectomy with splenectomy is recommended to assure adequate oncologic margins and to achieve lymph node clearance. However, for patients with benign or low-grade malignant tumors in the body/tail of the pancreas, conservation of the spleen preserves immune function and eliminates the risk of overwhelming postsplenectomy infection and other complications related to the splenectomy procedure itself. Established surgical techniques to preserve the spleen include the Warshaw procedure (WP) which includes ligation of splenic vessels with preservation of the short gastric and left gastroepiploic vessels. Another method is splenic vessel preservation (SVP, also known as a Kimura procedure), where sparing of the splenic vessels without ligation is performed, with meticulous ligation of small pancreatic branches; this latter technique is thought to provide better blood supply to the retained spleen. The method involving resection of the splenic vessels is easier and less labor-consuming, particularly in laparoscopic and robot-assisted resections. However, the Warshaw approach is associated with a risk of morbidity, such as splenic infarction and gastric/perigastric varices (a long-term complication of left-sided portal hypertension) [1]. In a meta-analysis by Elabbasy et al. [2], carried out to evaluate the postoperative clinical outcomes of patients undergoing minimally invasive spleen-preserving distal pancreatectomy with or without vessel preservation, the SVP procedure resulted in a lower incidence of splenic infarction (SVP vs. WP, 6% vs. 28%; RR – 0.17;

S. Alfieri (✉)
Digestive Surgery Unit, Fondazione Policlinico Universitario Agostino Gemelli,
Università Cattolica del Sacro Cuore
Rome, Italy
e-mail: sergio.alfieri@unicatt.it

U. Boggi (Ed), *Minimally Invasive Surgery of the Pancreas*,
Updates in Surgery
DOI: 10.1007/978-88-470-3958-2_22, © Springer-Verlag Italia 2018

P <0.001) and a decreased risk of postoperative gastric/perigastric varices (SVP vs. WP, 2% vs. 21%; RR = 0.16; P = 0.002). SVP patients had undergone intra/postoperative splenectomy in 0.6% of cases, which was significantly lower than among WP patients (7.9%, P <0.001). Meta-analysis of the data revealed no association between the two operative groups and operative time (P = 0.67), operative blood loss (P = 0.56), or length of hospital stay (P = 0.84). There was no difference between the two procedures in terms of the incidence of postoperative pancreatic fistula (SVP vs. WP, 23% vs. 24%; P = 0.37).

22.2 Robotic Distal Pancreatectomy

The da Vinci robotic surgical system was introduced to overcome the limitations of conventional laparoscopic approaches and has been actively applied in general surgery. The da Vinci system has unique characteristics that might represent major advantages for a safe and effective laparoscopic surgery. These are stable three-dimensional (3D) views, wrist-like movements of the effector instruments (seven degrees of freedom), and no fulcrum effect, tremor, or need for scale adjustment for instrument movement.

In comparison to the da Vinci Si platform, the new da Vinci Xi presents many advantages. The docking is simpler and designed to be user-friendly, guided by a port placement menu and a laser. The laparoscope has a digital, highly magnified, 3D, high-definition, end-mounted camera for improved vision; additionally, it requires no draping. The scope can be placed on any of the robotic arms and it autofocuses. Thanks to the improved design of the arms, the ports can be placed relatively close to each other and still avoid collision [3].

Since 2006 we have been collecting data for a multi-institutional Italian registry on robotic distal pancreatectomy (RDP) for benign, borderline and malignant diseases. One hundred forty-two RDP were performed for benign and borderline disorders; in 103 cases it was possible to preserve the spleen (73%) with splenic vessel conservation, in the remaining cases the reasons for splenectomy were tight adhesions between the pancreatic lesion and the splenic vessels or a suspicion of malignant transformation (in 7 cases with a preoperative diagnosis of pancreatic G1 or G2 neuroendocrine tumor and a subsequent definitive histology report of neuroendocrine carcinoma). In no case was splenectomy due to massive bleeding or irreversible injury of the splenic vessels. Our data indicate that the da Vinci robot surgical system might be very helpful for spleen preservation during distal pancreatectomy.

We have been using the new da Vinci Xi surgical system since 2015. However, despite the improvements experienced with this new system in performing a multiquadrant operation (rectal surgery), the stable operating field lessens this specific advantage for distal pancreatectomy, which, furthermore, requires a similar docking technique for both the platforms.

22.3 Surgical Technique

Under general anesthesia, the patient is placed in the supine position on the surgical table and then shifted into a reverse Trendelenburg position with the left side up, with arms tucked at sides and legs spread apart (Fig. 22.1). An intra-abdominal pressure is established at 14 mmHg using the Veress needle technique in the left upper quadrant (Palmer's point). A total of five ports are used. Among them, one 12-mm port is placed for the assistant surgeon's intervention during the procedure (suction, retraction, clip positioning and use of endoscopic stapler). The four 8-mm robotic ports are placed in supraumbilical fields: two ports in the right upper quadrant and two in the left upper quadrant. The 12-mm assistant port (A) is placed into the umbilicus or along the transverse umbilical line, between the two robotic ports in the left quadrant, 7 cm or more from adjacent da Vinci ports. We use a 30° telescope. The dissection is performed by ultrasonic knife (U) and fenestrated bipolar forceps (B), the stomach is pulled up by prograsp forceps (P). The patient cart is located on the right or left side of the patient,

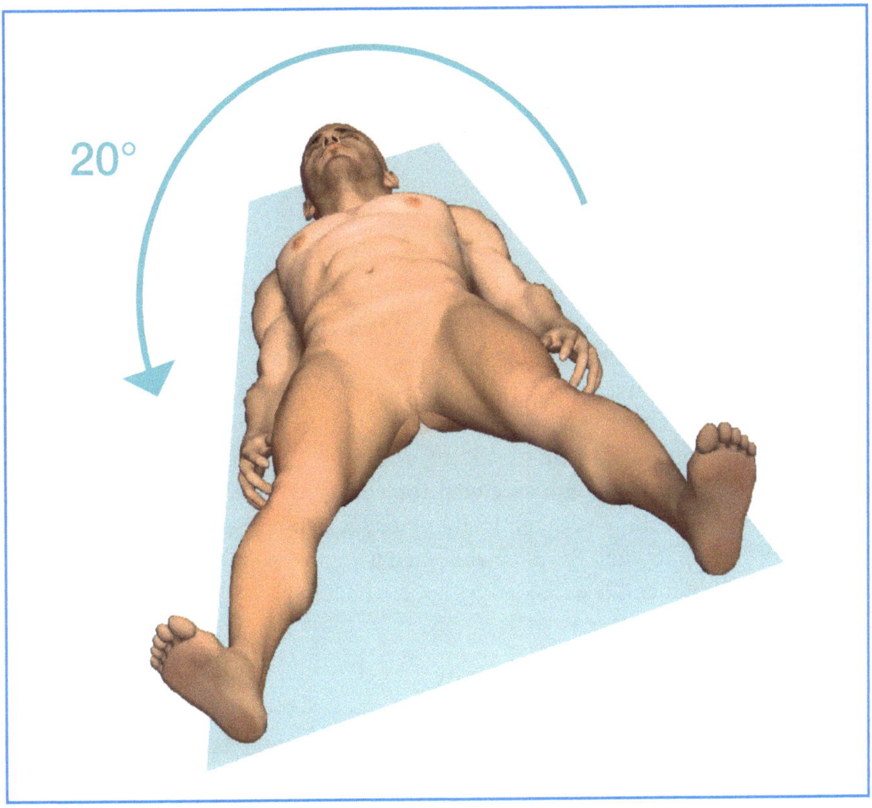

Fig. 22.1 Patient position in robotic spleen-preserving distal pancreatectomy

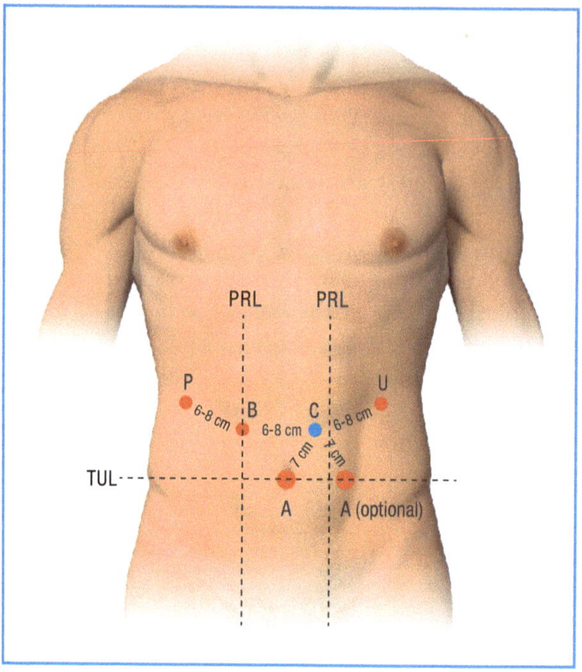

Fig. 22.2 Port placement in robotic spleen-preserving distal pancreatectomy: *TUL*, transverse umbilical line; *PRL*, pararectal line; *A* (and *A optional*) 12-mm assistant port; *P*, R1 for prograsp forceps; *B*, R2 for fenestrated bipolar forceps; *C*, R3 for 30° camera; *U*, R4 for ultrasonic knife

while the assistant is between the patient's legs. Port placement is described in Fig. 22.2. The lesser sac is entered by dividing the gastrocolic ligament with preservation of the gastroepiploic artery. During the division of the gastrocolic ligament, the splenocolic ligament is not mobilized to avoid division of the left gastroepiploic artery at the origin. The pancreas body-tail and the hilum of the spleen are then exposed and R1 (P) is used to pull up the stomach, which is a much more stable approach compared with laparoscopy, reducing the need for assistance. Intraoperative laparoscopic ultrasound examination is performed. The probe is inserted into the abdominal cavity through the assistant port (A) to seek for previously undetected lesions and to determine accurate surgical resection margins. Marks are made with an electrotome to define the margins. At the end of procedure one drain is systematically placed around the pancreas stump. The specimen is then extracted from the abdomen using a plastic bag: a port incision, generally the umbilical, is extended by approximately 1.2–3 cm.

22.3.1 Kimura Technique

In this technique [4], the superior and inferior borders of the body of the pancreas are the first to be dissected until a window between the splenic vessels and posterior border of the pancreas is visible on the right side of the tumor. This technique may be performed by first dissecting the vessels or by first transecting the pancreas.

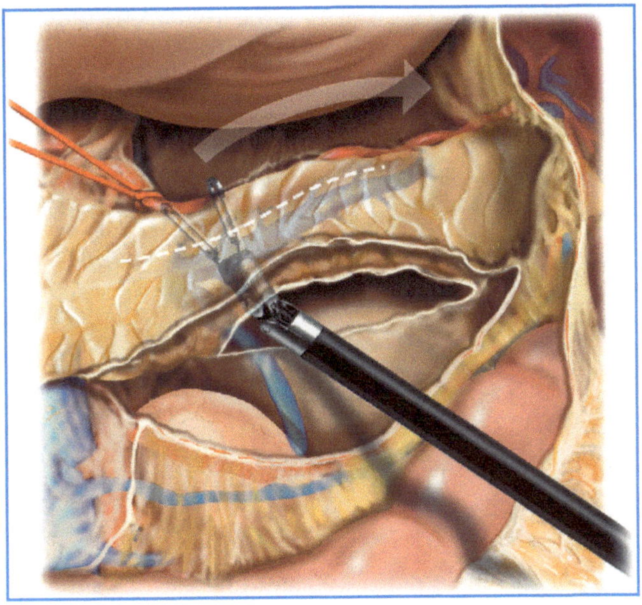

Fig. 22.3 The bipolar clamp pull-up the inferior border of the pancreas (previously freed by the trasversus mesocolon)

1. *Dissecting the vessels first* The proximal splenic artery is dissected from the superior pancreatic border and tied with a rubber band for vascular control (Fig. 22.3). The splenic vein is identified behind the pancreas and within the thin connective tissue membrane (fusion fascia of Toldt), which is cut longitudinally above the splenic vein. The splenic vein is situated fairly deep in the pancreatic parenchyma. In extended distal pancreatectomy, the lower border of the pancreas is freed from the transverse mesocolon and the superior mesenteric-portal vein by blunt dissection at the level of the neck, thereby creating a retropancreatic tunnel. An important step is the dissection of the splenic vein from the pancreas starting from the body towards the spleen (Fig. 22.4). It is very challenging to free the splenic vein in the opposite direction because it is difficult to discriminate the distal end of the pancreas from the fatty tissue in the hilum of the spleen. Moreover, in this area the splenic artery and vein are already divided into small vessels that can easily be injured. There are many branches originating from the splenic vein on both sides, and they should be carefully ligated and cut by using 5-mm endoclips and/or a harmonic scalpel [5]. Transfixation sutures or ligatures (easily performed in robotic surgery) are often used. After the pancreas has been freed from the splenic vein, it is dissected from the splenic artery in the opposite direction, starting from the spleen towards the head of the gland. This step is easier than separating the pancreas from the vein because all of the few arterioles originating from the splenic artery lie on one side, and the adhesions of the pancreas to the artery are very loose. Transection of the pancreas is then performed using an endoscopic stapler (with thick or very thick cartridge) or

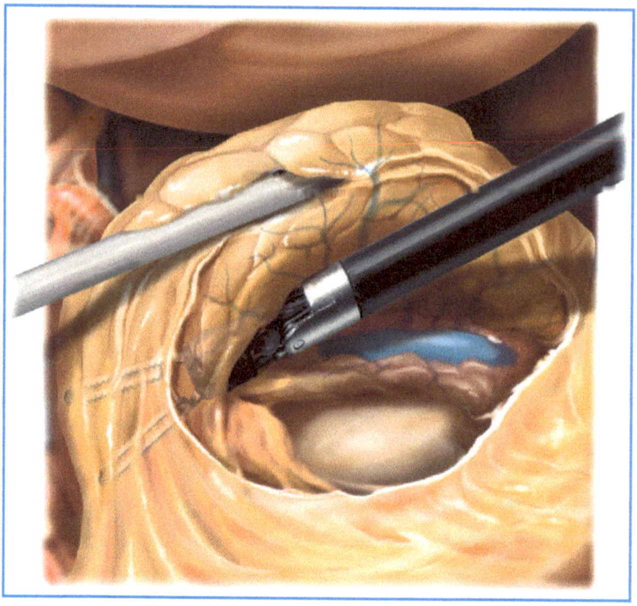

Fig. 22.4 The inferior border of the pancreas is completely mobilized from mesocolon and pulled up. The small branch from splenic vessels are dissected and tied with harmonic scalpel or clips

ultrasonic scalpel respecting a safe margin from the tumor. Hemostasis of the pancreatic stump is obtained by electrocautery or transfixation.

2. *Dividing the pancreas first* After identification and isolation of the splenic vessels at the superior and inferior borders of the pancreas and visualization of the posterior surface of parenchyma, a tape is applied around the pancreas, which is pulled up away from the vessels, and the transection is carried out by endoscopic stapler or harmonic scalpel without any previous vascular control. Then, the splenic vessels are dissected free from the pancreas towards the splenic hilum. The distal pancreas is lifted gently and the loose tissue between the pancreas and splenic vessels is separated using the ultrasound knife, thus freeing the splenic artery and vein from the pancreatic parenchyma. All small blood vessel branches are occluded.

22.3.2 Warshaw Technique

If the Warshaw technique is utilized [6], the spleen should be first assessed for color (as a baseline) and size (an enlarged spleen is less likely to survive on the reduced blood supply after resection of the main splenic vessels). The left gastroepiploic vessels should be identified and preserved as they leave the greater curve of the stomach and course through the omentum to join the main splenic vessels in the splenic hilum; these are in fact a noteworthy collateral blood supply to the spleen, in addition to the main blood supply, represented be the short gastric vessels. The peritoneum at the superior border of the pancreas is separated and the splenic artery is dissected and sectioned between clips and/or ligation. After the inferior border of the pancreas is freed, also the splenic vein is sectioned. Some authors cut the pancreatic parenchyma and the splenic vein together with an endoscopic stapler. As previously described in the Kimura technique, it is possible to transect the pancreas before ligation and section of the splenic artery and vein. The distal pancreas together with the splenic vessels are dissected in the right to left direction towards the tail of the gland; at this level, the splenic vessels are then ligated individually for completion of the distal pancreatectomy [5]. It is important to keep the dissection right at the border of the pancreas, especially around the tail, in order not to disrupt the network of short gastric and gastroepiploic collateral vessels anastomosing with the main splenic artery and vein at the splenic hilum.

22.4 Conclusions

Despite having the advantage of being more accurate during the surgical procedure, the robotic technique does not avoid the postoperative complications of a WP in the case of spleen-preserving distal pancreatectomy. If spleen preservation is planned, sparing of the splenic vessels is highly recommended.

References

1. Jain G, Chakravartty S, Patel AG (2013) Spleen-preserving distal pancreatectomy with and without splenic vessel ligation: a systematic review. HPB (Oxford) 15(6):403–410
2. Elabbasy F, Gadde R, Hanna MM et al (2015) Minimally invasive spleen-preserving distal pancreatectomy: does splenic vessel preservation have better postoperative outcomes? A systematic review and meta-analysis. Hepatobiliary Pancreat Dis Int 14(4):346–353
3. Cirocchi R, Partelli S, Coratti A et al (2013) Current status of robotic distal pancreatectomy: a systematic review. Surg Oncol 22(3):201–207
4. Kimura W, Yano M, Sugawara S et al (2010) Spleen-preserving distal pancreatectomy with conservation of the splenic artery and vein: techniques and its significance. J Hepatobiliary Pancreat Sci 17(6):813–823
5. Lee LS, Hwang HK, Kang CM, Lee WJ (2016) Minimally invasive approach for spleen-preserving distal pancreatectomy: a comparative analysis of postoperative complication between splenic vessel conserving and Warshaw's technique. J Gastrointest Surg 20(8):1464–1470
6. Warshaw AL (2010) Distal pancreatectomy with preservation of the spleen. J Hepatobiliary Pancreat Sci 17(6):808–812

Robotic Distal Pancreatectomy with En Bloc Splenectomy

23

Giovanni Butturini, Alessandro Giardino, Isacco Damoli, Alessandro Esposito, Isabella Frigerio, and Marco Ramera

23.1 Introduction

Since the first years of introduction and use of robotic systems for surgical operations it clearly appeared that distal pancreatic resections would be easily suitable for this innovative approach. In the last 20 years, laparoscopic distal pancreatectomy has assumed an increasingly important role and has rapidly become established as the procedure of choice in selected cases [1, 2]. However, the laparoscopic technique has some limitations: slight increase in tremor due to the rigid lever-fulcrum system, poor ergonomics for the surgeons associated with prolonged standing position, visual limitations of two-dimensional (2D) vision worsening the approach to the distal pancreas. Furthermore, in the most difficult cases and even worse, in pancreatic ductal cancer, these limitations are quite often overwhelming, making the minimally invasive approach rarely used or indicated [3, 4].

The da Vinci robotic system (Intuitive Surgical, Sunnyvale, CA, USA), with three-dimensional (3D) display, articulated devices and ergonomic position, is designed to address the limits of laparoscopy and is taking on an increasingly important role in distal pancreatectomies [5, 6].

23.2 Indications for Distal Pancreatectomy with En Bloc Splenectomy

Distal pancreatectomy with *en bloc* splenectomy, a common indication in pancreatic ductal adenocarcinoma [7], also plays an important role in distal

G. Butturini (✉)
Hepato-Pancreato-Biliary Unit, Pederzoli Hospital
Peschiera del Garda, Italy
e-mail: gbutturini@ospedalepederzoli.it

U. Boggi (Ed), *Minimally Invasive Surgery of the Pancreas*,
Updates in Surgery
DOI: 10.1007/978-88-470-3958-2_23,

neuroendocrine tumors more than 2 cm in diameter, even though recent evidence shows that, in asymptomatic patients, a parenchyma-sparing pancreatectomy may be suggested given the usually good prognosis [8]. Mucinous tumors, whether cystadenomas or intraductal papillary mucinous tumors, require a spleen-preserving resection because the lymph nodes are very rarely involved. In these cases, nodal sampling is usually recommended [9]. Moreover, in the case of splenic vein compression or large mucinous tumors, splenectomy should be considered so as to minimize the risk of rupture which rarely, but possibly, leads to pseudomixoma peritonei with serious late consequences. All the aforementioned considerations should be taken into account in a correct presurgical planning in order to rationalize the operation time and reduce the risk of damage to the nearby organs or the tumor itself. A presurgery imaging review in close collaboration with the radiologist is crucial for planning the surgical strategy. A contrast-enhanced, multislice computed tomography scan is the best modality to study the relations between the tumor and the splenic vessels [10]. Pancreatic metastases from renal cell carcinoma should be approached with anatomical resections including splenectomy and lymphadenectomy owing to the 20% risk of nodal spread [11]. Careful intraoperative ultrasound is mandatory because of frequent preoperatively undetected multiple nodules inside the gland which constitute an indication for total pancreatectomy.

Splenectomy has to be considered in the event of untreatable bleeding during spleen preservation resections, even when not planned preoperatively [12]. For these reasons, a splenic vessel loop should be positioned after careful dissection of the vessels during spleen-preserving pancreatectomies.

23.3 Surgical Technique

In this section, the main surgical steps [13] of distal pancreatectomy with *en bloc* splenectomy are described.

The patient is placed supine with legs spread apart in a 20° reverse Trendelenburg position. Trocars (n = 5) are inserted along a transverse umbilical line. The camera is placed in the umbilical port, the 3rd and 4th arms are placed in the right lateral and medial trocar, the 2nd arm is placed in the left lateral trocar, while the assistant trocar is placed between the camera and the left lateral trocar. We prefer to insert this last trocar 3 cm lower than the others. Visual exploration of the peritoneal cavity, to detect potential metastases, is mandatory as is intraoperative ultrasound, to better detect small intraparenchymal liver lesions and local vascular involvement at the primary site. All of the above preliminary assessments are very useful, if not mandatory, to ensure safety and rapidity and to avoid unnecessarily long and complex procedures.

The operating surgeon is at the console and cooperates closely with the table-side assistant so that two specialists are needed to perform the operation safely.

The tableside surgeon must be a minimally invasive specialist with a high level of skill in laparoscopic pancreatic surgery. The lesser sac must be entered with a wide dissection including all of the short gastric vessels. The more proximal gastric vessels can be interrupted at the very end, during spleen mobilization. The stomach can be lifted with a transabdominal stitch, which allows utilization of the 4th arm for dissection and pancreatic retraction.

The pancreatic superior and inferior margins must be dissected so as to lift up the neck and insert a vascular loop. First, the inferior margin of the pancreatic neck is dissected at the level of the superior mesenteric vein, then the superior margin is dissected soon after clearance of the hepatic artery lymph node (n. 8a), which allows a good view of the portal vein and the hepatic artery itself. The splenic artery must be dissected at the origin, in accordance with oncologic resection rules. This maneuver must be performed cautiously to identify the hepatic artery which should be clearly distinguished from the splenic artery before its section. To this end, the left gastric artery is a very important landmark. The splenic artery can be sutured and sectioned with hem-o-lok (Teleflex Inc., Morrisville, NC, USA) titanium endoclips or mechanical staplers. The robot platform also allows the choice of transfixed stitches, which are easy to perform. In the case of tumor involvement of the celiac trunk, distal pancreatectomy can be performed after sectioning the common hepatic artery and celiac trunk. In that case, gastroduodenal flow must be maintained in order to preserve arterial blood supply to the liver.

As soon as the splenic artery is ligated and sectioned, the subsequent step is to identify the splenic vein by dissecting the inferior margin of the pancreas at the neck. Pneumoperitoneum facilitates sharp dissections with monopolar forceps or Cadiere bipolar forceps (Intuitive Surgical, Sunnyvale, CA, USA), also useful for the management of small vein branches. Once vascular control has been secured, the pancreas is transected at the neck with a 60-mm endostapler or ultrasound dissector. In selected cases, it is difficult to recognize and dissect the splenic artery at the superior pancreatic margin because the artery dives into the pancreatic gland. To minimize the risk of accidental lesion in these patient subsets, a variation in the usual approach can be suggested and transection of the neck can be done first with the ultrasound forceps proceeding with caution to separate the gland gradually and recognize the artery at the cranial margin easily. During pancreatic neck transection, the assistant should gently retract the pancreatic distal portion on the left to open the space of the neck and facilitate identification of the splenic artery. Pancreatic tail dissection should be performed medial to lateral making sure to cauterize selectively the short posterior gastric vessels and infracolic veins that may have a large caliber. Sometimes it is necessary to perform the resection in the adipose tissue surrounding the kidney at the Gerota's fascia level beginning at the left lateral margin of the superior mesenteric artery. Whenever indicated, it is easy to gain access to the left adrenal gland, sectioning the main adrenal vein at the origin on the left renal vein and removing all the nodes of the para-aortic space (n. 16). Circumferential dissection of the superior mesenteric artery is not usually indicated because of the risk of long-standing diarrhea and the inability to achieve complete clearance of station 14 nodes without resection of the portal lamina. Splenectomy is the last step and should be performed with a counterclockwise approach. Initially the left colonic flexure has to be mobilized in order to lift the inferior splenic border. Once retracted with the 4th arm, the posterior ligaments can be easily dissected up to the superior border. The spleen can be ultimately twisted to access the posterior adhesions with the retroperitoneum. The specimen is introduced in a 15-cm plastic bag and extracted through a 3-cm Pfannenstiel incision. Smaller bags available on the market should be avoided to reduce the risk of bag rupture during specimen extraction, an important step not to be underestimated: caution is needed to avoid spreading of tumor cells, also by changing gloves at the end of the maneuver. A soft drain is placed on the pancreatic remnant through the most caudal trocar. It is recommended to obtain the frozen section margin examination as in open resections.

23.3.1 Surgical Equipment

Distal pancreatectomy with *en bloc* splenectomy is a complex procedure which requires high-level skills and surgical devices. A Maryland forceps (Intuitive Surgical, Sunnyvale, CA, USA) is useful for dissection and coagulation, a curved scissor or hook with monopolar energy is used for sharp and blunt dissection, a Cadiere forceps is used as a retractor and a ultrasound dissector is useful for fat tissue coagulation and small vessel hemostasis. An intraoperative ultrasound probe must be available for every procedure. In addition, hem-o-lok endoclips or alternatively mechanical vascular staplers are mandatory for clipping large vessels. Transection of pancreatic parenchyma can be performed both with a mechanical stapler or ultrasound dissector.

23.3.2 Postoperative Management

The nasogastric tube, useful to deflate the stomach during the operation, is removed at the end of the operation. Oral free fluid is allowed in the afternoon and a light breakfast on the first postoperative day [14]. Drain amylases are sampled on day 1 and 3. The drains are removed on day 3 if amylase content is negative (<200 U/mL) and if associated with benign appearance and/or good clinical condition; otherwise the test is repeated on day 5 [15]. No proper prospective randomized trials are available to support this approach. Free oral diet is allowed on day 2 or 3 depending on clinical condition and compliance. Discharge may be considered from day 5 in the absence of complications. No postoperative imaging is required in the absence of clinical indications.

23.4 Early and Late Complications

Postoperative pancreatic fistula (POPF) represents the more frequent complication after distal pancreatectomy occurring in approximately one-third of patients in high-volume centers [16–18]. A conservative approach is usually the treatment with the better results despite a small number of patients requiring percutaneous drainage and rarely repeat surgery, usually for vascular rather than septic complications. The surgical drains can be held in place in the case of POPF, especially if infected, regardless of clinical condition. Antibiotics are reserved for clinically relevant POPF although a bacterial and/or fungal overinfection of drained fluid is very common.

Early postoperative bleeding occurs with an incidence of 5% of patients and may be caused by either pancreatic stump bleeding, easily managed via laparoscopy with a stitch or clip, or by severe acute pancreatitis, a dramatic event which can lead to more complex reoperation.

Pancreatic stump fluid collections are frequent and in the vast majority of patients are self-limiting and indolent. Rarely, it is necessary to perform an endoscopic drainage of long-standing and symptomatic postsurgical pseudocysts [19].

Other rare abdominal complications can be: bowel or gastric perforations, late bleeding caused by splenic artery stump pseudoaneurysms, and bowel occlusion for adhesions or strangulation in misrecognized transverse mesocolon hole. All the above should be promptly recognized and treated laparoscopically or with angiographic embolization [20].

Late postsplenectomy complications deserve special attention. Patients must be aware of the possible late consequences: increased exposure to infections (overwhelming infections) [21, 22] and persistent thrombocytosis [23]. Vaccination against *Haemophilus influenzae*, pneumococcus and meningococcus is mandatory so to minimize capsulated bacteria infection [24]. Other infections, less common and always misunderstood, may be related to pet bites (*Capnocytophaga canimorsus*) [25]. Persistent thrombocytosis [1] can occur in a 14% of patients and salicylate acid (100 mg) is indicated to reduce platelet aggregation [26].

References

1. Malleo G, Damoli I, Marchegiani G et al (2015) Laparoscopic distal pancreatectomy: analysis of trends in surgical techniques, patient selection, and outcomes. Surg Endosc 29(7):1952–1962
2. Ricci C, Casadei R, Taffurelli G et al (2016) Laparoscopic distal pancreatectomy: many meta-analyses, few certainties. Updates Surg 68(3):225–234
3. Anderson B, Karmali S (2014) Laparoscopic resection of pancreatic adenocarcinoma: dream or reality? World J Gastroenterol 20(39):14255–14262

4. Mehrabi A, Hafezi M, Arvin J et al (2015) A systematic review and meta-analysis of laparoscopic versus open distal pancreatectomy for benign and malignant lesions of the pancreas: it's time to randomize. Surgery 157(1):45–55
5. Damoli I, Butturini G, Ramera M et al (2015) Minimally invasive pancreatic surgery – a review. Wideochir Inne Tech Maloinwazyjne 10(2):141–149
6. Wright GP, Zureikat AH (2016) Development of minimally invasive pancreatic surgery: an evidence-based systematic review of laparoscopic versus robotic approaches. J Gastrointest Surg 20(9):1658–1665
7. Parikh PY, Lillemoe KD (2015) Surgical management of pancreatic cancer – distal pancreatectomy. Semin Oncol 42(1):110–122
8. Falconi M, Eriksson B, Kaltsas G et al; Vienna Consensus Conference participants (2016) ENETS consensus guidelines update for the management of patients with functional pancreatic neuroendocrine tumors and non-functional pancreatic neuroendocrine tumors. Neuroendocrinology 103(2):153–171
9. Tanaka M, Fernández-del Castillo C, Adsay V et al; International Association of Pancreatology (2012) International consensus guidelines 2012 for the management of IPMN and MCN of the pancreas. Pancreatology 12(3):183–197
10. D'Onofrio M, Capelli P, Pederzoli P (eds) (2015) Imaging and pathology of pancreatic neoplasms. A pictorial atlas. Springer, Milan
11. Tosoian JJ, Cameron JL, Allaf ME et al (2014) Resection of isolated renal cell carcinoma metastases of the pancreas: outcomes from the Johns Hopkins Hospital. J Gastrointest Surg 18(3):542–548
12. de Rooij T, Sitarz R, Busch OR et al (2015) Technical aspects of laparoscopic distal pancreatectomy for benign and malignant disease: review of the literature. Gastroenterol Res Pract 2015:472906
13. Napoli N, Kauffmann EF, Perrone VG et al (2015) The learning curve in robotic distal pancreatectomy. Updates Surg 67(3):257–264
14. Balzano G, Bissolati M, Boggi U et al; AISP Study Group on Distal Pancreatectomy (2014) A multicenter survey on distal pancreatectomy in Italy: results of minimally invasive technique and variability of perioperative pathways. Updates Surg 66(4):253–263
15. Bassi C, Dervenis C, Butturini G et al; International Study Group on Pancreatic Fistula Definition (2005) Postoperative pancreatic fistula: an international study group (ISGPF) definition. Surgery 138(1):8–13
16. Memeo R, Sangiuolo F, de Blasi V et al (2016) Robotic pancreaticoduodenectomy and distal pancreatectomy: state of the art. J Visc Surg 153(5):353–359
17. Boggi U, Napoli N, Costa F et al (2016) Robotic-assisted pancreatic resections. World J Surg 40(10):2497–2506
18. Gavriilidis P, Lim C, Menahem B et al (2016) Robotic versus laparoscopic distal pancreatectomy – The first meta-analysis. HPB (Oxford) 18(7):567–574
19. Butturini G, Damoli I, Crepaz L et al (2015) A prospective non-randomised single-center study comparing laparoscopic and robotic distal pancreatectomy. Surg Endosc 29(11):3163–3170
20. Ueda T, Murata S, Yamamoto A et al (2015) Endovascular treatment of post-laparoscopic pancreatectomy splenic arteriovenous fistula with splenic vein aneurysm. World J Gastroenterol 21(25):7907–7910
21. Theilacker C, Ludewig K, Serr A et al (2016) Overwhelming postsplenectomy infection: a prospective multicenter cohort study. Clin Infect Dis 62(7):871–878
22. Sinwar PD (2014) Overwhelming post splenectomy infection syndrome – review study. Int J Surg 12(12):1314–1316
23. Buzelé R, Barbier L, Sauvanet A, Fantin B (2016) Medical complications following splenectomy. J Visc Surg 153(4):277–286
24. Hammerquist RJ, Messerschmidt KA, Pottebaum AA, Hellwig TR (2016) Vaccinations in asplenic adults. Am J Health Syst Pharm 73(9):e220–e228

25. Taquin H, Roussel C, Roudière L et al (2017) Fatal infection caused by Capnocytophaga canimorsus. Lancet Infect Dis 17(2):236
26. Barbui T, Barosi G, Grossi A et al (2004) Practice guidelines for the therapy of essential thrombocythemia. A statement from the Italian Society of Hematology, the Italian Society of Experimental Hematology and the Italian Group for Bone Marrow Transplantation. Haematologica 89(2):215–232

Laparoscopic Pancreatoduodenectomy 24

Francesco Corcione, Diego Cuccurullo, and Pierluigi Angelini

24.1 Introduction

Laparoscopic pancreatoduodenectomy (LPD) is still a poorly diffused surgical procedure, even though the first report by Gagner [1] dates back to 1994. According to the US National Cancer Database (NCDB), only 10% of 8213 pancreatoduodenectomies for stage I–II pancreatic ductal adenocarcinoma (PDAC) performed between 2010 and 2013 were laparoscopic. Currently, there is no prospective multicenter report present in the literature. Nevertheless, implementation of LPD in the past five 5 years has been characterized by a sharp rise in interest, potentially as a result of a greater centralization of patients.

24.2 Patient Selection

LPD requires multiple complex reconstructions, with a high incidence of severe postoperative complications, particularly postoperative pancreatic fistula (POPF). The procedure is hampered by the anatomic location of the organ in the retroperitoneum and by its proximity to major blood vessels. Assessing surgical resectability with high-quality radiological imaging is therefore fundamental, and intraoperative ultrasound is a desirable diagnostic complement. Regarding the selection of patients, while few pioneering groups have pushed the boundaries of LPD into the field of major venous resections [2, 3], most authors [4, 5] still exclude LPD in cases of obesity, large (>3 cm) or borderline resectable disease, concomitant chronic pancreatitis, neoadjuvant radiotherapy or previous abdominal surgeries. The advanced laparoscopic skill and expensive sophisticated

F. Corcione (✉)
Department of General Surgery, Center of Laparoscopic and Robotic Surgery
V. Monaldi Hospital, A.O.R.N. dei Colli
Neaples, Italy
e-mail: francesco.corcione@ospedalideicolli.it

U. Boggi (Ed), *Minimally Invasive Surgery of the Pancreas*,
Updates in Surgery
DOI: 10.1007/978-88-470-3958-2_24,

medical facilities required to perform LPD are only present in a few subspecialty centers. Specialized training in open and minimally invasive pancreatic surgery favored by the centralization of caseloads has drastically reduced morbidity and mortality [6]. Unfortunately, the US NCDB data [7] show that in 2010-11 only 384 (9%) cases of PDAC were treated with LPD. Furthermore, 96.2% (369 out of 384 patients) of procedures were performed in low-volume centers (<10 LPD/year) with an alarming high mortality rate (7.5%).

24.3 Operative Data and Learning Curve

Minimally invasive pancreatoduodenectomy (MIPD) can be performed with various technical modalities ranging from pure LPD, hand- or laparoscopically assisted PD to robotic or robotically assisted PD. Recent reviews [8–10] consider studies with both benign and malignant tumors, different selection criteria and heterogeneous MIPD techniques; furthermore, the data are often affected by studies with a limited number of cases. Concerning pure LPD, Tables 24.1, 24.2, 24.3, and 24.4 report the data of 446 pure LPD collected from six single-institution reports [4, 5, 11–14] with more than 45 cases published in the last 3 years, including at least 70% of malignancies. Among these studies, the selection of patients for LPD (Table 24.2) varies widely, ranging from universal inclusion [11, 13] to more restrictive inclusion criteria [4, 5, 12]. However, interesting data

Table 24.1 Articles published in the last 3 years with >45 pure laparoscopic pancreatoduodenectomy procedures

Author	Year	Country	N. of cases	Age (years) mean±SD *or* mean (range)	BMI kg/m² mean±SD *or* mean (range)	Malignancy n. (%)	PDAC n. (%)
Croome et al. [11]	2014	UK	108	66.6±9.6	27.4±5.4	108 (100%)	108 (100%)
Dokmak et al. [5]	2015	France	46	60 (27–85)	22.6 (17–30)	36 (78.3%)	15 (32.6%)
Senthilnathan et al. [12]	2015	India	130	54 (28–76)	27.9 (22–33)	130 (100%)	58 (44.6%)
Delitto et al. [4]	2016	USA	52	65.3±1.7	26.3±0.8	52 (100%)	28 (53,8%)
Stauffer et al. [13]	2016	USA	58*	69.9 (40–84)	25.9 (17.7–49.6)	58 (100%)	58 (100%)
Wang et al. [14]	2017	China	52	57.8 (28–73)	N/A	46 (88%)	8 (15.3%)

* 7 (12.1%) total pancreatectomy
BMI, body mass index; *N/A*, not applicable; *PDAC*, pancreatic ductal adenocarcinoma.

Table 24.2 Exclusion criteria for laparoscopic pancreatoduodenectomy

Author	BMI	Borderline resectable	Pancreatic duct caliber	Evident vascular invasion	Previous surgical adhesions	Expected histology	Neo-adjuvant therapy
Croome et al. [11]*	–	–	–	–	–	No PDAC	–
Dokmak et al. [5]	–	–	–	Yes	–	CP/AP, IPMN	Yes
Senthilnathan et al. [12]	–	Yes	–	Yes	Yes	Benign	–
Delitto et al. [4]	>40	Yes, NCCN criteria [15]	–	–	Yes	Benign	–
Stauffer et al. [13]*	–	–	–	–	–	No PDAC	–
Wang et al. [14]	–	–	<1 mm	–	–	–	–

* Universal inclusion for PDAC

BMI, body mass index; *CP/AP*, chronic/acute pancreatitis; *IPMN*, intraductal papillary mucinous neoplasm; *NCCN*, National Comprehensive Cancer Network; *PDAC*, pancreatic ductal adenocarcinoma.

emerge from these six large series. Expressed as a weighted average, operating time (OT) is 359.7 minutes (range, 276–541); estimated blood loss (EBL) is 250.9 mL (range, 80–492); conversions to open surgery are 7.1% (range, 0–24.1%); conversions to hand- or robotically assisted LPD are 2.01% (0–5.6%); harvested lymph nodes (LN) are 21.1 (18.1–23.4) and the percentage of R0 resections is 82.8% (60–94.9%). In four of six series [4, 5, 11, 13] LPD results are compared with those of open pancreatoduodenectomy (OPD) in patients with similar demographic characteristics. In two cases [5, 13] OT is longer in LPD, while in all four series EBL is less, with fewer blood transfusions in two cases [11, 13]. Only in one case [13] are harvested LN statistically higher in LPD (27 vs. 17) and in another [4] LPD shows a higher percentage of R0 (90.4% vs. 74%).

Regarding training for LPD, Croome et al. [11] excluded from his study 10 patients undergoing LPD in the first 6 months of their experience in order to avoid the early segment of the learning curve. Comparing the results between the first 20 and the last 26 cases, Dokmak et al. [5] found a statistically significant decrease of OT, EBL and transfusion need. Similarly, in Corcione et al.'s study [16], OT and length of stay (LOS) decreased when comparing the first and the last 11 cases. A reduction in OT, EBL, clinically significant POPF [17] and LOS was found by Song et al. [18] when comparing the first 47 and the last 50 cases of their series. Several other studies [19–21] reported a significant decrease in OT and EBL after the first 10 cases, while greater experience [18, 22] proved vital for achieving improvements in major postoperative morbidity (Table 24.5).

Table 24.3 Operative data for open and laparoscopic pancreatoduodenectomy

Author		N. of cases	OT (min)	EBL (mL)	Conversion n. (%)	Conversion to hybrid n. (%)	Vascular resection n. (%)	Pancreatic stump	Pylorus preservation	Harvested lymph nodes mean±SD *or* mean (range)	R0 %
Croome et al. [11]	LPD	108	379	492.4	7 (6.4%)	5 (4.6%) RA	22 (20.4%)	Two-layer duct-to-mucosa PJ	N/A	21.4±8.1	77.8%
	OPD	214	387	866.7	–	–	51 (23.8%)	–	–	20.1±7.5	76.6%
	P value		ns	<0.001			ns			ns	ns
Dokmak et al. [5]	LPD	46	342	368	3 (6.5%)	1 (2.2%)	0	One-layer PJ 4/0 polyglactin interrupted suture	0	20 (8–59)	60%
	OPD	46	264	293	–	–	N/A	–	–	25 (8–47)	50%
	P value		<0.001	ns						ns	ns
Senthilnathan et al. [12]	LPD	130	310	110	1 (0.7%)	0	1 (0.7%)	Two-layer duct-to-mucosa PJ	85 (57%)	18.15±4.73	90.8%
Delitto et al. [4]	LPD	52	361	260	7 (9%)	0	0	End-to-end intussuscepting PJ running suture	N/A	23	90.4%
	OPD	50	360	518	–	–	–	–	–	20.8	73%
	P value		ns	<0.001						ns	0.03
Stauffer et al. [13]	LPD	58*	518	250	14 (24.1%)	3 (5.2%) HA	20 (34.5%)	Two-layer duct-to-mucosa PJ	58 (100%)	27 (9–70)	84.5%
	OPD	193	375	600	–	–	60 (31.1%)	–	–	17 (1–63)	79.8%
	P value		<0.001	<0.001			ns			<0.001	ns
Wang et al. [14]	LPD	52	276	80	0	0	0	Embedding end-to-side PJ with 4-layers of mattress sutures	0	N/A	N/A

* 7 (12.1%) total pancreatectomy

EBL, estimated blood loss; *GJ*, gastrojejunostomy; *HA*, hand-assisted; *LPD*, laparoscopic pancreatoduodenectomy; *N/A*, not applicable; *ns*, not significant; *OPD*, open pancreatoduodenectomy; *OT*, operating time; *PJ*, pancreatojejunostomy; *RA*, robotic-assisted.

Table 24.4 Short- and long-term outcomes for open and laparoscopic pancreatoduodenectomy

Author		N. of cases	Major complications* n. (%)	Reoperations n. (%)	LOS (days)	Mortality n. (%)	POPF B+C n. (%)	DGE n. (%)	DFS % at 20 months	OS (months)
Croome et al. [11]	LPD	108	6 (5.6%)	N/A	6	1 (1%)	12 (11%)	10 (9%)	32%	25.3
	OPD	214	29 (13.6%)	N/A	9	4 (2%)	26 (12%)	39 (18%)	24.8%	21.8
	P value		ns		<0.001	ns	ns	0.03	0.03	ns
Dokmak et al. [5]	LPD	46	13 (28%)	11 (24%)	25	1 (2%)	9+11 (44%)	8 (17%)	N/A	N/A
	OPD	46	9 (20%)	5 (11%)	23	0	12+3 (32%)	7 (15%)	N/A	N/A
	P value		ns	ns	ns	ns	0.007 (grade C)	ns		
Senthilnathan et al. [12]	LPD	130	14 (10.8%)	5 (3.8%)	8	2 (1.5%)	6+5 (8.4%)	14 (10.7%)	N/A	33
Delitto et al. [4]	LPD	52	13 (25%)	–	9	1 (2%)	6 (12)	NA	N/A	27.9
	OPD	50	16 (32%)	–	11.9	0	13 (26%)	NA	N/A	23.5
	P value		ns		0.025	ns	ns			ns
Stauffer et al. [13]	LPD	58**	13 (22.4%)	1 (1.7%)	6	2 (3.4%)	4+0 (7.8%)	10 (17.2%)	N/A	18.5
	OPD	193	32 (30.1%)	12 (6.2%)	9	10 (5.2%)	9+5 (8.6%)	28 (14.5%)	N/A	20.3
	P value		ns	ns	<0.001	ns	ns	ns		ns
Wang et al. [14]	LPD	52	N/A	0	12	0	1+0 (1.9%)	2 (3.8%)	N/A	N/A

* Clavien-Dindo grade >II
** 7(12.1%) total pancreatectomy
DFS, disease-free survival; *DGE*, delayed gastric emptying; *LOS*, length of hospital stay; *LPD*, laparoscopic pancreatoduodenectomy; *OPD*, open pancreatoduodenectomy; *OS*, overall survival; *N/A*, not applicable; *ns*, not significant; *POPF B+C*, postoperative pancreatic fistula grades B+C.

Table 24.5 Outcomes of the learning curve for laparoscopic pancreatoduodenectomy

Author	Year	Total cases	Types	Statistical method	Cases to achieve the learning curve	Outcomes
Corcione et al. [16]	2013	22	LPD	Cases split into predefined segment	11	OT
Kuroki et al. [19]	2014	30	LPD	Cases split into predefined segment	10	OT, EBL
Speicher et al. [20]	2014	56	LPD+ Hybrid	Cases split into predefined segment	10–50	OT, EBL
Dokmak et al. [5]	2015	46	LPD	Cases split into predefined segment	20	OT, EBL
Paniccia et al. [21]	2015	30	LPD	Cases split into predefined segment	15	OT, EBL
Song et al. [18]	2015	97	LPD	Cases split into predefined segment	47	OT, EBL, CsPOPF, LOS, ReAl, OvCompl
Wang et al. [22]	2016	57	LPD+ HALPD	CUSUM and RA-CUSUM	38	OT, EBL, H LN, more challenging cases

CUSUM, cumulative sum; *EBL*, estimated blood loss; *HALPD*, hand-assisted laparoscopic pancreatoduodenectomy; *LOS*, length of hospital stay; *HLN*, harvested lymph nodes; *LPD*, laparoscopic pancreatoduodenectomy; *CsPOPF*, clinically significant postoperative pancreatic fistula; *OT*, operating time; *OS*, overall survival; *OvCompl*, overall complications; *RA-CUSUM*, risk-adjusted CUSUM; *ReAl*, realimentation.

24.4 Surgical Technique

Most authors report the use of 5 or 6 ports varying the site of the optical port from the umbilicus to the supraumbilical or umbilical region, the right paraumbilical or right pararectal position. Some authors [23] vary the position of the camera among different ports in the subsequent steps of LPD.

Laparoscopic Whipple procedures are usually fairly similar to the open surgical procedure. Different strategies are adopted to evaluate resectability such as preliminary laparoscopic ultrasound [16] or different kinds of initial approach to the superior mesenteric artery (SMA) [23]. Concerning the pancreatic transection, there is wide use of ultrasonic coagulating shears but the majority of surgeons prefers to transect the duct with cold scissors 2–3 mm from the right side of the parenchymal transection line. Treatment of the pancreatic stump is the real key point of the entire procedure. Duct occlusions, sometimes adopted at the beginning of the learning curve [16], were characterized by an excessively high

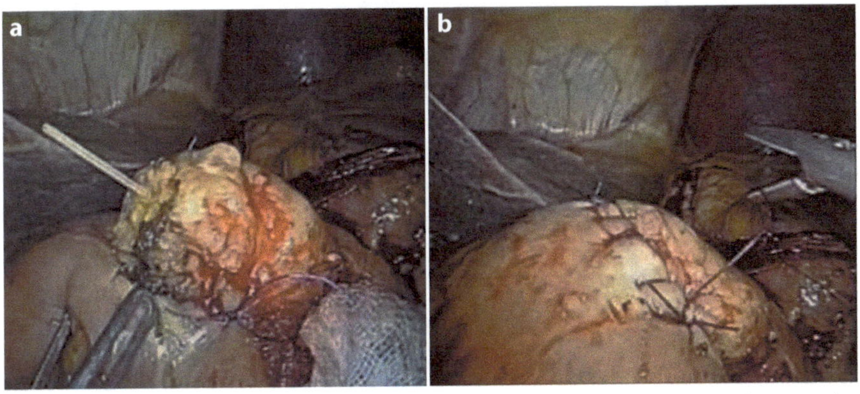

Fig. 24.1 Two-layer end-to-side pancreatojejunostomy (stented small Wirsung). **a** First posterior layer between the jejunal serosa and pancreatic capsule. **b** Final appearance of second anterior layer between the jejunal serosa and pancreatic capsule

percentage of fistulae. Most surgeons prefer to perform a pancreatojejunostomy (PJ) (Fig. 24.1) over a pancreatogastrostomy (PG). A recent meta-analysis [24] showed evidence of a lower complication rate of PG compared to PJ in terms of a reduced rate of POPF in open surgery. However, laparoscopic PG is not a common technique because the specific anatomic relationship between the stomach and pancreatic remnant makes PG more difficult under laparoscopic procedure. It is also more difficult to perform a gastrointestinal anastomosis after PG. In Boggi et al.'s review [8], among 682 LPD, 573 (84%) pancreatic remnants were drained into the jejunum and most pancreatic anastomosis were stented either routinely or selectively.

In all LPD reported in Table 24.3, a PJ was carried out with some technical variants. Regarding pylorus preservation, the literature data vary from 350 cases (55%) of preservation to 286 antrectomies (44.9%) for a total of 636 in Boggi et al.'s review [8]. Finally, the possibility to perform a "tangential" or complete vascular resection during LPD is clearly expressed in the experience of Croome et al. [11], Senthilnathan et al. [12] and Stauffer et al. [13] (Table 24.3).

24.5 Postoperative Outcomes

Considerable variability in morbidity and mortality still persists in LPD between low- and high-volume hospitals. Data from six tertiary centers (Table 24.4) showed evidence of major complications (Clavien-Dindo grade >II) ranging from 5.6% to 28% and there was no statistical difference with OPD in the four series [4, 5, 11, 13]. The mean mortality rate was 1.65% and the mean percentage of grade B+C POPF was 14.18%. Among the studies, only Dokmak et al. [5], despite more restrictive inclusion criteria than the other authors, found a statistically significant higher incidence of grade C POPF than in the OPD series (23.9% vs. 6.5%; $p = 0.007$). On the contrary, the original embedding end-to-side PJ with four layers of mattress sutures reported by Wang et al. [14] was followed by a very low percentage of POPF, with no grade C fistulae (0%). No difference with OPD was noted in delayed gastric emptying in any of the six series, varying from 3.8% to 17.2%.

All these satisfactory outcomes allowed the LOS following LPD to be contained within a weighted average of 10.4 days, statistically significantly shorter compared to the OPD in three series [4, 11, 13]. It should be noted that the shortest LOS (both 6 days) were those of the two large series [11, 13] including 100% of PDAC, as well as a significant number of vascular resections.

24.6 Oncologic Outcomes

Recent meta-analyses [6–10] evaluating intraoperative oncologic outcomes confirmed similar or better results in harvested lymph nodes and of R0 resection in LPD compared to OPD. Patient selection is probably responsible for the 100% rate of negative margins achieved in many LPD series, which is very different from the typical R0 margin rate of 70–80% in large OPD trials.

Patient selection similarly affected the scarce data available until a few years ago on disease-free survival and overall survival. Palanivelu et al. [25] in 2007 found a median survival rate of 46 months for their first 42 patients operated with LPD technique, with a 5-year overall survival of 19.1% for PDAC. The same group recently reported [12] a worse median survival rate of 33 months, most likely a consequence of expanded patient selection criteria for LPD with growing expertise.

To overcome this bias, the recent data from Croome et al. [11] and Stauffer et al. [13] (Tables 24.1 and 24. 2) in unselected patients affected by PDAC are compared to patients with similar characteristics who underwent OPD at their institutions during the same period of time. Croome et al. report fewer complications and shorter LOS in the LPD group with a significant difference in median time to commencement of adjuvant chemotherapy (LPD 48 days vs. OPD 59 days; $P < 0.001$) and a longer progression-free survival in the LPD group ($P = 0.03$). In Stauffer et al.'s study, the LPD group showed less EBL with lower transfusion rates and a larger number of harvested lymph nodes with higher lymph node ratio, but the postoperative outcomes were similar after LPD and OPD. Shorter LOS for LPD was not associated with a shorter time to start adjuvant therapy and the overall survival rate was similar to the OPD group. However, LPD was associated with a promising 32% at the Kaplan-Meier estimates of the 5-year survival rate.

24.7 Costs and Quality of Life

In 2013 Mesleh et al. [26] published the first detailed study analyzing the costs of LPD compared to OPD, showing no significant difference in overall costs (181 cost-units for LPD vs. 179 for OPD). Specifically, the higher surgical costs (65 vs. 48 cost-units) of LPD, due to longer OT and increased equipment costs, were offset by the lower admission costs of LPD (116 vs. 131 cost-units) incurred by the departments of anesthesia, critical care, pathology, pharmacy, nursing and radiology. Tran et al.'s analysis [27] of 15,574 patients who underwent PD from 2000 to 2010 included in the Nationwide Inpatient Sample database showed that the 681 (4.4%) LPD had a lower cumulative morbidity rate (39.4% vs. 46%; $p = 0.001$) and similar mortality rate (3.8% vs. 5%) compared to OPD. LOS was slightly longer in OPD (12 vs. 11 days; $p < 0.001$). Median hospital charge rate was similar in both groups, but when stratifying outcome by hospital volume, at high-volume centers LPD resulted in shorter LOS (9 vs. 13 days; $p < 0.001$) with significantly lower median hospital charges (76,572 vs. 106,367 US dollars; $p < 0.001$).

Only a few studies consider the value of LPD for patients beyond the mere economic cost. It is interesting to note that Langan et al. [28] found a better quality of life in the first 6 months after LPD than after OPD (median Karnofsky scores at 6 months, 92% vs. 66%; $p = 0.003$) but they did not find any significant difference 6 months after surgery.

24.8 Conclusions

More than 20 years after its introduction, pure LPD remains a challenging procedure with a steep learning curve. Its results and costs are clearly demonstrated to be better at high-volume hospitals, where some surgical groups were recently able to validate the safeness and feasibility of LPD also when requiring major vascular resection. If performed by well-experienced surgeons, the short- and long-term oncologic outcomes seem to be similar to those of open surgical procedures with the advantage of reduced intraoperative blood loss and a shorter LOS.

In order to fully understand the potential and the limitations of LPD, in the next few years we should strive to increase the centralization of patients, start the first multicenter randomized trials, and set up, in high-volume hospitals for PDAC, training programs able to shorten the LPD learning curve for dedicated surgeons, as stated at the first international state-of-the-art conference on minimally invasive pancreatic resection [29].

References

1. Gagner M, Pomp A (1994) Laparoscopic pylorus-preserving pancreatoduodenectomy. Surg Endosc 8(5):408–410
2. Kendrick ML, Sclabas GM (2011) Major venous resection during total laparoscopic pancreaticoduodenectomy. HPB (Oxford) 13(7):454–458
3. Khatkov IE, Izrailov RE, Khisamov AA et al (2017) Superior mesenteric-portal vein resection during laparoscopic pancreatoduodenectomy. Surg Endosc 31(3):1488–1495
4. Delitto D, Luckhurst CM, Black BS et al (2016) Oncologic and perioperative outcomes following selective application of laparoscopic pancreaticoduodenectomy for periampullary malignancies. J Gastrointest Surg 20(7):1343–1349
5. Dokmak S, Ftériche FS, Aussilhou B et al (2015) Laparoscopic pancreaticoduodenectomy should not be routine for resection of periampullary tumors. J Am Coll Surg 220(5):831–838
6. Gooiker GA, van Gijn W, Wouters MW et al (2011) Systematic review and meta-analysis of the volume-outcome relationship in pancreatic surgery. Br J Surg 98(4):485–494
7. Sharpe SM, Talamonti MS, Wang CE et al (2015) Early national experience with laparoscopic pancreaticoduodenectomy for ductal adenocarcinoma: a comparison of laparoscopic pancreaticoduodenectomy and open pancreaticoduodenectomy from the national cancer data base. J Am Coll Surg 221(1):175–184
8. Boggi U, Amorese G, Vistoli F et al (2015) Laparoscopic pancreaticoduodenectomy: a systematic literature review. Surg Endosc 29(1):9–23
9. de Rooij T, Klompmaker S, Abu Hilal M et al (2016) Laparoscopic pancreatic surgery for benign and malignant disease. Nat Rev Gastroenterol Hepatol 13(4):227–238
10. Coppola A, Stauffer JA, Asbun HJ (2016) Laparoscopic pancreatoduodenectomy: current status and future directions. Updates Surg 68(3):217–224
11. Croome KP, Farnell MB, Que FG et al (2014) Total laparoscopic pancreaticoduodenectomy for pancreatic ductal adenocarcinoma: oncologic advantages over open approaches? Ann Surg 260(4):633–638; discussion 638–640
12. Senthilnathan P, Srivatsan Gurumurthy S, Gul SI et al (2015) Long-term results of laparoscopic pancreaticoduodenectomy for pancreatic and periampullary cancer-experience of 130 cases from a tertiary-care center in South India. J Laparoendosc Adv Surg Tech A 25(4):295–300
13. Stauffer JA, Coppola A, Villacreses D et al (2017) Laparoscopic versus open pancreatico-duodenectomy for pancreatic adenocarcinoma: long-term results at a single institution. Surg Endosc 31(5):2233–2241
14. Wang M, Xu S, Zhang H et al (2017) Embedding pancreaticojejunostomy used in pure laparoscopic pancreaticoduodenectomy for nondilated pancreatic duct. Surg Endosc 31(4):1986–1992
15. Tempero MA, Malafa MP, Behrman SW et al (2014) Pancreatic adenocarcinoma, version 2.2014: featured updates to the NCCN guidelines. J Natl Compr Canc Netw 12(8):1083–1093
16. Corcione F, Pirozzi F, Cuccurullo D et al (2013) Laparoscopic pancreaticoduodenectomy: experience of 22 cases. Surg Endosc 27(6):2131–2136
17. Bassi C, Dervenis C, Butturini G et al (2005) Postoperative pancreatic fistula: an international study group (ISGPF) definition. Surgery 138(1):8–13
18. Song KB, Kim SC, Hwang DW et al (2015) Matched case-control analysis comparing laparoscopic and open pylorus-preserving pancreaticoduodenectomy in patients with periampullary tumors. Ann Surg 262(1):146–155
19. Kuroki T, Kitasato A, Adachi T et al (2014) Learning curve for laparoscopic pancreaticoduo-denectomy: a single surgeon's experience with consecutive patients. Hepatogastroenterol-ogy 61(131):838–841
20. Speicher PJ, Nussbaum DP, White RR et al (2014) Defining the learning curve for team-based laparoscopic pancreaticoduodenectomy. Ann Surg Oncol 21(12):4014–4019

21. Paniccia A, Schulick RD, Edil BH (2015) Total laparoscopic pancreaticoduodenectomy: a single-institutional experience. Ann Surg Oncol 22(13):4380–4381
22. Wang M, Meng L, Cai Y et al (2016) Learning curve for laparoscopic pancreaticoduodenectomy: a CUSUM analysis. Gastrointest Surg 20(5):924–935
23. Azagra JS, Arru L, Estévez S et al (2015) Laparoscopic pancreatoduodenectomy with initial approach to the superior mesenteric artery. Wideochir Inne Tech Maloinwazyjne 10(3):450–457
24. Hallet J, Zih FS, Deobald RG et al (2015) The impact of pancreaticojejunostomy versus pancreaticogastrostomy reconstruction on pancreatic fistula after pancreaticoduodenectomy: meta-analysis of randomized controlled trials. HPB (Oxford) 17(2):113–122
25. Palanivelu C, Jani K, Senthilnathan P et al (2007) Laparoscopic pancreaticoduodenectomy: technique and outcomes. J Am Coll Surg 205(2):222–230
26. Mesleh MG, Stauffer JA, Bowers SP et al (2013) Cost analysis of open and laparoscopic pancreaticoduodenectomy: a single institution comparison. Surg Endosc 27(12):4518–4523
27. Tran TB, Dua MM, Worhunsky DJ et al (2016) The first decade of laparoscopic pancreaticoduodenectomy in the United States: costs and outcomes using the nationwide inpatient sample. Surg Endosc 30(5):1778–1783
28. Langan RC, Graham JA, Chin AB et al (2014) Laparoscopic-assisted versus open pancreaticoduodenectomy: early favorable physical quality-of-life measures. Surgery 156 (2):379–384.
29. Vollmer CM, Asbun HJ, Barkun J et al (2017) Proceedings of the first international state-of-the-art conference on minimally-invasive pancreatic resection (MIPR). HPB (Oxford) 19(3):171–177

Hybrid Laparoscopic Pancreatoduodenectomy

25

Dirk Bausch and Tobias Keck

25.1 Introduction

Pancreatic surgery is technically complex and requires considerable expertise. Laparoscopy adds the need for considerable experience with advanced laparoscopic techniques. Laparoscopic distal pancreatectomy has rapidly become the procedure of choice for the treatment of small benign premalignant pancreatic lesions of the pancreatic tail owing to its relative simplicity. In contrast, the widespread use of laparoscopic pancreatoduodenectomy has been precluded by its technical difficulty, given that it requires extensive dissection near the mesenteric-portal axis, and reconstruction with laparoscopic suturing is challenging.

The procedure was first described 1994 by Gagner and Pomp [1] but the first larger series of patients who underwent laparoscopic pancreatoduodenectomy was published more than a decade later [2]. In this series, however, the authors performed full laparoscopic reconstruction in only 13 of 25 patients. For the remaining nine patients, the resection was performed laparoscopically and the reconstruction was performed through a small midline incision [2]. This hybrid laparoscopic pancreatoduodenectomy offers several advantages over a fully laparoscopic procedure.

1. Proper laparoscopic dissection can be evaluated prior to open reconstruction via the minilaparotomy.
2. The additional complexity of laparoscopic reconstruction can be avoided for initial cases and acquired after familiarity with the procedure is obtained.
3. The advantages of laparoscopy, such as the magnified view during resection, are combined with the safety of conventional reconstruction.

T. Keck (✉)
Klinik für Chirurgie, Universitätsklinikum Schleswig-Hosltein, Campus Lübeck
Lübeck, Germany
e-mail: tobias.keck@uksh.de

U. Boggi (Ed), *Minimally Invasive Surgery of the Pancreas*,
Updates in Surgery
DOI: 10.1007/978-88-470-3958-2_25, © Springer-Verlag Italia 2018

4. The minilaparotomy needed for reconstruction is not much larger than the incision required to remove the specimen.
5. Portal-vein resection, a procedure only selected centers worldwide perform fully laparoscopically, can usually be accomplished through the minilaparotomy.
6. Operating times similar to open surgery can be achieved after relatively few cases.
7. The long and flat learning curve of a fully laparoscopic pancreatoduodenectomy can be shortened considerably [3].

25.2 Indications and Preoperative Assessment

Originally, minimally invasive pancreatoduodenectomy was predominantly used to treat small premalignant lesions of the pancreatic head, such as cystic or neuroendocrine tumors [4]. Since 2014, retrospective analysis of long-term survival after oncologic laparoscopic pancreatoduodenectomy is available (Table 25.1) and demonstrates no significant difference in median survival compared to conventional surgery [5–7]. Despite the lack of prospective data, it thus seems feasible to perform the procedure for malignant lesions in specialized centers.

The imaging gold standard prior to pancreatic surgery is computed tomography with vascular assessment (angio-CT). Magnetic resonance imaging with simultaneous cholangiopancreatography (MRCP) is a valid alternative, especially for cystic pancreatic tumors. These modalities permit the detection of anatomic vascular variants, such as a replaced right hepatic artery, and help to establish the relation of the lesion to the mesenteric-portal axis. This is of importance for laparoscopic procedures since anatomic variants or adhesions to the mesenteric-portal axis are the most common cause of conversion to open surgery [8]. Careful evaluation of preoperative imaging may thus reduce the rate of unplanned conversions.

Table 25.1 Current retrospective studies comparing long-term survival after laparoscopic and open pancreatoduodenectomy for pancreatic cancer

Author	Year	Number of patients		Median survival (months)	
		laparoscopic	open	laparoscopic	open
Croome et al. [5]	2014	108	214	25,3	21,8
Stauffer et al. [6]	2016	58	193	18,5	20,3
Kantor et al. [7]	2016	828	7385	20,9	20,7

25.3 Patient Positioning and Technical Requirements

The procedure is performed with the patient in a modified beach-chair position: half-sitting with spread legs and raised upper body. Both arms are placed next to the body to prevent plexus lesions. If necessary, the right arm can be positioned at a 90° angle using an armrest. To permit sufficient intraoperative gravity displacement, the patient needs to be firmly secured to the operating table.

During the procedure, the surgeon is standing to the right of the patient, the first assistant between the patient's legs and the second assistant to the left of the patient. The nurse is standing next to the surgeon (Fig. 25.1a).

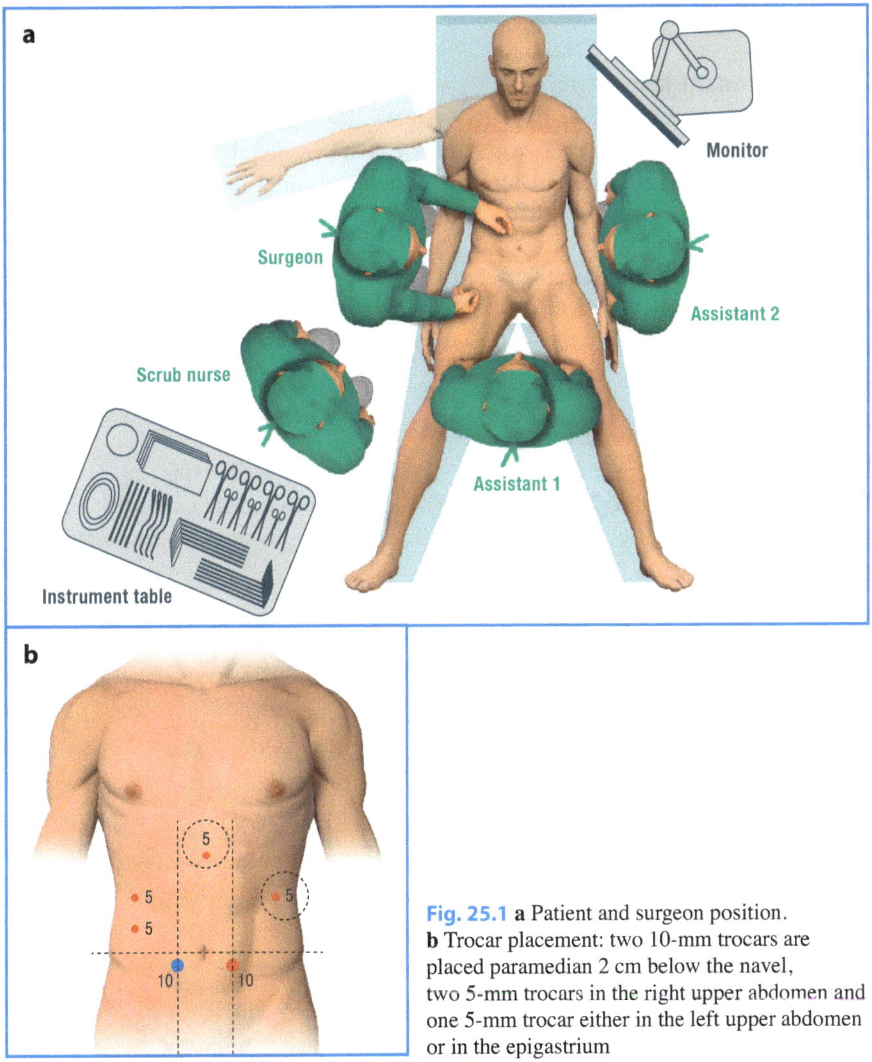

Fig. 25.1 **a** Patient and surgeon position. **b** Trocar placement: two 10-mm trocars are placed paramedian 2 cm below the navel, two 5-mm trocars in the right upper abdomen and one 5-mm trocar either in the left upper abdomen or in the epigastrium

The following specialized instruments are needed for the procedure in addition to commonly used simple laparoscopic instruments:

- a dissection device that permits both dissection and vessel sealing;
- laparoscopic bulldog clamps and applicator;
- bipolar laparoscopic scissors and Overholt clamp;
- titanium and polydioxanone (PDS) clips;
- a laparoscopic retractor, such as Goldfinger (OB Tech) or Endo Paddle Retract (Medtronic).

25.4 Surgical Procedure

25.4.1 Initial Steps

25.4.1.1 Trocar Placement

We commonly use a total of five trocars: two 10-mm trocars are placed paramedian 2 cm below the navel, two 5-mm trocars in the right upper abdomen, and one 5-mm trocar either in the left upper abdomen or in the epigastrium (Fig. 25.1b).

25.4.1.2 Access to the Bursa Omentalis

After exploration of the abdomen, the bursa omentalis is opened close to the gastroepiploic arcade while carefully preserving the latter. This permits gravity displacement of the omentum majus using a reverse Trendelenburg position.

25.4.1.3 Intraoperative Sonography

Small lesions in the pancreatic head can then be located using laparoscopic sonography to determine their relation to the mesenteric-portal axis and/or celiac trunk if needed. This helps in preventing injury of the aforementioned vessels.

25.4.2 Kocher Maneuver

The next step is a Kocher maneuver, which can easily be performed laparoscopically up to the origin of the superior mesenteric artery at the aorta. Usually, the ligament of Treitz can be fully dissected during the laparoscopic Kocher maneuver. This renders later dissection of the first jejunal loop from the left unnecessary. To facilitate the Kocher maneuver, mobilization of the right colonic flexure may be helpful, albeit not necessary (Fig. 25.2a).

25.4.3 Exposure of Superior Mesenteric Vein

The superior mesenteric vein is then exposed. Henle's loop, in particular the right gastroepiploic vein, serves as a guiding structure for finding the vein. The

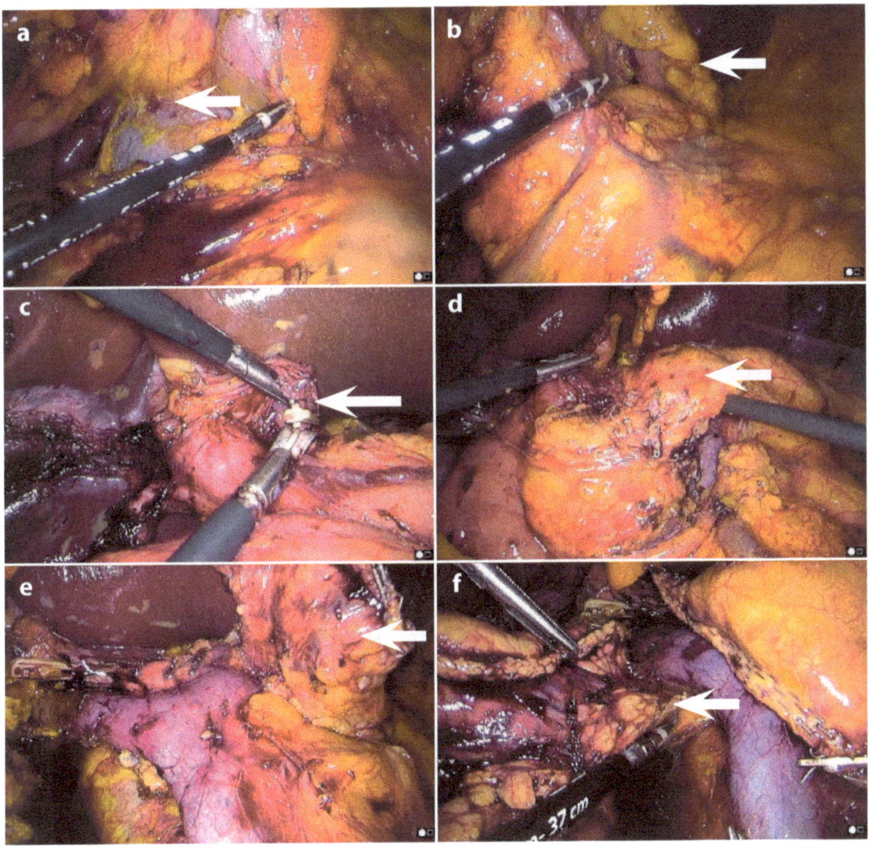

Fig. 25.2 Hybrid laparoscopic pancreatoduodenectomy. **a** Kocher maneuver (*arrow*, left renal vein). **b** Exposure of the superior mesenteric vein (*arrow*, right gastroepiploic vein). **c** Dissection of the hepatoduodenal ligament (*arrow*, hepatic and gastroduodenal artery). **d** Tunnel above the superior mesenteric vein (*arrow*, pancreas). **e** Mobilization of pancreatic remnant (*arrow*, pancreas). **f** Transection of the mesopancreas (*arrow*, mesopancreas)

right gastroepiploic vein is then clipped with titanium clips close to the superior mesenteric vein. In the case of larger tumors, branches of the superior mesenteric vein in the mesenteric root may serve as alternate guiding structures. After exposure of the superior mesenteric vein, dissection continues a few centimeters along the inferior pancreatic border towards the pancreatic tail (Fig. 25.2b).

25.4.4 Dissection of the Hepatoduodenal Ligament

Dissection then continues at the hepatoduodenal ligament. Complete lymphadenectomy is performed and the common hepatic duct, proper, left and right hepatic artery, gastroduodenal artery and portal vein are dissected. At this point, resectability can finally be assessed and stenosis of the common hepatic artery ruled out by clamping the gastroduodenal artery. The gall bladder is then mobilized and remains on the specimen side of the bile duct after transection of the latter. Prior to transection of the bile duct, the presence of a replaced right hepatic artery should be ruled out. After transection of the bile duct, the gastroduodenal artery is ideally exposed and it can be transected between PDS clips. We usually place an additional silk ligature on the side of the hepatic artery to prevent bleeding in case of slippage of the clip. Lymphadenectomy is then continued towards the pancreatic tail along the upper border of the pancreas and celiac trunk (Fig. 25.2c). After circumferential dissection of the portal vein in the hepatoduodenal ligament, a tunnel can be completed above the vein below the pancreas (Fig. 25.2d).

25.4.5 Transection of Duodenum and Jejunum

After transecting the right gastroepiploic artery, dissection of the pylorus is performed and the duodenum is transected using a laparoscopic linear stapler 1 cm distal to the pylorus.

If the first jejunal loop has already been freed during the Kocher maneuver, it is pulled to the right and transected using a laparoscopic linear stapler. Otherwise, the Kocher maneuver is completed to the left, and transection of the first jejunal loop is performed.

25.4.6 Transection of the Pancreas

The pancreas is then transected. This can be either performed using a dissection device that permits both dissection and vessel sealing or using a laparoscopic linear stapler. To avoid thermal injury, we prefer using a stapling device followed by reopening the staple line at the main pancreatic duct. If another dissection device is used, identification and preservation of the main pancreatic duct is mandatory. Thereafter, the pancreatic remnant is mobilized along the splenic vein for 3 cm to permit a pancreatogastrostomy (Fig. 25.2e). If the pancreas is transected to the left of the mesenteric-portal axis, it can be dissected up to the origin of the splenic artery. Usually, two small arterial branches arising from the mesenteric and splenic artery are encountered during dissection and should be clipped with titanium clips prior to their transection.

25.4.7 Transection of the Mesopancreas

The resection is then completed by transecting the mesopancreas following the first venous jejunal branch and later the superior mesenteric artery up to its origin at the aorta. The first assistant retracts the superior mesenteric vein to the left using a cotton swab during transection. Larger branches of the superior mesenteric artery to the pancreas are clipped using titanium clips prior to their transection (Fig. 25.2f). After its complete release, the specimen is placed in a specimen removal bag and removed via an epigastric median minilaparotomy (5–8 cm long).

25.4.8 Reconstruction

After placing a wound retractor in the minilaparotomy, the hepaticojejunostomy is usually performed first. The first jejunal loop can be brought either through a retrocolic window or through the former ligament of Treitz. We usually perform the hepaticojejunostomy using interrupted 5-0 or 6-0 PDS C1 sutures, depending on the size of the hepatic duct.

The pancreatic anastomosis is usually performed as an invagination pancreatogastrostomy. After a small dorsal gastrostomy for the insertion of the pancreatic remnant, a somewhat larger ventral gastrostomy is performed to access the stomach. A 2-0 PDS SH purse string suture is placed around the dorsal gastrostomy (Fig. 25.3a). A PDS 4-0 suture is placed at the upper and lower border of the pancreatic remnant. This facilitates insertion of the pancreas into

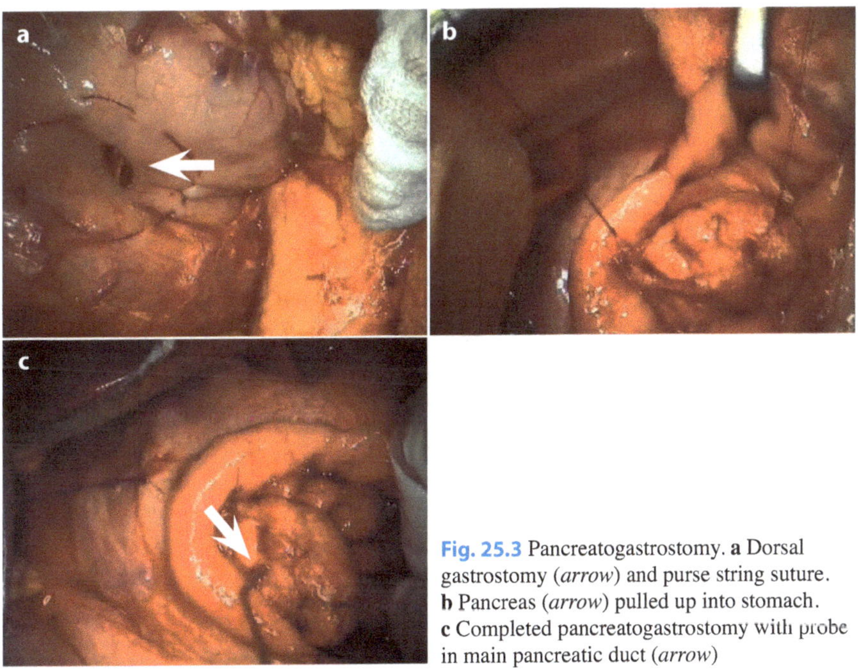

Fig. 25.3 Pancreatogastrostomy. **a** Dorsal gastrostomy (*arrow*) and purse string suture. **b** Pancreas (*arrow*) pulled up into stomach. **c** Completed pancreatogastrostomy with probe in main pancreatic duct (*arrow*)

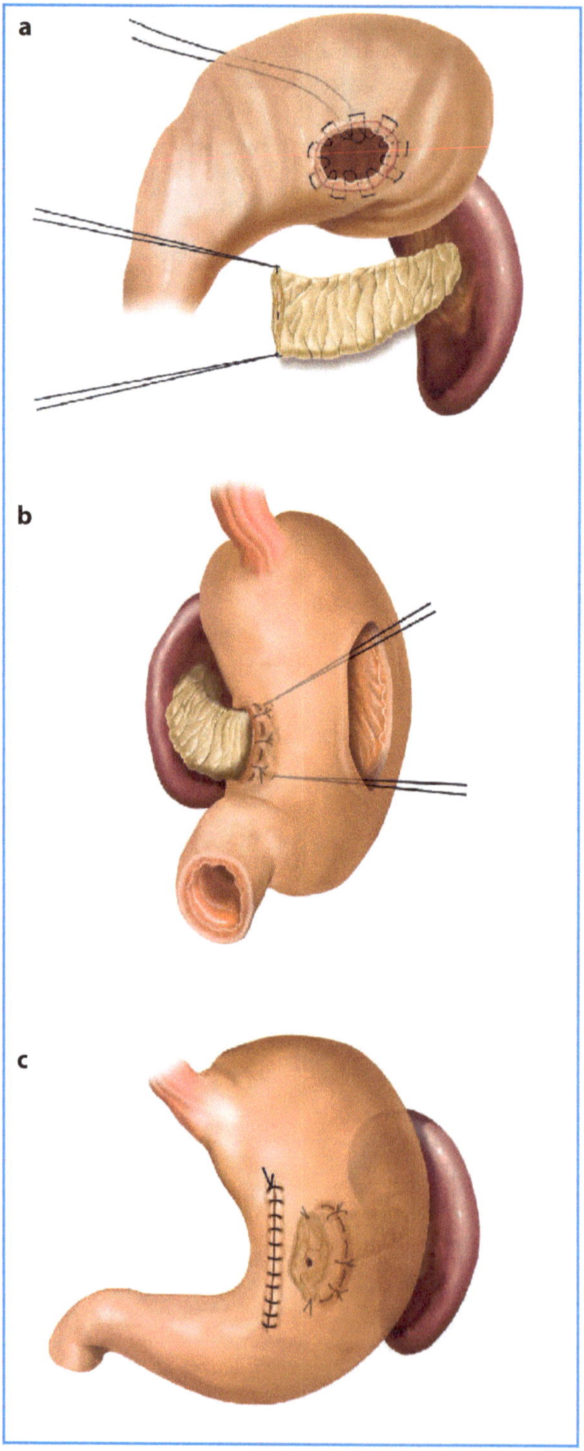

Fig. 25.4 Technical approach to pancreatogastrostomy. **a** A posterior small incision in made in the stomach and a purse-string suture is placed (2-0 PDS). **b**. The well mobilized pancreatic stump is invaginated in the stomach through an additional ventral gastrostomy and the purse-string suture is closed. Additional single sutures are placed to secure the pancreas in the stomach. **c** The ventral gastrostomy is closed with a single-layer running suture (4-0 PDS)

the stomach and further prevents bleeding from the two small arteries in this area. The pancreatic remnant is then inserted into the stomach and the purse string suture is tied (Fig. 25.3b). While this is sufficient, we usually place additional 4-0 PDS SH interrupted sutures to perform an inner anastomosis (Fig. 25.3c). Thereafter, the ventral gastrostomy is closed using a running suture.

The duodenojejunostomy is performed as a retrocolic end-to-side anastomosis with continuous 4-0 PDS sutures. Two of the trocar insertion sites are then used to place one drain at the hepaticojejunostomy and one drain at the pancreatic anastomosis. The median laparotomy is then closed with a running suture of the fascia and an intracutaneous skin suture.

25.5 Specific Intraoperative Complications and their Management

Despite extensive dissection close to the mesenteric-portal axis, relevant intraoperative bleeding is rare during laparoscopic pancreatic surgery in our experience. However, bleeding control can be difficult if bleeding occurs. Early visualization of the superior mesenteric vein at the inferior border of the pancreas facilitates placement of a laparoscopic bulldog clamp if bleedings occurs during the procedure. In such a case, uncontrolled coagulation should be avoided. Temporary increase of intra-abdominal pressure and compression with a cotton swab can reduce portal venous bleeding prior to placement of a suture to control it. In the case of venous bleeding, suction should be avoided as it tends to increase bleeding due to a reduction of intra-abdominal pressure.

Bleeding of the stapler line after pancreatic transection can be controlled by bipolar coagulation and temporary placement of a gauze.

Thermal injury of arteries, especially during transection of the mesopancreas can also lead to bleeding. We therefore prefer the use of titanium clips for larger arteries arising from the superior mesenteric artery. In cases of complex arterial injury, conversion to open surgery is usually required.

25.6 Conclusions

Overall, a hybrid approach to pancreatoduodenectomy circumvents the time-consuming and technically difficult full laparoscopic reconstruction but retains the advantages commonly associated with laparoscopic procedures, such as decreased postoperative pain, narcotic use and length of hospital stay [2, 9, 10].

References

1. Gagner M, Pomp A (1994) Laparoscopic pylorus-preserving pancreatoduodenectomy. Surg Endosc 8(5):408–410
2. Dulucq JL, Wintringer P, Mahajna A (2006) Laparoscopic pancreaticoduodenectomy for benign and malignant diseases. Surg Endosc 20(7):1045–1050
3. Speicher PJ, Nussbaum DP, White RR et al (2014) Defining the learning curve for team-based laparoscopic pancreaticoduodenectomy. Ann Surg Oncol 21(12):4014–4019
4. Siech M, Bartsch D, Beger HG et al (2012) Indications for laparoscopic pancreas operations: results of a consensus conference and the previous laparoscopic pancreas register. Chirurg 83(3):247–253 [Article in German]
5. Croome KP, Farnell MB, Que FG et al (2014) Total laparoscopic pancreaticoduodenectomy for pancreatic ductal adenocarcinoma: oncologic advantages over open approaches? Ann Surg 260(4):633–638; discussion 638–640
6. Stauffer JA, Coppola A, Villacreses D et al (2017) Laparoscopic versus open pancreaticoduodenectomy for pancreatic adenocarcinoma: long-term results at a single institution. Surg Endosc 31(5):2233–2241
7. Kantor O, Talamonti MS, Sharpe S et al (2017) Laparoscopic pancreaticoduodenectomy for adenocarcinoma provides short-term oncologic outcomes and long-term overall survival rates similar to those for open pancreaticoduodenectomy. Am J Surg 213(3):512–515
8. Wellner UF, Küsters S, Sick O et al (2014) Hybrid laparoscopic versus open pylorus-preserving pancreatoduodenectomy: retrospective matched case comparison in 80 patients. Langenbecks Arch Surg 399(7):849–856
9. Lee JS, Han JH, Na GH et al (2013) Laparoscopic pancreaticoduodenectomy assisted by mini-laparotomy. Surg Laparosc Endosc Percutan Tech 23(3):e98–e102
10. Keck T, Kuesters S, Wellner U et al (2011) Laparoscopic pylorus-preserving pancreatic head resection and hybrid open reconstruction via pancreatogastrostomy. J Gastrointest Surg 15(2):373–377

Robotic Pancreatoduodenectomy

26

Ugo Boggi, Vittorio G. Perrone, and Fabio Vistoli

26.1 Introduction

First performed by Codivilla in 1898, pancreatoduodenectomy (PD) has intrinsic challenges and, despite improvements, continues to be associated with high rates of postoperative complications. While several authors have reported large series with no postoperative mortality at 30 days [1], a realistic appraisal shows an operative mortality rate of between 2% and 5% [2] with morbidity in 40–50% of the patients [3]. These figures are expected be even higher if outcomes are measured at 90 days instead of at 30 days, because it is known that the absolute number of adverse events increases by 30% between index discharge and 90 days and by 10% between 30 and 90 days. The number of severe adverse events increases in even greater percentages either between discharge and 90 days or between 30 and 90 days [4].

According to these figures, minimally invasive PD (MIPD) is confronted with the unique challenge of improving the outcome of a still imperfect open operation. In particular, in open PD no technique was shown to be ideal [5] and the development of postoperative pancreatic fistula (POPF) cannot be completely prevented [6].

Despite all these difficulties, MIPD is gaining momentum [7]. A recent worldwide survey of opinions and use of minimally invasive pancreatic resection showed that 29% of responding surgeons performed MIPD, and that the most common reasons for not performing MIPD were lack of specific training (62%), difficulty of surgical technique (44%) and lack of time in surgical schedule (37%). Interestingly enough, while the current value of MIPD was deemed superior to that of open PD only by 17% and 7% of surgeons performing and not performing

U. Boggi (✉)
Division of General and Transplant Surgery, University of Pisa
Pisa, Italy
e-mail: u.boggi@med.unipi.it

U. Boggi (Ed), *Minimally Invasive Surgery of the Pancreas*,
Updates in Surgery
DOI: 10.1007/978-88-470-3958-2_26, © Springer-Verlag Italia 2018

MIPD, respectively, equivalent figures for the future value of MIPD were 53% and 23% [8].

The enhanced surgical dexterity offered by robotic assistance [9] is expected to be particularly rewarding in a procedure such as MIPD, because of difficult dissection and need for complex digestive reconstruction. At the time of this writing robotic pancreatic surgery has employed only the da Vinci Surgical System (dVss) (Intuitive Surgical, Sunnyvale, CA, USA) because, until recently, this was the only available system. Recently, another robotic platform was launched, the Telelap ALF-X (SOFAR S.p.A., ALF-X Surgical Robotics Department, Trezzano Rosa, Milan, Italy) [10]. Other robotic systems are under development.

When considering the potential of robotic PD (RPD) as compared to laparoscopic PD a couple of important considerations apply.

First, after more than two decades of evolution in instruments and ancillary technologies, laparoscopic techniques are likely to have reached a development plateau. On the other hand, robotic assistance is still in its infancy and, so far, the only manufacturer (Intuitive Surgical) has dedicated no specific attention to the needs of pancreatic surgery, probably because of economic considerations based on anticipated market profits in other surgical specialties.

Second, the real advantage of robotic assistance when compared to standard laparoscopy is to have placed a computer between the surgeon and the patient. Basically, robotic surgery is computer-assisted surgery. Future developments are expected to provide the surgeon with more information, like aircraft pilots in their cockpits, and could eventually lead to the implementation of artificially intelligent systems with the ability to automatically perform an entire procedure, or part of it.

26.2 Selection of Patients for Robotic Pancreatoduodenectomy

There is no general agreement on selection criteria for MIPD, in general, and for RPD, in particular. Some authors are rather inclusive, as they believe that most procedures feasible through an open approach can be performed also using minimally invasive techniques. Other authors are more selective. Selection criteria are also expected to evolve with experience, so that beginners are more likely to select good-risk patients with low-grade tumors, while more expert surgeons could also accept patients at higher medical risk with pancreatic cancer. Our current selection criteria are reported in Table 26.1.

It is important to note that indications for surgery must not be expanded because of the availability of robotic assistance. Likewise, cosmesis should play no role in the decision regarding surgical technique.

Table 26.1 Selection criteria for robotic pancreatoduodenectomy at the University of Pisa

General criteria	Availability of robotic system Suitability for laparoscopy		
Specific criteria		≤40 procedures	BMI: Males: ≤28 kg/m^2; Females: ≤30 kg/m^2 No need for concurrent procedures No visceral involvement No vein involvement
		41–80 procedures	BMI: Males: ≤30 kg/m^2; Females: ≤35 kg/m^2 Consider patients needing concurrent procedures, if manageable No vein involvement No visceral involvement
		>80 procedures	Do not accept patients with central obesity Consider patients needing concurrent procedures, if manageable Consider patients needing visceral resections, if manageable Consider patients needing vein resection, if manageable
Histology criteria	***Pancreatic cancer***	≤40 procedures	Do not accept
		41–80 procedures	Accept if clear surgical margins can be defined. Be more selective for cancers in the uncinate process
		>80 procedures	Accept if clear surgical margins can be defined
	Other histology	≤40 procedures	Do not accept large tumors Do not accept duodenal cancer Do not accept chronic pancreatitis
		41–80 procedures	Accept larger tumors Consider accepting duodenal cancer, if no extravisceral growth Do not accept chronic pancreatitis
		>80 procedures	Accept all tumor sizes, if manageable Accept duodenal cancer, if manageable Accept chronic pancreatitis, if manageable

26.3 Techniques for Robotic Pancreatoduodenectomy

The first RPD was performed by Giulianotti at the Misericordia Hospital in Grosseto (Italy) and was reported in 2003 [11]. After this initial report, a handful of groups have implemented programs for RPD worldwide.
We herein describe the technique developed in Pisa [9, 12, 13].

Patient position, sites for port placement, and operating room setup are shown in Fig. 26.1. Five ports are used. With the Si system, ports are placed along a smiling line, with the Xi systems they are placed along a straighter line.

After tumor resectability is confirmed, the liver is hung to the anterior abdominal wall by several sutures (Fig. 26.2). This technique avoids the use of a liver retractor and makes the fourth robotic arm fully available for surgical assistance.

Dissection begins from the hepatoduodenal ligament. The gallbladder is not removed until the end of the procedure as it is used to retract the liver. The common bile duct, the hepatic artery, and the portal vein are identified and exposed. The presence of anatomic variations in arterial liver supply should be defined at preoperative computed tomography to reduce the possibility of surgical misadventure. The lymph node stations to be cleared depend on tumor type, but lymph nodes 8a are always removed for safe visualization of the common hepatic artery. The gastroduodenal artery is identified, dissected, double-ligated using 0 linen sutures, and divided with a safety margin. The duct is also divided between ligatures or clips, to avoid bile spillage during the procedure, and a swab is taken for culture. The duct margin is sent for frozen-section histology, if required.

Next, the gastrocolic ligament is opened proceeding from left to right until the right colonic flexure is mobilized. The right gastroepiploic vessels are identified, dissected off, clipped by hem-o-lok (Teleflex Medical, Research Triangle Park, NC, USA) and divided. During this procedure, the fourth robotic arm is used to elevate the gastric antrum thus opening the dissection plane (Fig. 26.3). The first part of the duodenum is then divided with a laparoscopic stapler loaded with a vascular cartridge.

The pancreatic neck is separated from the superior mesenteric/portal vein (SM/PV), and stay sutures are placed at the inferior and superior border of the gland. While dividing the neck of the pancreas, the main pancreatic duct must be identified and cut sharply. Since at this level the duct is typically located in the upper third of the neck and division proceeds upwards, the harmonic scalpel can be used to divide the first few centimeters of the gland. As the anticipated position of the duct is approached, robotic scissors are used until the duct is visualized and divided. The pancreatic margin is sent for frozen-section histology, if required.

To proceed with duodenal kocherization, the duodenum is grasped with the fourth robotic arm and handled as required. During dissection of the posterior margin, the duodenum will be suspended to the right side of the patient and elevated so that the dissection line along the right side of the superior mesenteric artery will come into clearer view (Fig. 26.4). Additionally, in order to facilitate safer dissection around large peripancreatic vessels, the hepatic artery and the portal vein are looped (Fig. 26.5).

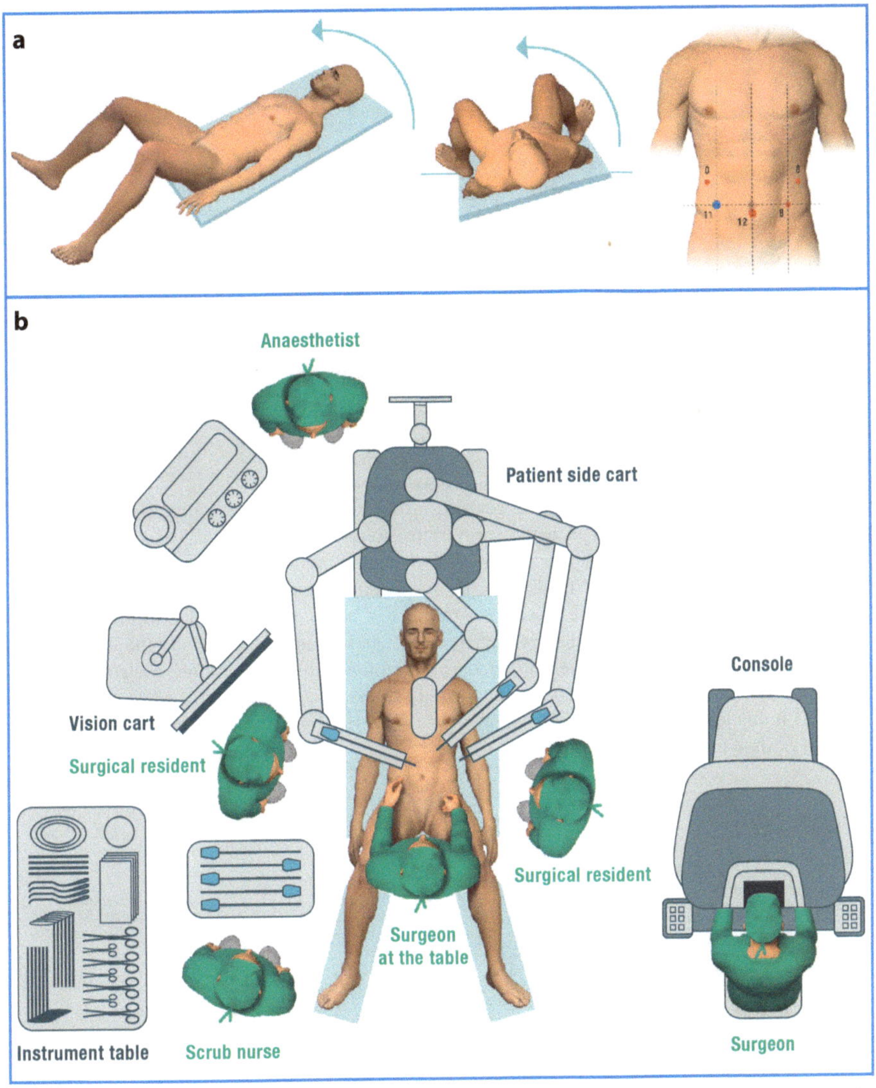

Fig. 26.1 **a** The patient is positioned supine with the legs parted, and the table is oriented 25° in reverse Trendelenburg and tilted to the left. Using the Si system, the 11-mm optic port is placed along the right midclavicular line at the level of the umbilicus (*blue circle*). The 12-mm assistant port is placed immediately below or above the umbilicus, depending on the distance between the xiphoid and the umbilicus (*large red circle*). One 8-mm robotic port is placed on the right side along the anterior axillary line 3 to 4 cm cephalad to the optic port. The other two 8-mm robotic ports are placed specular to the right-sided ports on the left side (*small red circles*). **b** Operating room setup. The console is placed at the feet of the patient, so that the operating surgeon can stay in direct visual contact with the surgeons at the table. The assistant surgeon stands between the patient's legs. One or two surgical assistants or residents help with the exchange of instruments. The scrub nurse and the instrument table are placed to the right of the patient, making this part of the operating room "clean". With the Si system, the robotic tower is placed over the head the patient

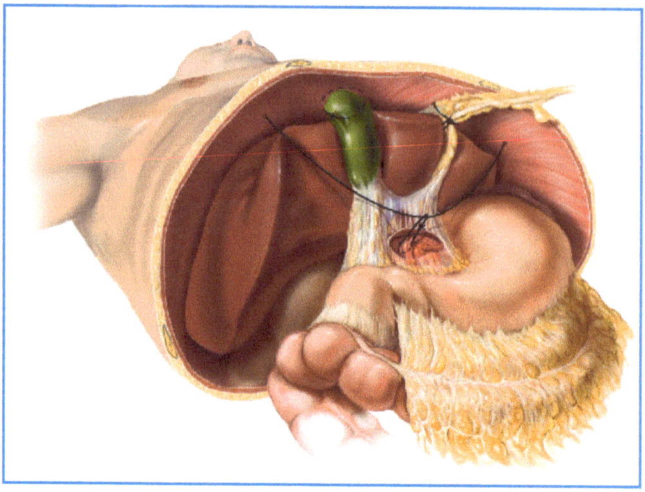

Fig. 26.2 Methods for instrumentless liver suspension during robotic pancreatoduodenectomy. The round ligament of the liver is suspended using a transparietal suture. Segment 5 and 6 are elevated by hanging the fundus of gallbladder to the right diaphragmatic dome, using an intracorporeal suture. A V-shaped sling is used to elevate the left lateral segment of the liver. The V-shaped sling is created using a transabdominal suture brought in below the costal margin along the left pararectal line, passed through the diaphragmatic crus, and brought out again at the level of the right pararectal line, immediately below the costal margin. Because the straight needle required to transfix the abdominal wall cannot be easily passed through the right diaphragmatic crus, a loop is created at this level using an intracorporeal suture. The transfixed suture is then passed through the loop, as shown in the figure

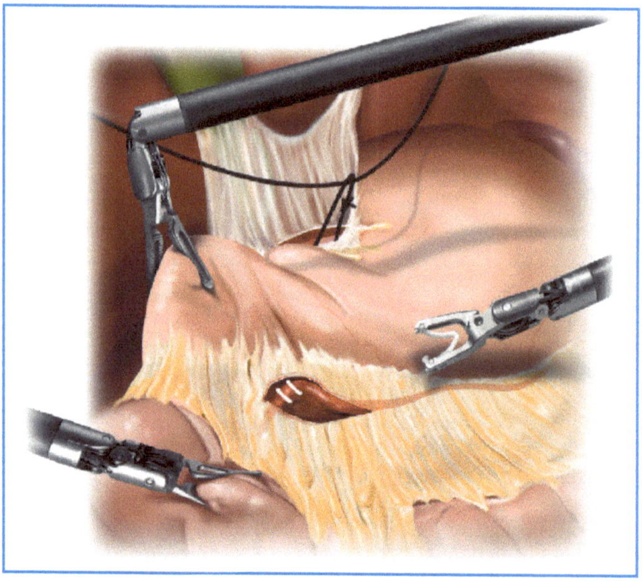

Fig. 26.3 After division of the gastrocolic ligament, the right gastroepiploic vessels are divided between hem-o-lok clips

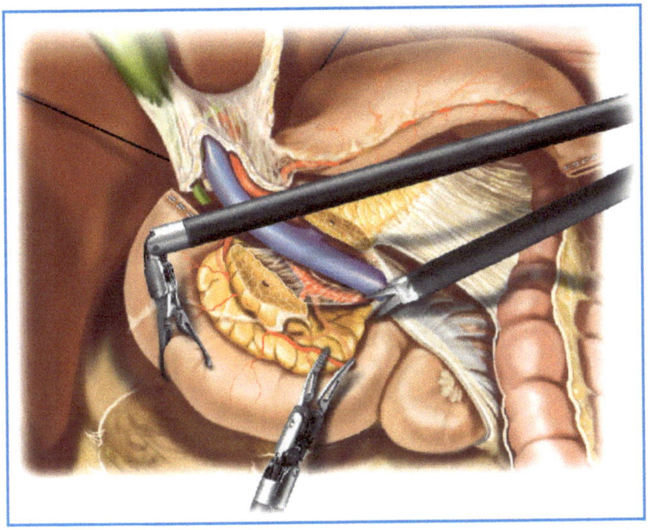

Fig. 26.4 Using a prograsp forceps handled by the robotic arm placed on the left subcostal area, the second portion of the duodenum is grasped, elevated and pulled to the right side of the patient. This maneuver, known as "duodenal hanging", pulls the uncinate process away from the superior mesenteric/portal vein thus exposing the resection line along the right side of the superior mesenteric artery

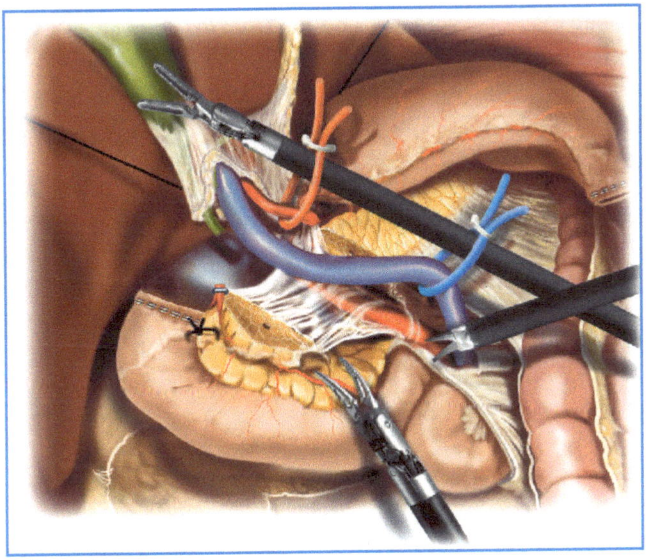

Fig. 26.5 The hepatic artery and the superior mesenteric/portal vein are encircled using vessel loops. The loops are closed by clips, so that the fourth robotic arm can be passed through the loops to facilitate exposure of the posterior margin, while still retaining the possibility to be used as a surgical instrument

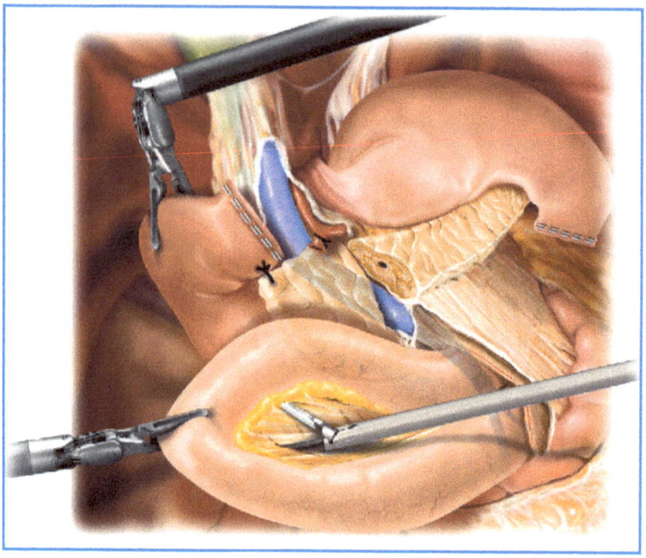

Fig. 26.6 Duodenal hanging brings the ligament of Treitz behind the superior mesenteric vessels. Incision of the ligament of Treitz exposes the proximal jejunum and allows the division of the mesentery of the proximal jejunum from the right side of the mesenteric vessels without additional intestinal mobilization

After a wide Kocher maneuver the posterior peritoneal layer is opened and the first jejunal loop is retracted to the right of the superior mesenteric vessels. The jejunal mesentery is divided from this perspective (i.e., from the right side of the superior mesenteric vessels), using a Harmonic scalpel (Ethicon Endo-Surgery, Johnson & Johnson, Somerville, NJ, USA). The bowel is not immediately divided to facilitate rotation around the mesenteric vessels at the time of reconstruction (Fig. 26.6). Dissection of the posterior margin proceeds along the periadvential plane of the superior mesenteric artery. The pancreaticoduodenal arteries and veins are identified and ligated or clipped. The use of energy devices at this level is minimized to avoid the risk of thermal injury to the wall of major vessels. Likewise, large retroperitoneal lymphatics are clipped to reduce the occurrence and amount of retroperitoneal fluid collections.

For pancreatic cancer, great attention is paid to achieve radical *en bloc* clearance of peripancreatic node stations and the lympho-neural tissue corresponding to the plexus capitalis (or extrapancreatic nerve plexus) and often referred as to "mesopancreas". Overall, the following stations are cleared: 12a–c, 8a, 8p, 9, 14a–d (see Chapter 27, Fig. 27.3).

Although all types of pancreatic anastomoses can be performed under robotic assistance, our preference goes to a duct-to-mucosa anastomosis with the jejunum. However, when the pancreas is thought to be at exceedingly high risk of POPF, we prefer to avoid suturing the gland and elect to construct a pancreaticocutaneous fistula (Fig. 26.7).

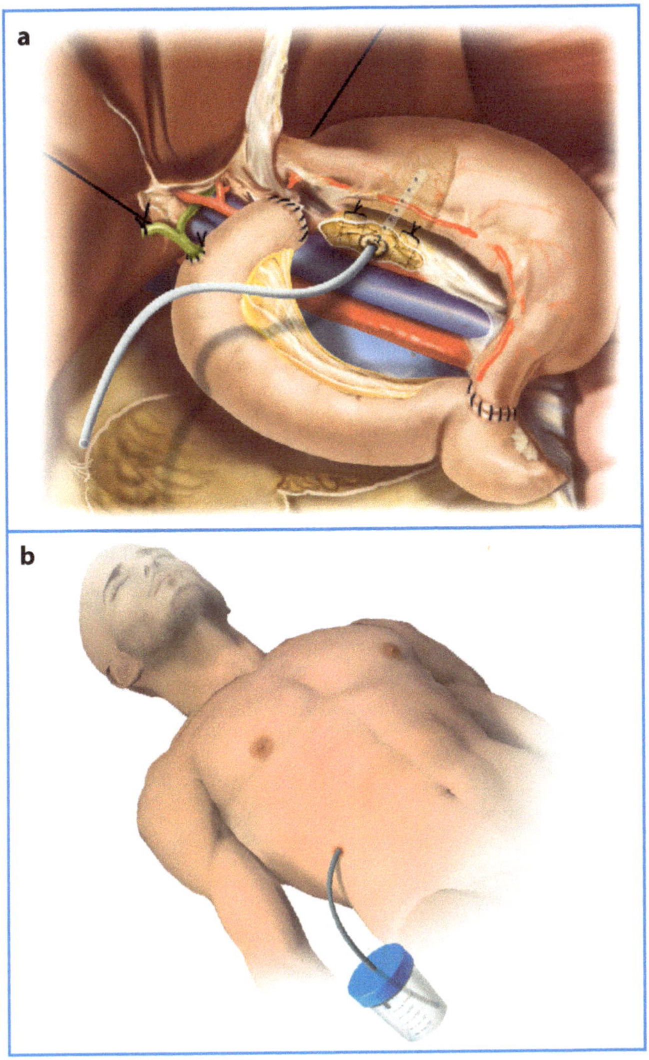

Fig. 26.7 A pancreaticocutaneous fistula is created by threading back into the main pancreatic duct a catheter of suitable caliber with side holes (**a**). The catheter is then brought outside the abdominal wall through a small stab wound (**b**). The large vessels are protected using the round and falciform ligaments, and one or two drains are placed near the pancreatic stump

Reconstruction is typically performed using a single jejunal loop passed behind the superior mesenteric vessels.

In nearly all patients we currently employ a modified Blumgart duct-to-mucosa pancreatojejunostomy [14]. This anastomosis consists of 2 to 4 U-shaped transfix sutures (4-0 expanded polytetrafluoroethylene [ePTFE]) that are passed to wrap the pancreas with the intestine, while avoiding the duct.

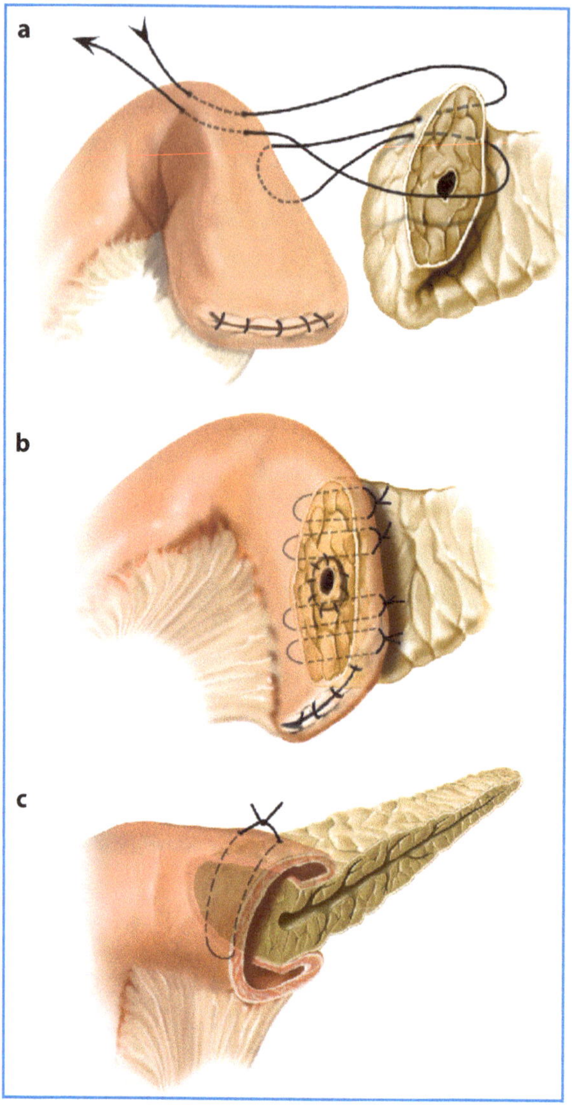

Fig. 26.8 The modified Blumgart anastomosis consists of 2 to 4 U-sutures that transfix the jejunum, the pancreas, and again the jejunum. In detail, a long (20 cm) 4-0 ePTFE suture is passed through the seromuscular layer of the jejunum at the antimesenteric level (**a**). This suture is transfixed through the pancreas (anterior to posterior), avoiding the duct, and passed again through the seromuscular layer of the jejunum near the mesentery. The suture is then passed all the way back (posterior to anterior) through all layers. When this type of suture is tied, the jejunum moves to wrap over the pancreatic stump (**b**). The pancreatojejunostomy needs to be perfected at the upper and lower margins by standard transfix sutures to close the corners of the anastomosis (**c**)

Anastomotic disruption is barely possibly with these anchoring sutures, unless the pancreatic stump becomes necrotic as a result of ischemia or pancreatitis. Before ligating the sutures, the duct-to-mucosa anastomosis is performed using interrupted 5-0 polydioxanone sutures. A duct stent is used when the duct is small (<4 mm), to facilitate the suture, and up to 12 sutures are placed (Fig. 26.8). The hepaticojejunostomy is performed end-to-side, approximately 7–10 cm downstream from the pancreatojejunostomy in a double layer, using half running 5-0 polydioxanone sutures. The duodenojejunostomy is done in two layers 10–15 cm distal from the hepaticojejunostomy [9, 12].

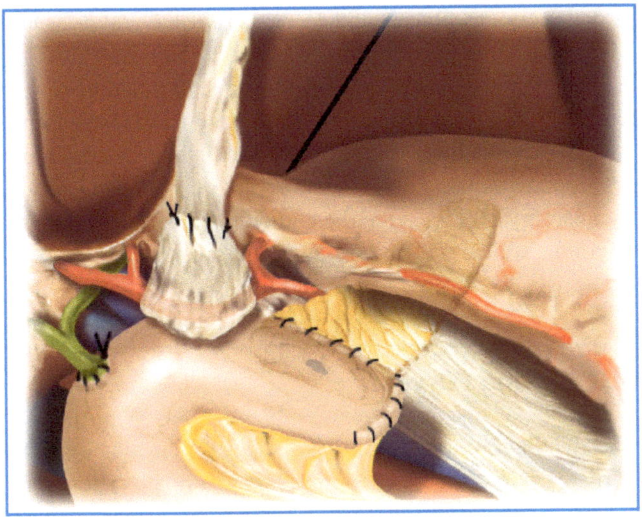

Fig. 26.9 The round and falciform ligaments of the liver are mobilized and wrapped around the hepatic artery, to cover the stump of the gastroduodenal artery

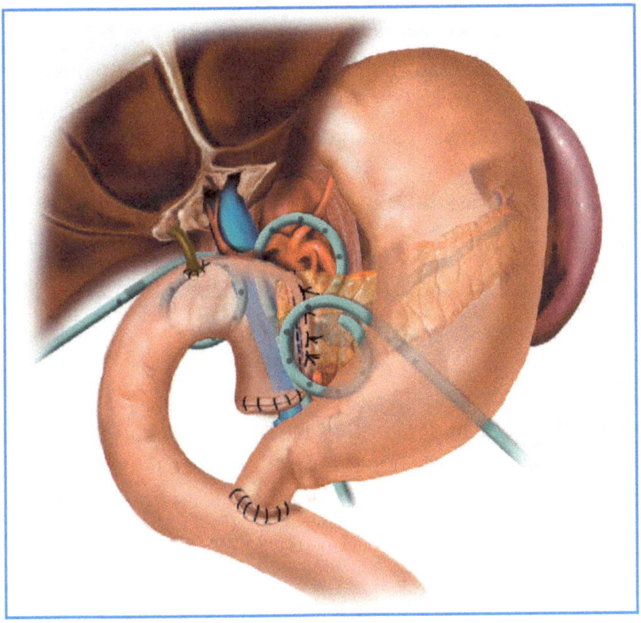

Fig. 26.10 Final position of surgical drains at the end of the procedure

At the end of the procedure, the specimen is extracted in an endoscopic jar via a small transverse suprapubic incision and the round ligament is mobilized to wrap the hepatic artery (Fig. 26.9).

Three 14-Fr pig-tail catheters are placed and left to drain by gravity. One catheter is placed in Morrison's pouch, behind the hepaticojejunostomy. The other two catheters are placed in front and behind the pancreatojejunostomy, respectively (Fig. 26.10). The catheter placed behind the pancreatojejunostomy is advanced through a small dedicated incision, placed between the two left-sided robotic ports, and is positioned immediately after completion of the posterior layer of the pancreatojejunostomy. At this stage the catheter can be easily passed behind the anastomosis without undue traction or manipulation.

26.4 Training and Learning Curve

At high-volume centers (>100 PD per year) when proficient pancreatic surgeons implemented RPD, the learning curve was defined in approximately 40 procedures per surgeon [15, 16]. This number of RPD seems reasonable considering that the learning curve for open PD and laparoscopic PD consisted in 60 operations each [17, 18]. Robotic assistance is indeed expected to improve surgeon dexterity in laparoscopic operations, thus potentially shortening the learning curve by some 20 procedures.

A training curriculum for the safe diffusion of MIPD has been recently proposed after the international "State-of-the-Art" conference held during the 12th annual International Hepato-Pancreato-Biliary Association World Congress in São Paulo, Brazil, on April 20th, 2016 [19]. The proposed path includes several steps: (1) a proficiency-based virtual reality simulation curriculum, (2) inanimate biotissue curriculum, (3) HPB video library, (4) intraoperative evaluation, and (5) skills maintenance with ongoing assessment.

26.5 Results of Robotic Pancreatoduodenectomy

RPD is a relatively young procedure. Initial results have shown the feasibility of RPD [9]. Larger experiences have also shown that RPD is reasonably safe and could be even convenient in selected patient populations. In our most recent report on 112 RPD, including the initial learning curve, we reported no grade C POPF in the last 72 consecutive patients and an overall 90-day mortality rate of 3.6% [12]. Additionally, we showed a strikingly low conversion rate of 2.7% (3/112). Conversion was never required because of technical problems in completing the procedure but for factors unrelated to robotic assistance (pneumoperitoneum intolerance in two patients, and vascular injury following port insertion).

A recent systematic review and meta-analysis by Peng et al. [20] analyzed a total of nine non-randomized observational clinical studies involving 680 patients: 245 RPD and 435 open PD. There were no randomized controlled trials. When these studies were assessed using the Newcastle–Ottawa Scale one study received a score of 6, five studies received a score of 7, two received a score of 8, and one received a score of 9. RPD versus open PD was associated with higher margin negativity (OR, 0.40; 95% CI, 0.20–0.77; $P = 0.006$), lower overall complication rate (OR, 0.65; 95% CI 0.47–0.91; $P = 0.012$), fewer wound infections (OR, 0.18; 95% CI, 0.06–0.53; $P = 0.002$), shorter length of hospital stay (WMD, –6.00; 95% CI, –9.80 to –2.21; $P = 0.002$). There was no significant difference in number of harvested lymph nodes, operative time, reoperation rate, incidence of delayed gastric emptying, bile leakage, pancreatic fistula and clinically significant pancreatic fistula, as well as in mortality [20].

26.6 Conclusions

MIPD is here to stay. The results achieved at several institutions worldwide show that patients can benefit from this innovative approach. Although the value of RPD versus laparoscopic PD was not addressed in this chapter, there is currently no sound evidence that robotic assistance is superior to conventional laparoscopy in MIPD. At this stage, this comparison could be biased by the fact that both procedures still need to be refined and that large series were collected by champions of robotics and laparoscopy. The results of these pioneers do not necessarily reflect the value of the respective procedures in daily practice. With a greater diffusion of MIPD a difference between RPD and laparoscopic PD could become evident as robotic surgery is known to enhance surgical dexterity and there is no logical reason why laparoscopy should be superior to robotics in the setting of PD. Indeed, while both procedures are laparoscopic operations that share all the benefits of the minimally invasive approach, the advantages associated with the use of a robot at the time of suturing are expected to become evident when MIPD starts to be performed by less gifted laparoscopic surgeons and/or by surgeons with less extensive experience with advanced laparoscopic procedures.

References

1. Aranha GV, Hodul PJ, Creech S, Jacobs W (2003) Zero mortality after 152 consecutive pancreaticoduodenectomies with pancreaticogastrostomy. J Am Coll Surg 197(2):223–231
2. Ho V, Heslin MJ (2003) Effect of hospital volume and experience on in-hospital mortality for pancreaticoduodenectomy. Ann Surg 237(4):509–514
3. van Heek NT, Kuhlmann KF, Scholten RJ et al (2005) Hospital volume and mortality after pancreatic resection: a systematic review and an evaluation of intervention in the Netherlands. Ann Surg 242(6):781–788
4. Schwarz L, Bruno M, Parker NH et al (2015) Active surveillance for adverse events within 90 days: the standard for reporting surgical outcomes after pancreatectomy. Ann Surg Oncol 22(11):3522–3529

5. Shrikhande SV, Sivasanker M, Vollmer CM et al; International Study Group of Pancreatic Surgery (ISGPS) (2017) Pancreatic anastomosis after pancreatoduodenectomy: a position statement by the International Study Group of Pancreatic Surgery (ISGPS). Surgery 161(5):1221–1234
6. Vollmer CM Jr, Sanchez N, Gondek S et al (2012) A root-cause analysis of mortality following major pancreatectomy. J Gastrointest Surg 16(1):89–102
7. Boggi U, Amorese G, Vistoli F et al (2015) Laparoscopic pancreaticoduodenectomy: a systematic literature review. Surg Endosc 29(1):9–23
8. van Hilst J, de Rooij T, Abu Hilal M et al (2017) Worldwide survey on opinions and use of minimally invasive pancreatic resection. HPB (Oxford) 19(3):190–204
9. Boggi U, Signori S, De Lio N et al (2013) Feasibility of robotic pancreaticoduodenectomy. Br J Surg 100(7):917–925
10. Stark M, Pomati S, D'Ambrosio A et al (2015) A new telesurgical platform – preliminary clinical results. Minim Invasive Ther Allied Technol 24(1):31–36
11. Giulianotti PC, Coratti A, Angelini M et al (2003) Robotics in general surgery: personal experience in a large community hospital. Arch Surg 138(7):777–784
12. Napoli N, Kauffmann EF, Menonna F et al (2016) Indications, technique, and results of robotic pancreatoduodenectomy. Updates Surg 68(3):295–305
13. Kauffmann EF, Napoli N, Menonna F et al (2016) Robotic pancreatoduodenectomy with vascular resection. Langenbecks Arch Surg 401(8):1111–1122
14. Fujii T, Sugimoto H, Yamada S et al (2014) Modified Blumgart anastomosis for pancreaticojejunostomy: technical improvement in matched historical control study. J Gastrointest Surg 18(6):1108–1115
15. Napoli N, Kauffmann EF, Palmeri M et al (2016) The learning curve in robotic pancreaticoduodenectomy. Dig Surg 33(4):299–307
16. Boone BA, Zenati M, Hogg ME et al (2015) Assessment of quality outcomes for robotic pancreaticoduodenectomy: identification of the learning curve. JAMA Surg 150(5):416–422
17. Fisher WE, Hodges SE, Wu MF et al (2012) Assessment of the learning curve for pancreaticoduodenectomy. Am J Surg 203(6):684–690
18. Speicher PJ, Nussbaum DP, White RR et al (2014) Defining the learning curve for team-based laparoscopic pancreaticoduodenectomy. Ann Surg Oncol 21(12):4014–4019
19. Hogg ME, Besselink MG, Clavien PA et al; Minimally Invasive Pancreatic Resection Organizing Committee (2017) Training in minimally invasive pancreatic resections: a paradigm shift away from "See one, do one, teach one". HPB (Oxford) 19(3):234–245
20. Peng L, Lin S, Li Y, Xiao W (2016) Systematic review and meta-analysis of robotic versus open pancreaticoduodenectomy. Surg Endosc [Epub ahead of print] doi:10.1007/s00464-016-5371-2

Robotic Pancreatoduodenectomy for Pancreatic Cancer with Superior Mesenteric/ Portal Vein Resection and Reconstruction

27

Ugo Boggi, Carlo Lombardo, and Niccolò Napoli

27.1 Introduction

Most patients with seemingly localized pancreatic cancer will eventually die because of growth of metastasis missed during the initial diagnostic work-up [1]. However, radical surgery – the surgeon's contribution to cure [2] – remains the only possibility to consistently prolong survival [3] and improve quality of life as compared to overtly palliative procedures [4]. For cancer of the head of the pancreas radical surgery means a margin-negative resection [5], an adequate number of examined lymph nodes [6], and *en bloc* clearance of the extrapancreatic nerve plexus (often referred to as "mesopancreas") [7, 8] (Fig. 27.1). These principles were established after decades of studies and constitute the oncologic benchmark against which any new surgical procedure must be confronted. Other major factors known to affect the oncologic outcome of pancreatoduodenectomy (PD) are low surgical morbidity [9], avoidance of blood transfusions [10], and the ability of patients to receive medical treatments and to tolerate their full course [9].

Robotic PD (RPD) is gaining momentum, as several pioneer surgeons have shown that it is feasible with a safety profile similar to the "gold standard" open PD [11–14]. A recent meta-analysis shows that RPD is associated with distinct advantages when compared to open PD [15].

Considering that up to 30% with otherwise resectable pancreatic cancers show signs of suspected involvement of the large peripancreatic vessels [16], the value of RPD needs also to be assessed in the setting of resection and reconstruction of the superior mesenteric/portal vein (SM/PV). After

U. Boggi (✉)
Division of General and Transplant Surgery, University of Pisa
Pisa, Italy
e-mail: u.boggi@med.unipi.it

U. Boggi (Ed), *Minimally Invasive Surgery of the Pancreas*,
Updates in Surgery
DOI: 10.1007/978-88-470-3958-2_27, © Springer-Verlag Italia 2018

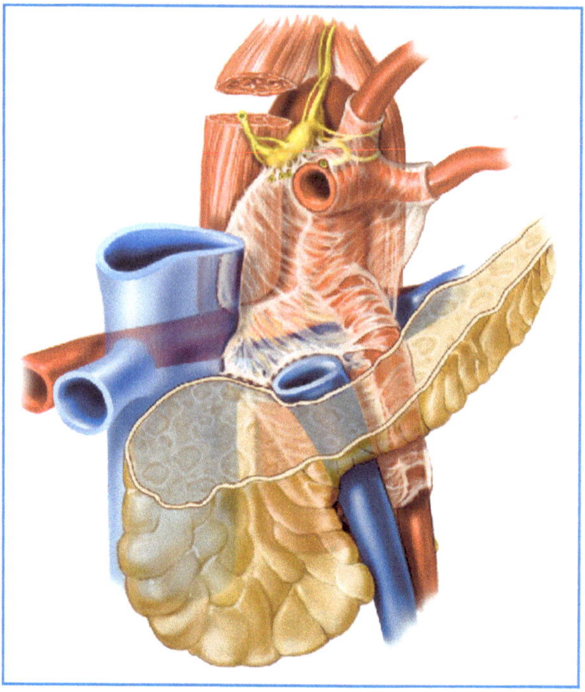

Fig. 27.1 The mesopancreas is the anatomical area, largely corresponding to the extrapancreatic nerve plexus, that extends posterior and medial to the head/uncinate process of the pancreas. Being mostly made up of lymphatic channels and nerve plexuses, and containing also lymph nodes, the mesopancreas has to be resected *en bloc* with the head of the pancreas because of the high frequency of neural and lymphatic spread of pancreatic cancer. Despite lacking well-defined anatomic boundaries the mesopancreas is limited medially by the right margin of the superior mesenteric artery, laterally by the medial/posterior aspect of the head of the pancreas and uncinate process, inferiorly by the left renal vein, and posteriorly by the space between the left margin of the inferior vena cava and the right diaphragmatic crus. Overall, the mesopancreas has the shape of a prism ending at the right celiac ganglion

a long debate, current guidelines indicate that vein involvement is not a contraindication to surgery [17, 18].

We have recently shown the feasibility of RPD with SM/PV resection and reconstruction and have provided a literature review on this issue [19]. In this chapter we present our technique and a summary of available results.

27.2 Indications to RPD with SM/PV Resection and Reconstruction

We have progressively expanded our indications for RPD (see Chapter 26), but overt vein involvement remains a contraindication in our hands. RPD could indeed be feasible in most of these patients but we still prefer to manage complex vascular scenarios through an open approach, because of anticipated longer operative times and associated technical challenges [19].

On the contrary, when tumor adhesion to the SM/PV is incidentally discovered during surgery or when there is limited contact between the tumor and the vein at preoperative work-up (≤180° in circumference and ≤2 cm in length) we keep pursuing RPD. Assessment of feasibility of SM/PV resection and reconstruction accept no compromise with respect to the golden principles established in open PD since the aim of the procedure is to avoid a positive tumor margin at the level of the vein groove [20]. Turrini et al. showed that survival is improved in patients with negative vein histology as compared to matched patients undergoing no vein resection with a positive vascular margin [21]. To achieve a true R0 resection it is key to use an artery-first approach and to proceed with *en bloc* resection of the vein. Indeed, if the tumor has been breached, a more extended resection is unlikely to improve survival. Respecting these principles requires segmental vein resection in most, if not in all, patients since side wall resections, with either immediate venorrhaphy or patch interposition, necessarily brings dissection closer to tumor margins [19, 20].

Even respecting these rather restrictive selection criteria, RPD with *en bloc* resection and reconstruction of SM/PV remains a formidable operation that neither accepts improvisation nor is a venue to nourish surgical ego. We have decided to accept this challenge very prudently and after an experience with over 400 open PD with *en bloc* resection and reconstruction of the SM/PV. We also had experience with vascular procedures, including reconstruction of the portal vein, in thousands of solid organ transplants.

27.3 Surgical Technique

The technique for RPD was presented in Chapter 26. Here we present only the details of the additional surgical maneuvers that are required for SM/PV resection and reconstruction.

It is key to have high-quality contrast-enhanced computer tomography not only to stage the tumor, but also to define individual vascular anatomy. Information on arterial anatomy is used to reduce the possibility of iatrogenic vascular injury, especially in cases of variation in arterial liver supply, as well as to plan for the most convenient route for the artery-first approach to the superior mesenteric artery (SMA) [22].

As in open PD, an artery-first approach to the SMA is employed in every patient [20]. An uncinate-first approach, followed by a bottom-up dissection, is also employed [13, 14].

Depending on tumor location and size, the SMA can be approached through different routes [22]. An anterior approach, often combined with a medial

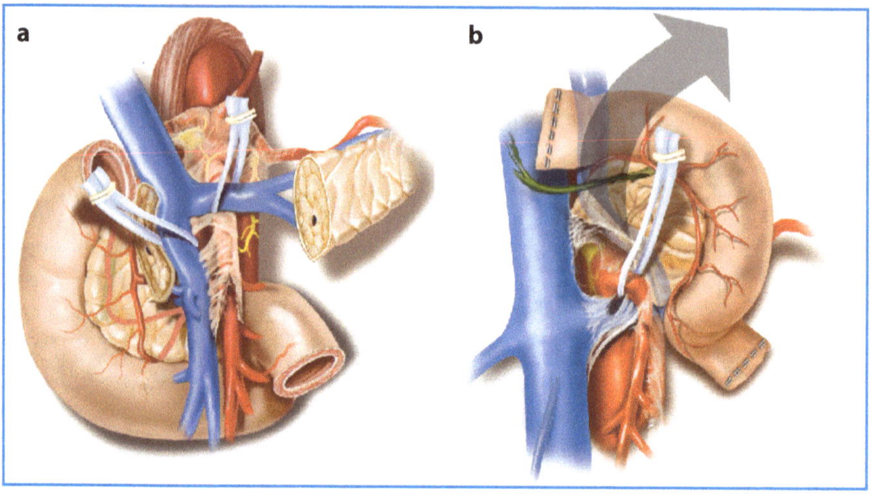

Fig. 27.2 Artery-first approach to the superior mesenteric artery. **a** Anterior approach. **b** Posterior approach

approach to the uncinate process, is feasible in most of the patients. After division of the pancreatic neck, the splenic vein is encircled with a vessel loop and elevated. Because of the endoscopic view and the need for limited working space, division of the splenic vein is not required to improve accessibility to the SMA. Starting from the level of the inferior margin of the uncinate process, dissection is carried out proximally, until the origin of the SMA from the aorta is reached, leaving the specimen attached only to the involved venous segment (Fig. 27.2a). The pancreaticoduodenal arteries are identified and individually ligated or clipped.

When required, a posterior approach to the SMA can also be used [19] (Fig. 27.2b). When the tumor originates from the dorsal portion of the head or from the neck of the pancreas, a superior approach may also be used to address the issue of resectability before proceeding with irreversible maneuvers.

Lymph node stations that are removed are shown in Fig. 27.3. Nodes are removed as much as possible *en bloc* with the specimen.

Once the specimen is completely freed from all its attachments but the involved vein segment, the vessels are cross-clamped using laparoscopy bulldog clamps operated by the surgeon at the table. As in open PD [20], the SMA is clamped first to reduce intestinal congestion during vein occlusion. The SMV is clamped next. If possible, based on the site planned for vascular resection, the splenoportal junction is not immediately occluded in order to maintain some portal blood flow during construction of the proximal anastomosis. Indeed, in most RPD, a jump graft is required because the Trendelenburg position makes a direct anastomosis unfeasible. Autologous vein grafts can be obtained from several sites. Our preference goes to one of the internal jugular veins. We do not use vascular prostheses [23], because of concerns about infection in the

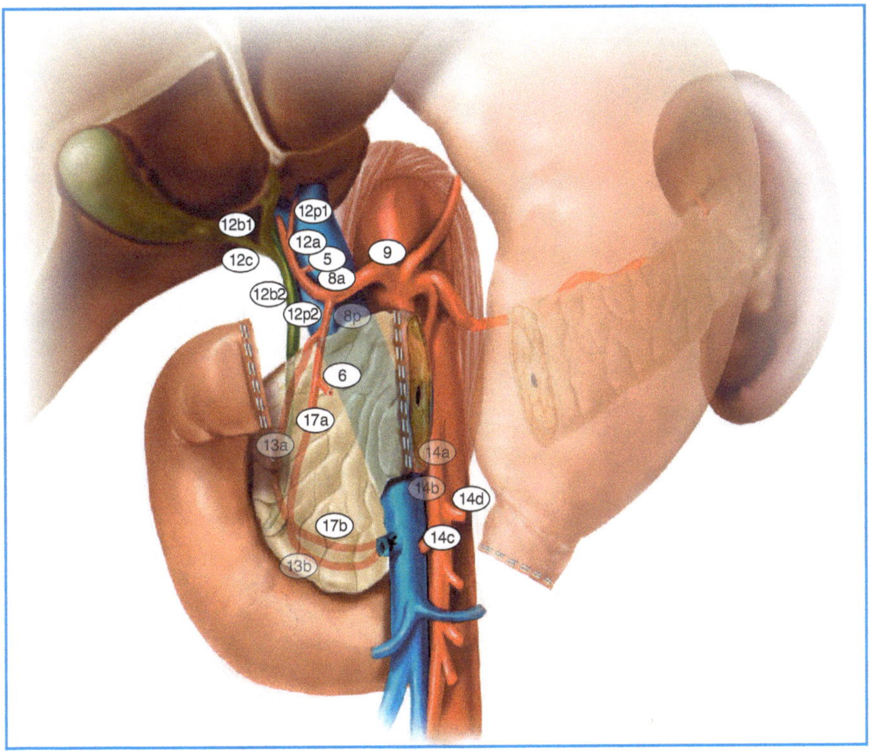

Fig. 27.3 Lymph node stations removed during robotic pancreatoduodenectomy with resection and reconstruction of the superior mesenteric/portal vein

setting of gastrointestinal surgery. We have also never used a patch of parietal peritoneum [24], but we are aware of this technique that could be employed when no vascular segment is available or suitable. The use of cold-stored vein allografts from deceased organ donors is an additional option [25].

Before completing the division of the SM/PV a tag suture is placed for proper vascular alignment. A tag suture is also placed on the jump graft to ensure correct orientation of the flow. Vascular anastomoses are carried out using two half-running sutures of 6/0 expanded polytetrafluoroethylene (ePTFE) of approximately 12 cm in length, using two black diamond microforceps.

The posterior row of the anastomosis is sutured from within the lumen. If necessary to improve exposure, stay sutures can be placed on the anterior walls of the veins and held using the fourth robotic arm.

When the portomesenteric junction is included in the resected segment, the splenic vein is always reimplanted after completion of the cranial anastomosis to the PV. When closing the sutures, attention is paid to avoid the purse string effect by leaving a small growth factor. Before the last suture is tied, the SM/PV is flushed with heparinized saline solution using a Bracci's catheter. The clamp placed cranially on the PV is released first so that the integrity of the vascular anastomoses

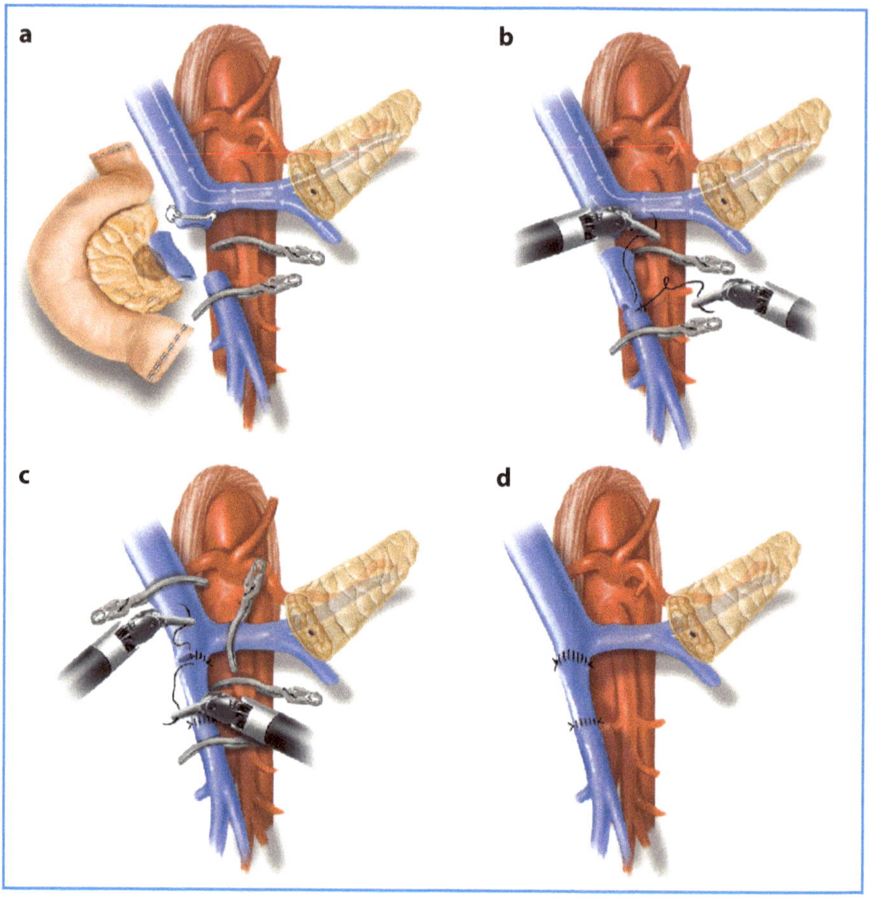

Fig. 27.4 Segmental superior mesenteric/portal vein resection and reconstruction using an interposition graft. **a** When vein resection involves the proximal part of the superior mesenteric vein, so that a short segment of the vein is available for cross-clamping before the splenoportal junction, portal flow to the liver can be maintained through the splenic vein (*arrows*) during construction of the proximal anastomosis. A bulldog clamp is placed also on the superior mesenteric artery to reduce intestinal congestion. **b** The resected vein segment is reconstructed using an interposition graft. **c** Construction of the distal anastomosis. **d** Reconstruction completed

is checked at a lower pressure. Bleeding sites are addressed, as required, and all clamps are eventually released. In patients requiring resection of shorter vein segments, a direct end-to-end anastomosis can be performed (Fig. 27.4).

27.4 Results

Resection and reconstruction of the SM/PV during PD is feasible using minimally invasive techniques, including laparoscopy [19, 26–29]. Although in published series selection criteria for vein resection are not always presented clearly, it is unlikely that all degrees of vascular involvement can be safely managed using minimally invasive techniques. On the other hand, it would not be wise to accept compromises on surgical technique or patient safety to pursue minimally invasive resection at all costs. As specifically regards RPD with SM/PV resection and reconstruction, there are a total of 22 cases reported in the literature, including 14 procedures described by our group [19].

27.4.1 Personal Experience

According to our last report, RPD with resection and reconstruction of the SM/PV was performed in 14 out of 130 patients (10.7%) undergoing RPD (either partial, n = 112, or total n = 18) [19]. There were no conversions to open surgery in patients requiring associated vascular procedures.

According to the International Study Group of Pancreatic Surgery (ISGPS) classification there were no type 1 resections (partial venous excision with direct venorrhaphy), one (7.1%) type 2 resection (partial venous excision using a patch), five (35.7%) type 3 resections (segmental resection with primary venovenous anastomosis), and eight (57.2%) type 4 resections (segmental resection with interposed venous conduit) [17]. No patient had clinical evidence of vein thrombosis, and long-term vein patency was demonstrated in 91.6% of the patients. RPD with SM/PV resection and reconstruction, when compared to standard RPD, was associated with longer mean operative time, higher median estimated blood loss, more frequent need for intraoperative blood transfusions. Postoperative complications, however, did not occur more frequently.

Regarding pathology parameters in patients diagnosed with pancreatic cancer, there was an equivalent mean number of examined lymph nodes (57.2±14.6 vs. 44.6±11) and a similar rate of margin positivity (16.7% vs. 26.1%). The mean length or the resected vein was 23.1±8.08 mm. Actual tumor infiltration was discovered in 10 patients (71.4%). Tumor involvement was limited to the adventitia in four patients (40.0%), reached the media in two patients (20.0%), and extended into the intima in the remaining two patients (40.0%). Circumferential tumor involvement was <180° in nine patients (90.0%) and ≥180° in one patient (10.0%). Mean length of the involved vein segment was 8.9±2.88 mm [19].

27.4.2 Literature Review

There are only two additional articles reporting on RPD with resection and reconstruction of the SM/PV.

Giulianotti et al. reported three cases of PV resection, including two RPD and one distal pancreatectomy. Of the two RPD, one patient received a stapled vein resection (type 1) and the other a partial venous excision with PTFE patch closure (type 2). The postoperative course was described as favorable in both patients, who were stage T2N1b and T3N0, respectively. Both resections were margin-negative [26].

Chen et al. reported five cases in the setting of a prospective matched comparison with open PD. The prevalence of vein resection was reported to be similar between RPD (5%) and open PD (6.7%) as was the mean length of the resected vein segment (3.8±0.8 cm vs. 3.9±1.0 cm). No specific details were provided on the type of vein resection [27].

27.5 Conclusions

RPD with resection and reconstruction of the SM/PV is feasible in selected patients and in the hands of trained and proficient robotic surgeons assisted by skilled laparoscopic tableside surgeons. Experience with vein resection and reconstruction in open PD and compliance with established oncologic principles are both mandatory. A low threshold for conversion to open surgery is also recommended.

The initial results of RPD with resection and reconstruction of the SM/PV are encouraging both in terms of safety and oncologic appropriateness, but further data are needed before final conclusions can be drawn.

References

1. Amikura K, Kobari M, Matsuno S (1995) The time of occurrence of liver metastasis in carcinoma of the pancreas. Int J Pancreatol 17(2):139–146
2. Imamura M, Doi R, Imaizumi T et al (2004) A randomized multicenter trial comparing resection and radiochemotherapy for resectable locally invasive pancreatic cancer. Surgery 136(5):1003–1011
3. Hartwig W, Hackert T, Hinz U et al (2011) Pancreatic cancer surgery in the new millennium: better prediction of outcome. Ann Surg 254(2):311–319
4. Nordby T, Ikdahl T, Bowitz Lothe IM et al (2013) Improved survival and quality of life in patients undergoing R1 pancreatic resection compared to patients with locally advanced unresectable pancreatic adenocarcinoma. Pancreatology 13(2):180–185
5. Howard TJ, Krug JE, Yu J et al (2006) A margin-negative R0 resection accomplished with minimal postoperative complications is the surgeon's contribution to long-term survival in pancreatic cancer. J Gastrointest Surg 10(10):1338–1345
6. Eskander MF, de Geus SW, Kasumova GG et al (2017) Evolution and impact of lymph node dissection during pancreaticoduodenectomy for pancreatic cancer. Surgery 161(4):968–976
7. Jin G, Sugiyama M, Tuo H et al (2006) Distribution of lymphatic vessels in the neural plexuses surrounding the superior mesenteric artery. Pancreas 32(1):62–66
8. Chowdappa R, Challa VR (2015) Mesopancreas in pancreatic cancer: where do we stand – review of literature. Indian J Surg Oncol 6(1):69-74

9. Kang CM, Kim DH, Choi GH et al (2009) Detrimental effect of postoperative complications on oncologic efficacy of R0 pancreatectomy in ductal adenocarcinoma of the pancreas. J Gastrointest Surg 13(5):907–914
10. Mavros MN, Xu L, Maqsood H et al (2015) Perioperative blood transfusion and the prognosis of pancreatic cancer surgery: systematic review and meta-analysis. Ann Surg Oncol 22(13):4382–4391
11. Giulianotti PC, Sbrana F, Bianco FM et al (2010) Robot-assisted laparoscopic pancreatic surgery: single-surgeon experience. Surg Endosc 24(7):1646–1657
12. Zureikat AH, Moser AJ, Boone BA et al (2013) 250 robotic pancreatic resections: safety and feasibility. Ann Surg 258(4):554–559
13. Boggi U, Signori S, De Lio N et al (2013) Feasibility of robotic pancreaticoduodenectomy. Br J Surg 100(7):917–925
14. Napoli N, Kauffmann EF, Menonna F et al (2016) Indications, technique, and results of robotic pancreatoduodenectomy. Updates Surg 68(3):295–305
15. Peng L, Lin S, Li Y, Xiao W (2016) Systematic review and meta-analysis of robotic versus open pancreaticoduodenectomy. Surg Endosc [Epub ahead of print] doi:10.1007/s00464-016-5371-2
16. Hidalgo M (2010) Pancreatic cancer. New Engl J Med 362(17):1605–1617
17. Bockhorn M, Uzunoglu FG, Adham M et al; International Study Group of Pancreatic Surgery (2014) Borderline resectable pancreatic cancer: a consensus statement by the International Study Group of Pancreatic Surgery (ISGPS). Surgery 155(6):977–988
18. Tempero MA, Malafa MP, Behrman SW et al (2014) Pancreatic adenocarcinoma, version 2.2014: featured updates to the NCCN guidelines. J Natl Compr Canc Netw 12(8):1083–1093
19. Kauffmann EF, Napoli N, Menonna F et al (2016) Robotic pancreatoduodenectomy with vascular resection. Langenbecks Arch Surg 401(8):1111–1122
20. Boggi U, Del Chiaro M, Croce C et al (2009) Prognostic implications of tumor invasion or adhesion to peripancreatic vessels in resected pancreatic cancer. Surgery 146(5):869–881
21. Turrini O, Ewald J, Barbier L et al (2013) Should the portal vein be routinely resected during pancreaticoduodenectomy for adenocarcinoma? Ann Surg 257(4):726–730
22. Sanjay P, Takaori K, Govil S et al (2012) 'Artery-first' approaches to pancreatoduodenectomy. Br J Surg 99(8):1027–1035
23. Liao K, Wang H, Chen Q et al (2014) Prosthetic graft for superior mesenteric-portal vein reconstruction in pancreaticoduodenectomy: a retrospective, multicenter study. J Gastrointest Surg 18(8):1452–1461
24. Dokmak S, Chérif R, Duquesne I et al (2016) Laparoscopic pancreaticoduodenectomy with reconstruction of the portal vein with the parietal peritoneum. Ann Surg Oncol 23(8):2664
25. Meniconi RL, Santoro R, Guglielmo N et al (2016) Pancreaticoduodenectomy with venous reconstruction using cold-stored vein allografts: long-term results of a single center experience. J Hepatobiliary Pancreat Sci 23(1):43–49
26. Giulianotti PC, Addeo P, Buchs NC et al (2011) Robotic extended pancreatectomy with vascular resection for locally advanced pancreatic tumors. Pancreas 40(8):1264–1270
27. Chen S, Chen JZ, Zhan Q et al (2015) Robot-assisted laparoscopic versus open pancreaticoduodenectomy: a prospective, matched, mid-term follow-up study. Surg Endosc 29(12):3698–3711
28. Croome KP, Farnell MB, Que FG et al (2014) Total laparoscopic pancreaticoduodenectomy for pancreatic ductal adenocarcinoma: oncologic advantages over open approaches? Ann Surg 260(4):633–638
29. Khatkov IE, Izrailov RE, Khisamov AA et al (2017) Superior mesenteric-portal vein resection during laparoscopic pancreatoduodenectomy. Surg Endosc 31(3):14

28 Minimally Invasive Total Pancreatectomy

Andrea Coratti and Mario Annecchiarico

28.1 Introduction

Pancreatic resection is one of the most complex and challenging abdominal procedures. In highly experienced centers, traditional open pancreatic surgery has a morbidity rate of about 30–40% and a mortality rate of approximately 2% [1, 2]. Therefore, in recent years some experienced centers have gradually introduced laparoscopic techniques in pancreatic surgery as an alternative to open traditional procedures, with the aim of reducing postoperative morbidity [3]. The potential benefits associated with the minimally invasive approach are multiple: laparoscopy can decrease pain and blood loss, resulting in fewer complications, faster recovery and shorter hospital length of stay [4, 5]. Early experiences have shown that laparoscopic pancreatic surgery is safe and feasible in selected patients, with a morbidity rate of 16% to 40% [6–10].

However, despite the many published studies, the laparoscopic approach to pancreatic resections has never gained wide acceptance and diffusion, especially as regards complex operations such as pancreatoduodenectomy (PD) or total pancreatectomy (TP). This is probably explained by the well-known limitations of conventional laparoscopic techniques, such as the restricted range of motion of the surgical instruments and the two-dimensional vision of the operative field, which make complex procedures difficult to perform with the laparoscopic approach.

The use of a robotic platform may overcome some of the difficulties experienced with standard laparoscopy in this kind of resection. Robot-assisted surgery provides a stable platform with high-definition and three-dimensional vision, magnified view of the operative field, and integration with other techniques of imaging. These advantages, combined with the increased freedom of movement of the surgical instruments and suppression of tremor, may lead to

A. Coratti (✉)
Division of Oncological and Robotic General Surgery, Careggi University Hospital
Florence, Italy
e-mail: corattian@gmail.com

U. Boggi (Ed), *Minimally Invasive Surgery of the Pancreas*,
Updates in Surgery
DOI: 10.1007/978-88-470-3958-2_28,

improved precision, accuracy and safety in performing some surgical procedures involved in pancreatic resections such as complex anastomoses or dissection. Moreover, the better ergonomics afforded to the surgeon by the robotic platform may reduce tiredness due to the position during the operation.

The first patient to undergo robot-assisted pancreatic surgery was reported in 2003 [11]. Since then, a small number of centers have adopted this technique and several small series have reported encouraging outcomes.

28.2 Procedure Overview

Our experience with robotic pancreatic surgery started about 10 years ago. The indications for robotic TP are limited in comparison with other kinds of pancreatic resection: the more common ones include extension of PD or distal pancreatectomy (DP) in cases of persistent positive margins in the pancreatic stump, multifocal tumors, intraductal pancreatic mucinous neoplasia (IPMN) involving the whole gland, chronic pancreatitis unresponsive to conservative treatment or unmanageable by other surgical approach.

The surgical technique involves two main steps developing around the division of the pancreatic neck: the first step is a PD, followed by a DP with or without splenectomy. In our experience, this two-step approach appeared easier and preferable to an *en bloc* TP because management of the entire pancreas during minimally invasive surgery may be very difficult.

28.3 Patient Position, Robotic Docking, and Port Placement

The patient is placed in a supine position with the legs spread apart. After placement of the ports, the patient is moved to a 10–15° reverse Trendelenburg position. A nasogastric tube is inserted to allow gastric decompression.

Using a da Vinci Si System (Intuitive Surgical Inc., Sunnyvale, CA, USA), the robotic cart is docked at the patient's head, making sure that the main axis of the cart coincides with the main working axis, coming from the opposite side. With the new Xi system, the robotic cart may be docked on the left or right side of the patient, and the final arrangement of the arms is obtained with a specific targeting procedure. Correct positioning of the robotic cart is fundamental because it cannot be changed after docking.

The camera port (8 mm or 12 mm on the Xi and Si systems, respectively) is placed approximately 2–3 cm to the right of the umbilicus: this position allows a perfect view of the hepatic hilum, portal vein and uncinate process, which represent the most important anatomical targets of TP. Three other 8-mm robotic ports and two assistant ports are placed as shown in Fig. 28.1. Independently of

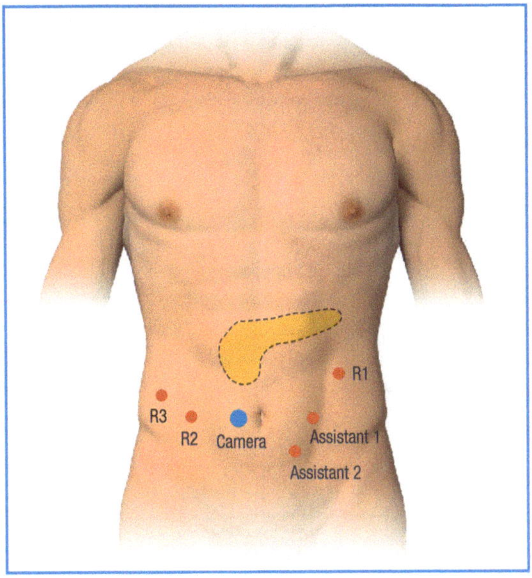

Fig. 28.1 Positioning of trocars and set-up

the robotic system, we use the fourth robotic arm in the right side of the abdomen as, in our experience, this position was preferable to the left side one.

28.4 Two-Step Robotic Technique

In our standard practice the robotic tools used for pancreatic surgery are monopolar scissors, bipolar Maryland forceps, a fenestrated grasper as a retractor, and harmonic shears.

28.4.1 First Step

The first step is PD. Surgery starts with sectioning of the gastrocolic ligament and opening the lesser sac: complete exposure and exploration of the pancreas is obtained, using also robotic intraoperative ultrasound, if necessary. The inferior pancreatic edge is mobilized and the superior mesenteric vein (SMV) is exposed below the glandular neck. Pancreatic mobilization proceeds on the right side: an extended take-down of the right colonic flexure and a Kocher maneuver (up to the left border of the aorta) are performed to expose the posterior surface of the pancreatic head and the uncinate process. The right colon mesentery is mobilized up to the origin of the right gastroepiploic vein, which is transected separately or together with Henle's venous trunk. In some cases, such as obese or overweight patients, it may be difficult to

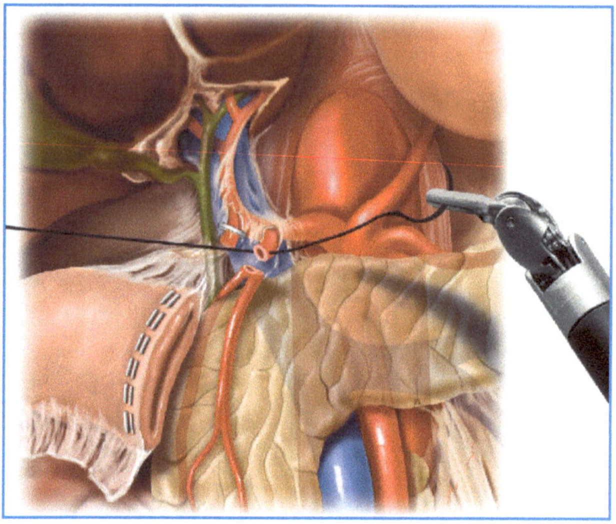

Fig. 28.2 Gastroduodenal artery ligation

complete Kocher maneuver during this step: a possible tip is to defer its completion until after transection of the bile duct, when duodenal mobility is greater and it is possible to have a better view behind the uncinate process.

The duodenum is prepared by opening the hepatoduodenal ligament and coagulating minor periduodenal vessels with the bipolar forceps. Duodenal transection is performed 2 cm from the pylorus using a standard laparoscopic stapler (only in selected cases do we sacrifice the pylorus by performing a distal gastric resection): transection of the duodenum opens a wide view on the hepatic hilum, hepatic artery, and splenic artery origin. At this point, the superior border of the pancreas, the common hepatic artery (CHA), and the splenic artery (SA) are exposed and, if necessary, the regional lymph nodes are harvested. However, we suggest achieving complete control of the CHA and SA in every case.

The right gastric artery is divided between metallic clips. The gastroduodenal artery (GDA) is cleared from the surrounding tissues and then transected, and the proximal stump is closed by a polypropylene suture and plastic clip (Fig. 28.2). The hepatic hilum is dissected, exposing the proper hepatic artery and its branches, the portal vein (PV) and the common bile duct (CBD): it is important to identify any aberrant anatomy, especially of the hepatic artery and biliary tree. A standard lymph node dissection is performed when necessary (Fig. 28.3). The gallbladder is removed separately, and the CBD is interrupted above the cystic duct. If necessary, the proximal margin of the CBD is sent to pathology for frozen-section; the distal stump is closed by suture.

When dissection of the hepatic hilum is completed, the tunnel between the pancreatic neck and the SMV-PV is completed taking care to avoid vascular injuries or bleeding from small venous branches. If the tunnel preparation proves difficult (e.g., presence of fibrotic adhesions between the pancreas and SMV/PV),

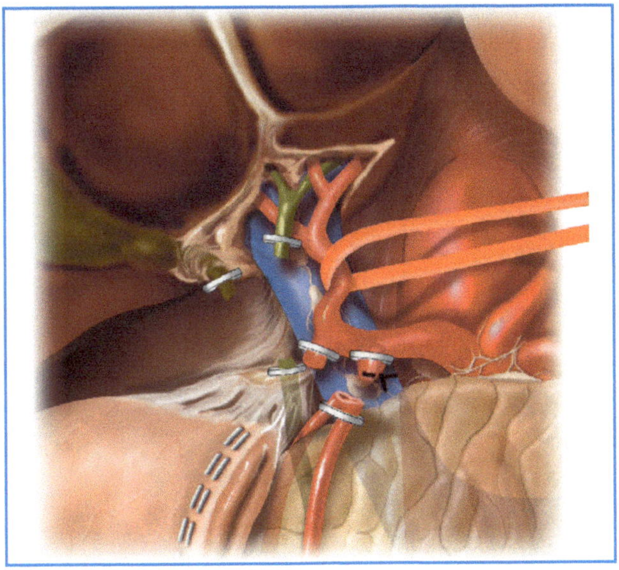

Fig. 28.3 Hepatic hilum dissection

we suggest completing it step-by-step jointly with the pancreatic transection, as an anterior approach: in this way, exposure of the venous mesenteric axis is gradual and safer. Pancreatic transection is performed by stapler or harmonic shears. In the latter case, two polypropylene sutures are placed on the left and right side of the pancreatic neck. Because harmonic shears lack the endowrist articulation, perfect retraction of the pancreatic margins is indispensable in order to achieve the best transection line.

After pancreatic transection, the first jejunal loop is prepared on the left side of the mesentery and divided distally to the Treitz ligament using a stapler. Then, the first jejunal loop is retracted and transposed on to the right side of the mesentery.

Dissection of the uncinate process represents the most difficult phase of right-side pancreatectomy. In our experience, the best exposure of the uncinate process and superior mesenteric artery (SMA) is obtained with two synchronous retractions: the first is carried out by the fourth robotic arm, which grabs the duodenum and pulls it sideways to the right; the second is done by the assistant surgeon, who retracts the SMV previously encircled with a vessel loop (Fig. 28.4). Dissection of the uncinate process is performed in a caudal to cephalic direction: the SMV and PV are progressively detached from the pancreas. Once the SMV-PV is reflected medially to the left, the SMA is identified and exposed posteriorly; in cancer cases, formal lymph node dissection has to be carried out up to its origin. Correct exposure of the SMA is mandatory in all cases before final detachment of the uncinate process, in order to avoid vascular injuries and major bleeding. The dissection proceeds bottom-up, dividing the inferior and superior pancreatoduodenal vessels between polypropylene ligatures or clips; tiny branches are divided

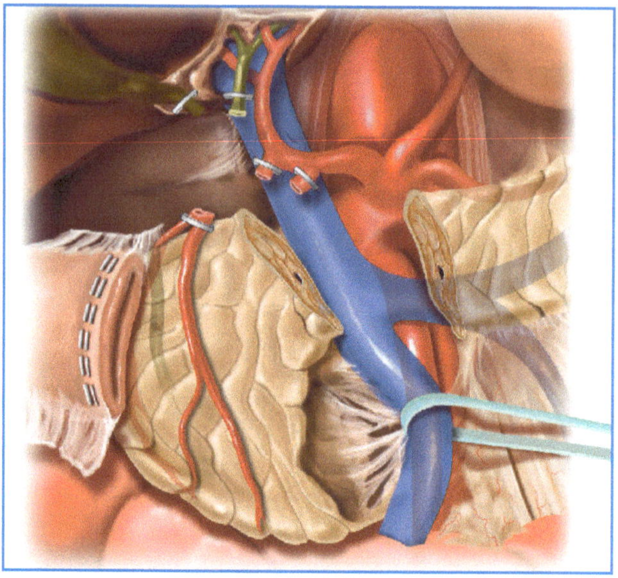

Fig. 28.4 Uncinate process dissection

with the Harmonic device. The aid of robotic technology is particularly evident during this step of the surgery: stability of the robotic platform, enhanced vision, and the Endowrist instruments allow precise dissection with minimal blood loss. Moreover, even in the case of bleeding, suturing can be performed as in open surgery and more easily than in standard laparoscopy.

At this point, the PD is completed and the first specimen is abandoned in the right hypochondrium.

28.4.2 Second Step

The second step of the surgery is DP. The splenic vein and artery are dissected and exposed. In the case of spleen-preserving surgery, the splenic vessels are controlled by vessel loops and dissected up to complete separation from the pancreatic parenchyma. Otherwise, if splenectomy is planned, they are transected by stapler or between plastic clips and/or sutures. Usually the splenic artery is ligated and divided first, followed by the splenic vein; however, this sequence may be inverted depending on the anatomy.

A medial-to-lateral dissection of the distal pancreas is completed, detaching the inferior pancreatic border from the mesentery of the transverse colon. The posterior dissection is carried out along the pancreas and Gerota's fascia: retroperitoneal and renal fatty tissue are removed *en bloc* in the case of neoplastic invasion (Fig. 28.5).

Finally, in the case of splenectomy, the short gastric vessels and lateral ligaments of the spleen are divided and the second specimen is removed *en bloc*.

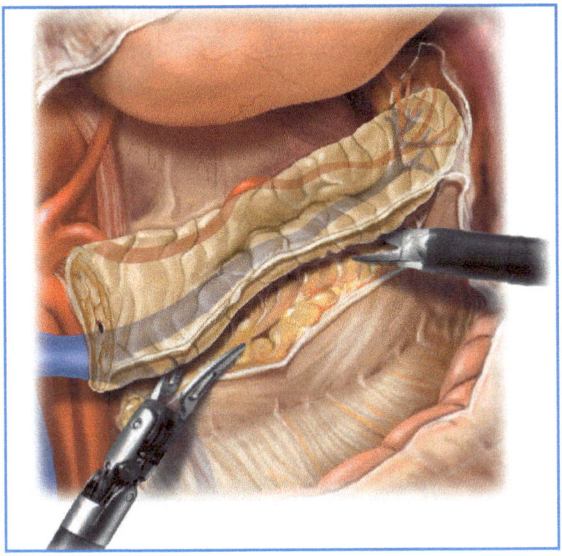

Fig. 28.5 Splenic artery and vein dissection

28.5 Reconstruction

The remnant jejunal stump is brought up to behind the root of the mesentery in a "neo-duodenal" position, and an end-to-side hepaticojejunostomy is performed using 4-0 or 5-0 absorbable sutures (Fig. 28.6). For medium to large ducts we use

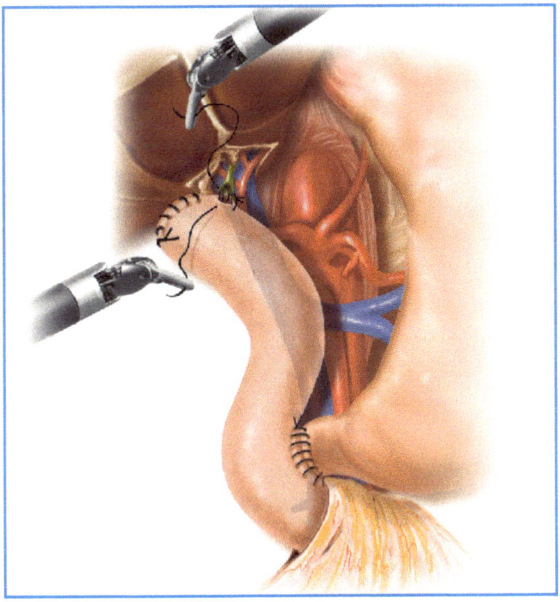

Fig. 28.6 End-to-side hepaticojejunostomy

two running sutures; in small ducts, we prefer interrupted stitches. A Hoffmeister type, hand-sewn, end-to-side duodenojejunostomy is performed using a single-layer 3-0 absorbable suture.

One or two drains are placed. The nasogastric tube is removed at the end of surgery.

28.6 Discussion

The application of minimally invasive techniques in pancreatic surgery has been delayed over the years due to the difficulty in approaching a deep organ positioned in the retroperitoneum and in close relation with major vascular structures. Furthermore, depending on the type of pancreatectomy, a complex reconstruction may be necessary after resection [12].

Only the laparoscopic approach for DP gained widespread popularity, and it is currently recognized as the gold standard of treatment for most diseases involving the distal portion of the gland [13]; however, only a small proportion of pancreatic diseases arise in the tail of the pancreas, and only 20% of adenocarcinomas. Contraindications to this procedure are prohibitive medical comorbidities and poor patient functional status [14]. As stated, the laparoscopic approach results in a shorter hospital stay, reduced blood loss, and fewer complications, with similar oncological outcomes in terms of lymph nodes harvested and R0 resection [15].

Conversely, laparoscopic PD had very limited diffusion because of long operative times, difficulties during reconstruction, and a higher risk of fistula and bleeding [16]. Moreover, open PD has a learning curve of about 60 procedures [17], a minimum of 10 hybrid procedures (laparoscopic resection and open reconstruction) are needed before starting a totally laparoscopic learning curve, and a high number of procedures are required to complete it [16]. These factors have limited the diffusion of laparoscopic PD, which has been applied in only very few high-volume centers and by experienced surgeons [18].

Laparoscopic TP is an infrequent procedure, usually performed in high-volume centers in a percentage between 5.6% and 6.4% [19]. General indications for TP are IPMN involving the whole gland [20, 21], hereditary pancreatic tumors (FAP, BRCA1, FAMM, HNPCC) [21, 22], multifocal pancreatic neuroendocrine tumors (P-NETs), extension of PD or DP in cases of persistent positive margins in the pancreatic stump [23], chronic pancreatitis with pain and unresponsive to other treatments [23–28], extensive adenocarcinoma [29] or extremely soft pancreatic tissue with a high-risk anastomosis [30]. Another indication for TP may be postoperative leakage from a pancreatic anastomosis after PD [31, 32].

Currently only few articles have been published about laparoscopic TP [33–36], and none of them have compared laparoscopic and open TP.

The robot-assisted approach to pancreatic resections has been gradually implemented and developed over the years: it has been supported not only by the scientific demonstration of its equivalent efficacy and safety, but also by the possibility to combine all the advantages of a minimally invasive approach with those of a robotic platform during resection and reconstruction [37]. The technical features of the robotic platform may overcome many of the shortcomings of traditional laparoscopy in difficult surgical steps, such as dissection and suturing, which are much easier to perform with robotics. Even the learning curve of robotic PD is reported to be likely similar to that of open PD [38].

A better view and increased dexterity could also help to reduce trauma to the tissues and to respect the anatomy, consequently decreasing the complication rate and improving the oncological adequacy of minimally invasive surgery. In fact, limited tissue trauma decreases the anti-TNF-mediated inflammatory response hence reducing cancer progression and leading to a shorter recovery after surgery: the consequence may be a greater percentage of patients fit for adjuvant therapy or being enrolled in clinical trials [14].

Robotic DP is demonstrated to be associated with a lower conversion rate (2%) and higher rate of spleen preservation [39] than laparoscopic DP, as a result of better control of vessels and easier management of bleeding [38].

On the contrary, robotic PD has been compared with the open procedure and the results do not demonstrate its superiority in terms of morbidity and fistula rates: furthermore, operative time is much longer with the robotic approach [14]. However, most of the series of robotic PD are probably influenced by two biases: the selection of patients and the learning curve. Usually, robotic PD series include a high percentage of benign or borderline lesions, or periampullary tumors, when it is well known that these cases are easier to resect but also associated with a higher risk of pancreatic fistula. The learning curve is another problem because the comparison between robotic and open PD is often made within surgical teams with extensive experience in open surgery, while robotic surgery has been approached more recently by the same teams [40, 41].

A systematic review and meta-analysis [37] comparing the robotic and open approach for all types of pancreatic resections (PD, DP, TP) showed no statistical differences in terms of postoperative pancreatic fistula, morbidity rate, reoperation rate; however, the trend was in favor of robotic surgery in terms of complication rate, number of positive margins at definitive histology, hospital stay, and blood loss. The mean conversion rate of robotic surgery to laparoscopic or open surgery was 10%, with bleeding, failure to progress, or visceral adhesions as the commonest reasons to convert [42].

Only small studies of robotic TP have been performed since the first experience [43], perhaps because of the relatively rare indication for minimally invasive TP, the long operative time, and the advanced technical skills required for this complex operation.

The possible advantages of robotic TP versus open TP have been described in a recent case-matched study [44]. Eleven patients undergoing robotic TP for benign or malignant disease were compared to 11 patients with similar indications, but without availability of the robotic system at the time of the scheduled surgery. Two vascular resections were performed in each group; no open conversion occurred for robotic TP, which presented longer operative time and lower blood losses than the open group. The length of hospital stay was similar between the two groups, but all the parameters evaluating the recovery were advantageous for robotic TP.

Recently other authors [45] have described their initial experience of 10 robotic TP, reporting long operative time (503 min), one conversion to open surgery (10%), Clavien-Dindo III-IV complications in 20% of cases, and no 90-day mortality. One patient also received pancreatic autologous islet cell transplantation using 225,000 unpurified islet equivalents infused by gravity through a sterile tube and a 14G needle inserted into the splenic vein stump.

Considering that many indications for TP concern benign or borderline diseases, frequently in young patients, robotics may have an important role in extending the minimally invasive approach to this specific operation, with consequent reduction of blood loss, faster postoperative recovery, and preservation of abdominal integrity and cosmesis. Some advantages could be demonstrated with the progressive increase of surgical experience, such as a reduction of operative time after the learning curve and a greater number of spleen-preserving procedures. At this time, the feasibility of robotic autologous islet cell transplantation has been demonstrated, but the efficacy of this procedure is necessary to eliminate postpancreatectomy deficits in endocrine and exocrine secretion and avoid another limiting factor to TP especially in the treatment of benign disease.

More studies will be necessary to compare robotic TP with laparoscopic and open techniques in terms of oncological and functional outcomes, and to define the real role of robotics in this complex surgery.

References

1. Kleeff J, Diener MK, Z'graggen K et al (2007) Distal pancreatectomy: risk factors for surgical failure in 302 consecutive cases. Ann Surg 245(4):573–582
2. Winter JM, Cameron JL, Campbell KA et al (2006) 1423 pancreaticoduodenectomies for pancreatic cancer: a single-institution experience. J Gastrointest Surg 10(9):1199–1210; discussion 1210–1211
3. Gagner M, Pomp A (1994) Laparoscopic pylorus-preserving pancreatoduodenectomy. Surg Endosc 8(5):408–410
4. Schwenk W, Haase O, Neudecker J, Müller JM (2005) Short-term benefits for laparoscopic colorectal resection. Cochrane Database Syst Rev (3):CD003145
5. Keus F, Gooszen HG, van Laarhoven CJ (2010) Open, small-incision, or laparoscopic cholecystectomy for patients with symptomatic cholecystolithiasis. An overview of Cochrane Hepato-Biliary Group reviews. Cochrane Database Syst Rev (1):CD008318
6. Ammori BJ, Ayiomamitis GD (2011) Laparoscopic pancreaticoduodenectomy and distal pancreatectomy: a UK experience and a systematic review of the literature. Surg Endosc 25(7):2084–2099

7. Borja-Cacho D, Al-Refaie WB, Vickers SM et al (2009) Laparoscopic distal pancreatectomy. J Am Coll Surg 209(6):758–765
8. Gagner M, Palermo M (2009) Laparoscopic Whipple procedure: review of the literature. J Hepatobiliary Pancreat Surg 16(6):726–730
9. Gumbs AA, Rodriguez Rivera AM, Milone L, Hoffman JP (2011) Laparoscopic pancreatoduodenectomy: a review of 285 published cases. Ann Surg Oncol 18(5): 1335–1341
10. Kooby DA, Gillespie T, Bentrem D et al (2008) Left-sided pancreatectomy: a multicentre comparison of laparoscopic and open approaches. Ann Surg 248(3):438–446
11. Melvin WS, Needleman BJ, Krause KR, Ellison EC (2003) Robotic resection of pancreatic neuroendocrine tumour. J Laparoendosc Adv Surg Tech A 13(1):33–36
12. Joyce D, Moris-Stiff G, Falk GA et al (2014) Robotic surgery of the pancreas. World J Gastroenterol 20(40):14726–14732
13. Liang S, Hameed U, Jayaraman S (2014) Laparoscopic pancreatectomy: indications and outcomes. World J Gastroenterol 20(39):14246–14254
14. Magge D, Zureikat A, Hogg M, Zeh HJ 3rd (2016) Minimally invasive approaches to pancreatic surgery. Surg Oncol Clin N Am 25(2):273–286
15. Kooby DA, Hawkins WG, Schmidt CM et al (2010) A multicenter analysis of distal pancreatectomy for adenocarcinoma: is laparoscopic resection appropriate? J Am Coll Surg 210(5):779–785
16 de Rooij T, Klompmaker S, Abu Hilal M et al (2016) Laparoscopic pancreatic surgery for benign and malignant disease. Nat Rev Gastroenterol Hepatol 13(4):227–238
17. Tseng JF, Pisters PW, Lee JE et al (2007) The learning curve in pancreatic surgery. Surgery 141(5):694–701
18. Cadière GB, Himpens J, Germay O et al (2001) Feasibility of robotic laparoscopic surgery:146 cases. World J Surg 25(11):1467–1477
19. Janot MS, Belyaev O, Kersting S et al (2010) Indications and early outcomes for total pancreatectomy at a high-volume pancreas center. HPB Surg doi:10.1155/2010/686702
20. Tanaka M, Chari S, Adsay V et al; International Association of Pancreatology (2006) International consensus guidelines for management of intraductal papillary mucinous neoplasms and mucinous cystic neoplasms of the pancreas. Pancreatology 6(1–2):17–32
21. Crippa S, Tamburrino D, Partelli S et al (2011) Total pancreatectomy: indications, different timing, and perioperative and long-term outcomes. Surgery 149(1):79–86
22. Heidt DG, Burant C, Simeone DM (2007) Total pancreatectomy: indications, operative technique, and postoperative sequelae. J Gastrointest Surg 11(2):209–216
23. Braasch JW, Vito L, Nugent FW (1978) Total pancreatectomy for end-stage chronic pancreatitis. Ann Surg 188(3):317–322
24. Warren KW, Poulantzas JK, Kune GA (1966) Life after total pancreatectomy for chronic pancreatitis: clinical study of eight cases. Ann Surg 164(5):830–834
25. Linehan IP, Lambert MA, Brown DC (1988) Total pancreatectomy for chronic pancreatitis. Gut 29(3):358–365
26. Stone WM, Sarr MG, Nagorney DM, McIlrath DC (1988) Chronic pancreatitis. Results of Whipple's resection and total pancreatectomy. Arch Surg 123(7):815–819
27. Easter DW, Cuschieri A (1991) Total pancreatectomy with preservation of the duodenum and pylorus for chronic pancreatitis. Ann Surg 214(5):575–580
28. Fleming WR, Williamson RC (1995) Role of total pancreatectomy in the treatment of patients with end-stage chronic pancreatitis. Br J Surg 82(10):1409–1412
29. Zakaria HM, Stauffer JA, Raimondo M et al (2016) Total pancreatectomy: short- and long-term outcomes at a high-volume pancreas center. World J Gastrointest Surg 8(9):634–642
30. Ross DE (1954) Cancer of the pancreas. A plea for total pancreatectomy. Am J Surg 87(1):20–33
31. Gueroult S, Parc Y, Duron F et al (2004) Completion pancreatectomy for postoperative peritonitis after pancreaticoduodenectomy: early and late outcome. Arch Surg 139(1):16–19

32 de Castro SM, Busch OR, van Gulik TM et al (2005) Incidence and management of pancreatic leakage after pancreatoduodenectomy. Br J Surg 92(9):1117–1123
33. Dallemagne B, de Oliveira AT, Lacerda CF et al (2013) Full laparoscopic total pancreatectomy with and without spleen and pylorus preservation: a feasibility report. J Hepatobiliary Pancreat Sci 20(6):647–653
34. Casadei R, Marchegiani G, Laterza M et al (2009) Total pancreatectomy: doing it with a mini-invasive approach. JOP 10(3):328–331
35. Galvani CA, Rodriguez Rilo H, Samamé J et al (2014) Fully robotic-assisted technique for total pancreatectomy with an autologous islet transplant in chronic pancreatitis patients: results of a first series. J Am Coll Surg 218(3):e73–e78
36. Choi SH, Hwang HK, Kang CM et al (2012) Pylorus- and spleen-preserving total pancreatoduodenectomy with resection of both whole splenic vessels: feasibility and laparoscopic application to intraductal papillary mucin-producing tumors of the pancreas. Surg Endosc 26(7):2072–2077
37. Zhang J, Wu WM, You L, Zhao YP (2013) Robotic versus open pancreatectomy: a systematic review and meta-analysis. Ann Surg Oncol 20(6):1774–1780
38. Boone BA, Zenati M, Hogg ME et al (2015) Assessment of quality of outcomes for robotic pancreaticoduodenectomy: identification of the learning curve. JAMA Surg 150(5):416–422
39. Chong CCN, Lee KF, Fong KA et al (2015) Robot-assisted laparoscopic spleen-preserving distal pancreatectomy. Surg Pract 19(1):40–41
40. Stafford AT, Walsh RM (2015) Robotic surgery of the pancreas: the current state of the art. J Surg Oncol 112(3):289–294
41. Shakir M, Boone BA, Polanco PM et al (2015) The learning curve for robotic distal pancreatectomy: an analysis of outcomes of the first 100 consecutive cases at high volume pancreatic centre. HPB (Oxford) 17(7):580–586
42. Zhou JY, Xin C, Mou YP et al (2016) Robotic versus laparoscopic distal pancreatectomy: a meta-analysis of short-term outcomes. PLoS One 11(3):e0151189
43. Giulianotti PC, Addeo P, Buchs NC et al (2011) Early experience with robotic total pancreatectomy. Pancreas 40(2):311–313
44. Boggi U, Palladino S, Massimetti G et al (2015) Laparoscopic robot-assisted versus open total pancreatectomy: a case-matched study. Surg Endosc 29(6):1425–1432
45. Zureikat AH, Nguyen T, Boone BA et al (2015) Robotic total pancreatectomy with or without autologous islet cell transplantation: replication of an open technique through a minimal access approach. Surg Endosc 29(1):176–183

Robotic Pancreas Transplantation

29

Ugo Boggi, Carlo Lombardo, and Fabio Vistoli

29.1 Introduction

Recent evidence shows that minimally invasive (MI) transplantation of the kidney [1–3] and the pancreas [4–6] is not just feasible but possibly convenient in selected patients [2].

Transplantation of the pancreas (PTx), either alone or in combination with a kidney, is an important therapeutic option in beta-cell-penic diabetic patients who, despite personalized and intensive insulin therapy, develop severe secondary diabetic complications and/or experience poor metabolic control [7]. This group of diabetic patients is particularly vulnerable to surgical complications because of the long-standing history of diabetes and secondary diabetic complications [7]. Sadly enough, PTx is associated with the highest rate of surgical complications among all solid organ transplantations [8]. The history of PTx has indeed been shaped by refinements in surgical techniques [9] but, despite improvements, surgical complications continue to occur frequently. Some of these complications, such as surgical site infection, wound dehiscence, and intestinal complications are among the problems that are expected to be reduced by MI surgery.

Robotic PTx was first performed in Pisa, by our group, on September 27, 2010 [4]. To the best of our knowledge, and according to published literature, our experience was duplicated only at the University of Illinois at Chicago [6].

29.2 Reasons Limiting Earlier Implementation of MI PTx

The reasons for the low use of MI PTx are multifactorial.

First, MI PTx was probably thought to be impossible on account of the complexity of the open procedure.

U. Boggi (✉)
Division of General and Transplant Surgery, University of Pisa
Pisa, Italy
e-mail: u.boggi@med.unipi.it

U. Boggi (Ed), *Minimally Invasive Surgery of the Pancreas*,
Updates in Surgery
DOI: 10.1007/978-88-470-3958-2_29X,

Second, advanced laparoscopic skills are required to complete PTx, but most transplant surgeons have not been trained in MI techniques.

Third, graft cooling is not immediately achieved during MI transplantation.

Fourth, pneumoperitoneum reduces renal perfusion [10]. Experimental evidence shows that also pancreatic perfusion is reduced by increased intra-abdominal pressure [11]. The impact of early impairment of graft microcirculation on the occurrence of vascular complications is not known, but vascular thrombosis is the leading cause of early graft failure in PTx [12].

Fifth, conventional laparoscopy has intrinsic limitations that have made the outcome of advanced laparoscopic surgery highly operator-dependent [13] and have restricted the range of complex operations for which laparoscopy is recommended [14].

29.3 Rationale for MI PTx

The technique for open PTx has several flaws that could be improved by MI surgery.

First, because of the size of the incision, the long history of diabetes, and the need for vigorous immunosuppression, wound complications occur frequently after PTx.

Second, the risk of perigraft fluid collections and intra-abdominal infection increases with the extent of intra-abdominal dissection and intestinal manipulation.

Third, gastroparesis occurs frequently in the PTx recipient as a result of the combination of surgical manipulation and autonomic neuropathy.

Fourth, reduced tissue handling is associated with lower activation of coagulation systems [15].

29.4 Practical Problems of Robotic PTx

From a technical point of view, the most striking difference between conventional and robotic PTx is the difficulty in keeping the graft cooled during construction of the vascular anastomoses. The temperature of renal grafts, for instance, is expected to increase according to a logarithmic curve, at the speed of 0.48° C per minute. Pre-reperfusion temperature depends on anastomotic time and is inversely proportional to graft weight [16]. A pre-revascularization graft temperature ≤15°C is considered protective [17]. Topical graft cooling using ice-slush solutions has been recently proposed for renal grafts during laparoscopic transplantation [18], although some practical problems could arise such as blurred vision and a need for more frequent suction, with the risk of pneumoperitoneum collapse. These additional difficulties could prolong anastomotic time, eventually leading to the same degree of graft rewarming despite topical ice cooling. Cooling kidney jackets have been described only in the experimental setting and for the kidney [19]. On the other hand, it is encouraging that renal transplantation through minimal skin incisions [20, 21], sharing with robotic PTx the issue of graft rewarming, was associated with good graft function.

The other main difference between open and robotic PTx is the need for pneumoperitoneum. Pneumoperitoneum is known to decrease graft perfusion. However, intravascular fluid expansion is known to reverse the effects of pneumoperitonuem on graft perfusion [22].

29.5 Requirements for Performing Robotic PTx

Advanced laparoscopic skills are required to face the challenges of MI PTx, even when using a robotic system.

The greatest challenges of robotic PTx are the necessity to create vascular anastomoses and the ability to deal with bleeding at the time of reperfusion. These skills should not be acquired during human PTx. The surgeon and the entire surgical team must be prepared beforehand. Training in dry and wet [23] labs is recommended. Preparatory human operations could involve procedures such as pyeloplasty and repair of splenic artery aneurysms. In these operations the surgeon is not placed under the pressure of time while refining his/her anastomotic technique.

For robotic PTx a dedicated operating room equipped with multiple high-definition screens is recommended. The operating table must be equipped with a heating blanket. The source of CO_2 should be centralized or two tanks should be placed in parallel and connected through a switching valve, so that CO_2 supply will never be discontinued during tank exchange. Two CO_2 insufflators should also be available to avoid pneumoperitoneum collapse, should intensive suction be required during control of major bleeding. A CO_2 heater must also be available. An alternative to the use of two standard insufflators is the use of a pressure barrier insufflator, such as the AirSeal system (Surgiquest, Milford, CT, USA).

Besides standard laparoscopic equipment, it is important to have a complete set of laparoscopic bulldog clamps as well as Satinsky-like laparoscopic vascular clamps, which require their associated trocars with flexible cannulas to permit introduction of curved jaw designs. Bracci or Fogarty catheters should also be available to flush the vessels.

Vascular anastomoses are performed using expanded polytetrafluoroethylene (ePTFE) (6-0 and 7-0) instead of polypropylene. Current robotic systems lack haptic feedback, so that repetitive needle driver manipulations weaken suture materials reducing maximal failure force of monofilaments by 35% as compared with 3% for braided sutures [24]. ePTFE shows no loss in strength after repetitive robotic manipulations, whereas polypropylene is weakened after three robotic manipulations at the same point [25]. Interrupted polypropylene sutures can be used to secure individual bleeding sites after graft reperfusion.

29.6 Surgical Technique

29.6.1 Donor Procedure

Pancreas grafts are procured from brain-dead multiorgan donors. When PTx is performed using the open technique we prefer to use a quick *en bloc* technique for graft procurement [26]. This technique requires quite complex bench surgery and, although major bleeding is not usually observed, the inability to fix small bleeding sites without an intact circulation is associated with the need to perfect the hemostasis in the recipient after graft reperfusion.

In robotic PTx we have preferred to dissect the pancreas entirely in the donor in order to make transplantation straightforward, optimize coordination between donor and recipient teams, and minimize the period of cold ischemia. Using this technique, at the back-table only the donor iliac Y-graft needs to be anastomosed to the superior mesenteric and splenic arteries, while bleeding in the recipient is minimized.

29.6.2 Recipient Procedure

The patient is positioned supine, with the right flank slightly elevated, and secured to the operating table using wide banding. Orientation of the operating table, position of ports, and site for placement of a GelPort device (Applied Medical, Rancho Santa Margarita, CA, USA) are depicted in Fig. 29.1a. This configuration refers to the use of the da Vinci Si robotic system (Intuitive Surgical Inc., Sunnyvale, CA, USA). The small midline incision is used to insert the graft and to provide hand assistance, if needed.

Using the Xi system, all robotic ports including the optic port are 8 mm in size. The optic port is placed in front of the target anatomy (i.e., the right common iliac vessels), basically in the same location as with the Si system. The other robotic ports are placed in a straighter configuration. With the Xi system, all four robotic arms are used.

Pneumoperitoneum is maintained between 10 and 12 mmHg until graft reperfusion, when it is decreased to 8–10 mmHg.

The tower of the robot is placed to the patient's right (Fig 29.1b). A 30° endoscope is used. As in the open procedure [27], dissection begins with mobilization of the right colon. The right common iliac artery and the proximal segment of the inferior vena cava are exposed. Dissection is performed using bipolar Maryland forceps and monopolar curved scissors. Large lymphatics are

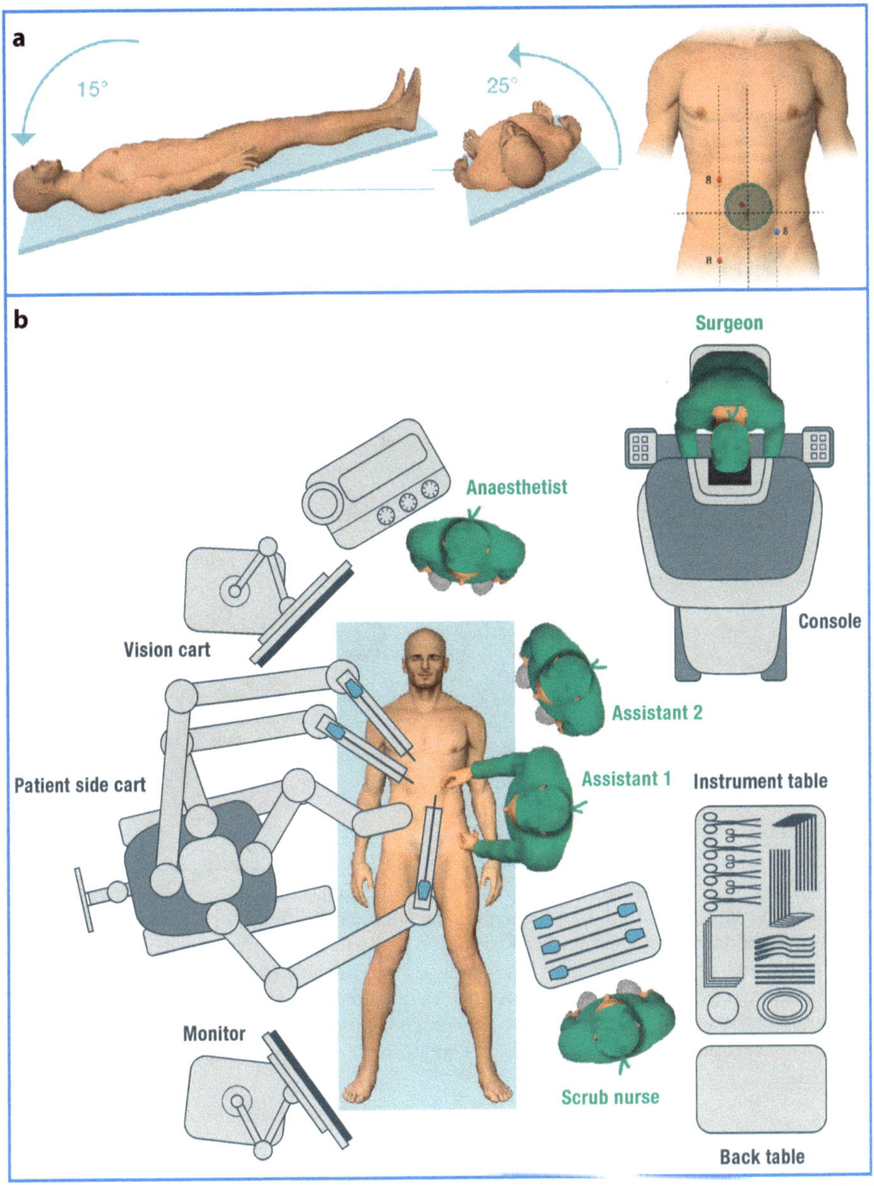

Fig. 29.1 **a** The patient is positioned supine and the table in a 15° Trendelenburg position and tilted some 25° to the left. A GelPort is placed in a small midline incision made just above the navel. The optic port is placed along the left pararectal line some 5 cm below the navel. Two 8-mm robotic ports are placed along the right pararectal line some 5 cm below the costal margin and 3 cm above the pubis, respectively. The assistant port is placed within the GelPort. **b** Operating room setup. The console is placed at the head of the patient, so that the operating surgeon can stay in direct visual contact with both the anesthesia team and the tableside surgeons. Surgical assistants, scrub nurse, instrument table, and back-table are all placed to the left of the patient making this part of the operating room "clean". The robotic tower is placed to the right of the patient

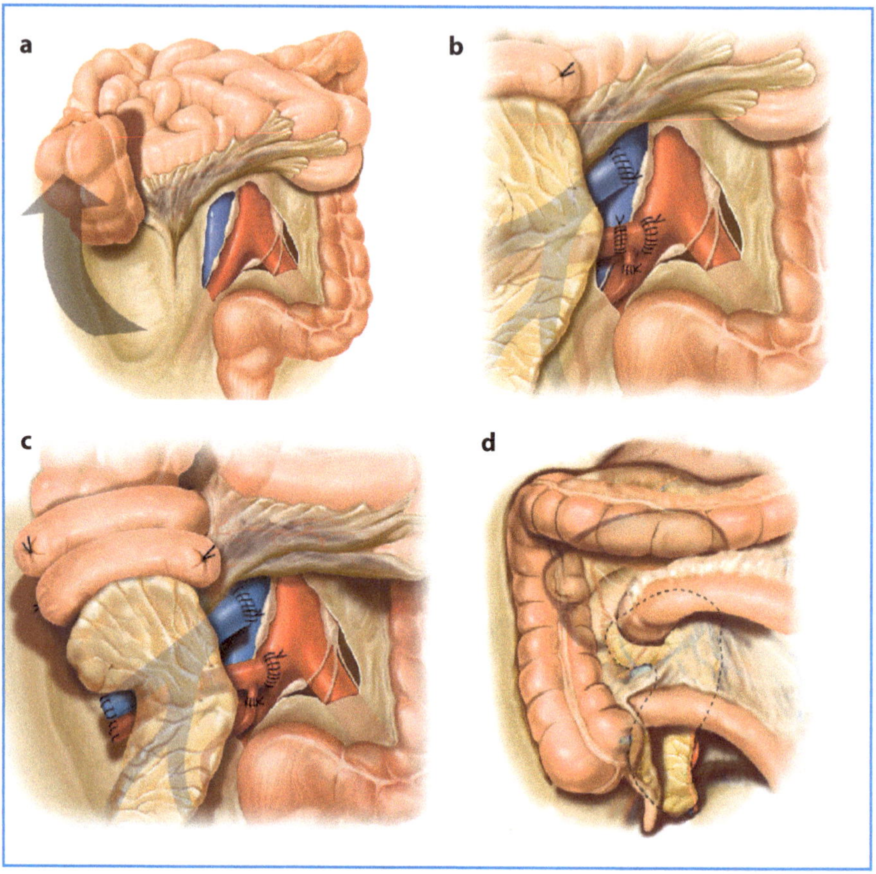

Fig. 29.2 Overview of surgical technique. **a** After mobilization of the cecum and ascending colon, the inferior vena cava and the right common iliac artery are exposed for vascular anastomosis. **b** The donor portal vein is anastomosed end-to-side to the recipient inferior vena cava. Similarly, the common limb of the donor Y-graft is anastomosed end-to-side to the right common iliac artery. **c** Exocrine drainage is achieved by duodenojejunal anastomosis. A Roux-en-Y limb is used and transferred to the site of graft transplantation through the mesentery of the right colon. **d** Finally, the right colon is placed over the pancreas making the graft a retroperitoneal organ

either ligated or clipped. Before vascular cross-clamping the patient is given 5000 units of sodium heparin. Bulldog clamps may be either placed manually, through the GelPort, or using laparoscopic appliers. The graft is then placed over the right psoas muscle in a "head-up" position. The inferior vena cava is unroofed and the donor portal vein is anastomosed end-to-side to the recipient inferior vena cava using two half-running sutures of 7-0 ePTFE. Next, the arterial anastomosis is fashioned, using 6-0 ePTFE, between the donor Y-graft and the recipient common iliac artery (Figs. 29.2 and 29.3). After graft reperfusion, hemostasis is perfected, as required. Heparin is not reversed since strong postoperative anticoagulation

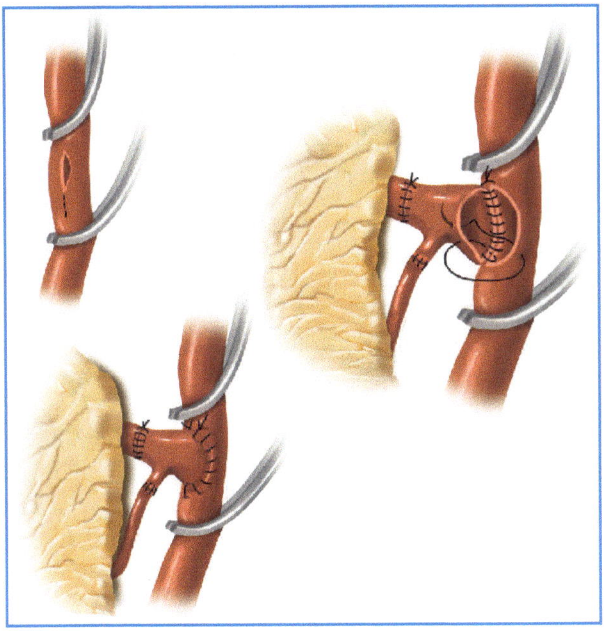

Fig. 29.3 Vascular anastomoses are performed using two half-running sutures. The posterior wall of each anastomosis is sutured from the inside

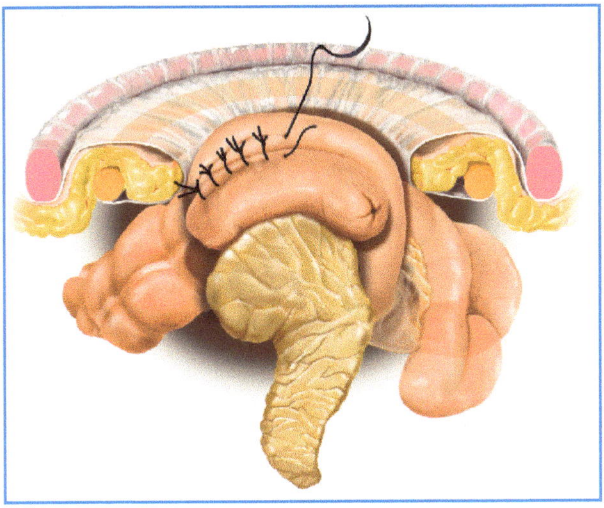

Fig. 29.4 With the head of the graft slightly elevated and rotated to the midline, the duodenojejunal anastomosis is performed manually through the small midline incision, protected by the Alexis wound retractor (Applied Medical, Rancho Santa Margarita, CA, USA)

is required to reduce the risk of vascular thrombosis, and we prefer to ensure hemostasis under these conditions.

Intestinal anastomoses can be easily performed using robotic assistance, but the availability of the small midline incision provides the opportunity to create a Roux-en-Y jejunal limb and to perform the duodenal anastomosis with ease using conventional techniques (Fig. 29.4) [27].

At the end, the operative field is inspected with the laparoscope and two drains are placed along the graft.

29.7 Other Techniques for Robotic PTX

To the best of our knowledge and according to published literature, robotic PTx has been duplicated only at the University of Illinois at Chicago (Chicago, USA).

Yeh et al. [6] described a case of robotic PTx after robotic kidney transplantation in an obese recipient. In contrast to the technique that we have presented, the pancreas was procured and prepared for transplantation according to standard techniques. To address the issue of postreperfusion bleeding, these authors decided to visualize leaking points by perfusing the graft with 500 cc of a vascular tracer composed of 1 liter of University of Wisconsin solution containing 1 mL of methylene blue. In the recipient, the graft was placed "head-down" in the left iliac fossa and exocrine drainage was created into the urinary bladder. The patient was placed in a severe Trendelenburg position. Two robotic ports (8 mm) were placed into the left subcostal and right lower quadrants. The optic port was inserted supraumbilically and the assistant port (12 mm) was placed between the right robotic arm and the camera trocar. A midline incision (7 cm) was made along the midline above the camera port and a GelPort placed. Vascular anastomoses were created using the same technique that we have described. The duodenobladder drainage was performed using a circular stapler. The anvil of the circular stapler was placed into the bladder through a small incision, while the shaft of the stapler was inserted into the fourth duodenal portion and threaded back to the second portion were the cartridge spike was deployed through the anterior wall. After firing the circular stapler the end of the duodenum was closed using an Endo GIA.

The patient achieved insulin independence which was maintained after 1 year of follow-up

29.8 Conclusions

So far, we have performed three robotic PTx, including a pancreas-after-kidney transplantation, a pancreas transplantation alone, and a simultaneous pancreas and kidney transplantation. We have not been able to perform more robotic PTx because of the rarity of suitable donors, the limited accessibility of the robotic system, and the high organizational needs of this complex procedure. Our experience, however, was extremely rewarding as all patients did impressively well, all achieved insulin-independence and all maintained this status at their longest follow-up. This favorable experience is supported also by the results we achieved in robotic kidney transplantation and the growing demand for this procedure among potential recipients. The robotic system clearly allows straightforward transplantation of solid organs as it enhances surgical dexterity, especially when fine sutures are required. What is key to the success of this procedure is to have a very efficient surgical team that must include a fully trained console surgeon, assistant tableside surgeons with laparoscopic skills, anesthetists able to maintain fluid and electrolyte balance with patients in Trendelenburg position, and scrub nurses familiar with the robotic system and with laparoscopic equipment.

References

1. Boggi U, Vistoli F, Signori S et al (2011) Robotic renal transplantation: first European case. Transpl Int 24(2):213–218
2. Garcia-Roca R, Garcia-Aroz S, Tzvetanov I et al (2017) Single center experience with robotic kidney transplantation for recipients with BMI of 40 kg/m2 or greater: a comparison with the UNOS registry. Transplantation 101(1):191–196
3. Frongia M, Cadoni R, Solinas A (2015) First robotic-assisted dual kidney transplant: surgical technique and report of a case with 24-month follow-up. Transplant Direct 1(9):e34
4. Boggi U, Signori S, Vistoli F et al (2012) Laparoscopic robot-assisted pancreas transplantation: first world experience. Transplantation 93(2):201–206
5. Boggi U, Signori S, Vistoli F et al (2011) Current perspectives on laparoscopic robot-assisted pancreas and pancreas-kidney transplantation. Rev Diabet Stud 8(1):28–34
6. Yeh CC, Spaggiari M, Tzvetanov I, Oberholzer J (2017) Robotic pancreas transplantation in a type 1 diabetic patient with morbid obesity: a case report. Medicine (Baltimore) 96(6):e5847
7. Boggi U, Vistoli F, Egidi FM et al (2012) Transplantation of the pancreas. Curr Diab Rep 12(5):568–579
8. Troppmann C, Gruessner AC, Dunn DL et al (1998) Surgical complications requiring early relaparotomy after pancreas transplantation. A multivariate risk factor and economic impact analysis of the cyclosporine era. Ann Surg 227(2):255–268
9. Boggi U, Amorese G, Marchetti P (2010) Surgical techniques for pancreas transplantation. Curr Opin Organ Transplant 15(1):102–111
10. Demyttenaere S, Feldman LS, Fried GM (2007) Effect of pneumoperitoneum on renal perfusion and function: a systematic review. Surg Endosc 21(2):152–160
11. Endo K, Sasaki T, Sata N et al (2014) Elevation of intra-abdominal pressure by pneumoperitoneum decreases pancreatic perfusion in an in vivo porcine model. Surg Laparosc Endosc Percutan Tech 24(3):221–225
12. Banga N, Hadjianastassiou VG, Mamode N et al (2012) Outcome of surgical complications following simultaneous pancreas–kidney transplantation. Nephrol Dial Transplant 27(4): 1658–1663
13. Bonrath EM, Zevin B, Dedy NJ, Grantcharov TP (2013) Error rating tool to identify and analyse technical errors and events in laparoscopic surgery. Br J Surg 100(8):1080–1088
14. Boggi U, Signori S, De Lio N et al (2013) Feasibility of robotic pancreaticoduodenectomy. Br J Surg 100(7):917–925
15. Diamantis T, Tsiminikakis N, Skordylaki A et al (2007) Alterations of hemostasis after laparoscopic and open surgery. Hematology 12(6):561–570
16. Feuillu B, Cormier L, Frimat L et al (2003) Kidney warming during transplantation. Transpl Int 16(5):307–312

17. Szostek M, Pacholczyk M, Lagiewska B et al (1996) Effective surface cooling of the kidney during vascular anastomosis decreases the risk of delayed kidney function after transplantation. Transpl Int 9(Suppl 1):S84–S85
18. Menon M, Abaza R, Sood A et al (2014) Robotic kidney transplantation with regional hypothermia: evolution of a novel procedure utilizing the IDEAL guidelines (IDEAL phase 0 and 1). Eur Urol 65(5):1001–1009
19. Navarro AP, Sohrabi S, Colechin E et al (2008) Evaluation of the ischemic protection efficacy of a laparoscopic renal cooling device using renal transplantation viability assessment criteria in a porcine model. J Urol 179(3):1184–1189
20. Park SC, Kim SD, Kim JI, Moon IS (2008) Minimal skin incision in living kidney transplantation. Transplant Proc 40(7):2347–2348
21. Øyen O, Scholz T, Hartmann A, Pfeffer P (2006) Minimally invasive kidney transplantation: the first experience. Transplant Proc 38(9):2798–2802
22. London ET, Ho HS, Neuhaus AM et al (2000) Effect of intravascular volume expansion on renal function during prolonged CO2 pneumoperitoneum. Ann Surg 231(2):195–201
23. Khanna A, Horgan S (2011) A laboratory training and evaluation technique for robot assisted ex vivo kidney transplantation. Int J Med Robot 7(1):118–122
24. Diks J, Nio D, Linsen MA et al (2007) Suture damage during robot-assisted vascular surgery: is it an issue? Surg Laparosc Endosc Percutan Tech 17(6):524–527
25. Ricchiuti D, Cerone J, Shie S et al (2010) Diminished suture strength after robotic needle driver manipulation. J Endourol 24(9):1509–1513
26. Boggi U, Vistoli F, Del Chiaro M et al (2004) A simplified technique for the en bloc procurement of abdominal organs that is suitable for pancreas and small-bowel transplantation. Surgery 135(6):629–641
27. Boggi U, Vistoli F, Signori S et al (2005) A technique for retroperitoneal pancreas transplantation with portal-enteric drainage. Transplantation 79(9):1137–1142

FSC®
www.fsc.org
MIX
Papier | Fördert gute Waldnutzung
FSC® C083411

Kolibri 360 GmbH
Ferdinand-Jühlke-Straße 7
99095 Erfurt, Deutschland
produktsicherheit@kolibri360.de